ALLE · ZEIT · WACH
SJ
1842

H. Göppinger

Life Style and Criminality

Basic Research and Its Application: Criminological Diagnosis and Prognosis

With Collaboration of
Michael Bock Jörg-Martin Jehle
Werner Maschke

With a Foreword by Peter P. Lejins

Springer-Verlag
Berlin Heidelberg New York
London Paris Tokyo

Professor Dr. med. Dr. jur. Dr. h. c. Hans Göppinger
Institute of Criminology, University of Tübingen
Corrensstrasse 34, D-7400 Tübingen

Professor Dr. rer. soz. Dr. jur. Michael Bock
University of Mainz, Saarstrasse 21, D-6500 Mainz

Direktor Dr. jur. Jörg-Martin Jehle
Kriminologische Zentralstelle e. V.
Adolfs-Allee 32, D-6200 Wiesbaden

Dr. jur. Werner Maschke
Institute of Criminology, University of Tübingen
Corrensstrasse 34, D-7400 Tübingen

Translator: Ina Kraan, certificated interpreter
Schreinerstrasse 43, CH-8004 Zürich

ISBN-13:978-3-642-71324-8 e-ISBN-13:978-3-642-71322-4
DOI: 10.1007/978-3-642-71322-4

Softcover reprint of the hardcover 1st edition 1987

2119/3140-543210

Foreword

It is with distinct pleasure that I accepted the invitation by Professor Göppinger to write a foreword to *Life Style and Criminality,* which is the English-language report on the comparative study of young offenders conducted by the Institute of Criminology of Tübingen University, and a rendition of the content of two of the author's works based on this study and bearing the German titles *Der Täter in seinen sozialen Bezügen* (The Offender in his Social Relationships) and *Angewandte Kriminologie* (Applied Criminology).

I consider that the availability in English translation of these Tübingen studies by Professor Göppinger should be of considerable interest to American criminologists. Professor Göppinger is a well-known criminologist in his country, whose voluminous textbook in criminology recently appeared in its fourth edition. Professor Göppinger holds degrees in law and medicine, and throughout his life has made use of both of these background orientations and competencies in his work. Scores of well-known German criminologists are Professor Göppinger's students, who pursue their careers in academia, in research, in governmental agencies and in a wide variety of private crime-related enterprises. In spite of the fact that his criminology text testifies to a thorough familiarity with the pertinent literature and research of world-wide scope, his general orientation and style of thinking and writing remain typically European and specifically German. The American reader of criminological literature has ample access to the current trends, fads, methodological refinements and ideologies of contemporary criminal justice and criminological writings in the United States. Works which are the outcome of a different scholarly tradition and at the same time address the same general problems that are of concern in the United States should be of special and potentially significant heuristic value to the American scholar. The Tübingen study is one of such works.

The specific subject of the research reported in Professor Göppinger's work is very familiar to American criminologists. At the risk of the usual dangers of oversimplification, it can be described as a comparison of a population of convicted young criminal offenders with a control group from the general normal population for the purpose of establishing the potential differences between the two, and by that means gaining an insight into the factors which might be those that lead to criminal behavior. The study, which started in 1965, deals with a group of 200 twenty to thirty year-old offenders who served at least a six months institutional sentence, and a similar-size control group. The author stresses the interdisciplinary nature of the study and of the elaborate methodology developed for the comparison of the two groups.

It is important to point out that in structuring the analysis of the data, the author makes extensive use of the concept of the ideal type as initiated by Max Weber and as further developed by Karl Jaspers. The reader should give careful attention to the function of this type of analysis, which permeates this study.

A major item of importance emerging from these Tübingen studies is the finding that it is the social settings and social relationships of the individual that are of primary importance in differentiating criminal offenders from nonoffenders. This finding is especially impressive, since the reading of Professor Göppinger's study creates the impression that he and his collaborators gave full and impartial attention to all other factors that came to the fore in this truly interdisciplinary study and could potentially also emerge as substantial differences between the two populations. And yet, the just mentioned social factors clearly seemed to be the principal ones in the background of the individuals in the two groups that distinguish one from the other. Here one should note the meticulously worked interview technique used throughout these studies, which, while carefully structured, is flexible enough to be adjusted to subtle idiosyncracies of each individual case. The data thus obtained and their analysis, consisting of a comparison of "ideal-typical behavior patterns", as Professor Göppinger refers to them, of the subjects in the two groups studied, is in many ways the key element in this research project. Analysis of the social aspects is accompanied by similar comparisons with regard to many additional factors.

In line with my personal interests and biases, I would like to call the reader's attention to the persuasive and persistent way in which the author, throughout his books, stresses the importance of criminology as an independent academic or scientific discipline. In spite of his ready recognition of the contributions of other disciplines such as psychiatry, psychology, sociology, medicine, etc., Professor Göppinger feels that criminology, because of its specific subject, *i.e.* criminal behavior, should stand independently - "eigenständige Wissenschaft" - while making use for its purposes of the results of a wide variety of other fields of study. The criminological study of criminal behavior is the basis for the applied development of preventive and crime-control programs. Professor Göppinger's repeated demonstration of how he arrives at this perspective on criminology makes good reading for those who are looking for a way out of the confusion caused by a plethora of academic disciplines attempting to colonize the phenomenon of crime for their own purposes and insisting on practical solutions for the crime problem exclusively in terms of their own field, which has been a futile and misleading attempt.

In reading Professor Göppinger's book, one should not lose sight of the author's dedication to the idea of *Applied* Criminology. Clearly, his goal in initiating and conducting the Tübingen studies is not only a contribution to the body of criminological theory, but at the same time also the development of a practical tool for the practitioners in their daily work of managing the problem of crime. As a matter of fact, Professor Göppinger cites instances of the use of the analytical findings of this research in practice, as this is reflected in a number of his publications which appeared in the course of the twenty years spent in developing and refining the analyses emanating from this study.

Translation of a foreign-language text, especially a scientific text, which by necessity contains a very sensitive scientific terminology, is always a very difficult task. The linguistic difficulty of finding the terms which accurately transmit the meaning intended by the author, is further complicated by the fact that the terminologies are deeply anchored in the general cultural setting of the country or the continent from which they stem. The differences in cultural, philosophical, or ideological settings, whichever term is more appropriate, especially in the realm of social science, convey different meanings to seemingly identical words and concepts, all of which must be accounted for in a translation. The reader must be aware of this natural difficulty. I know that Professor Göppinger has given utmost attention to assuring that these difficulties of presenting his study in a different language, to be read in different cultural settings, are properly overcome, so that the reader can readily follow his research designs and their execution.

I would like to conclude by reiterating once more that the English publication of *Life Style and Criminality* is a positive and refreshing contribution to the enhancement of research and study of crime and can well serve also as a springboard for devising better remedies for coping with the crime problem: the task for Applied Criminology.

College Heights Estades,
May 1987

PETER P. LEJINS, Ph. D., LLD h. c.
Professor Emeritus of Sociology
Professor Emeritus of Criminal Justice and Criminology
University of Maryland

Preface

The present volume deals with the most important results of the retrospective stage of the Tübingen Comparative Study of Young Offenders and the knowledge obtained that is of relevance for a practically oriented criminology. A future publication will present the results of the (prospective) follow-up study.

When the *Tübingen Comparative Study of Young Offenders* was initiated during the mid-1960s, long-term studies conceived as basic research and not directly geared to issues of crime policy or current needs were of great scientific interest and thus found the necessary support. The aim of the Tübingen study was to obtain broad basic knowledge about recidivist offenders as compared with the general population and, on the basis of this knowledge, to draw conclusions related to both the theoretical and practical aspects of criminology.

Such basic research, however, could not draw on a German criminological tradition such as the Anglo-American tradition of multifactorial studies exemplified by the studies of the GLUECKS. Therefore, *new methods* were implemented to allow the comprehensive study of a control group from the general population and to facilitate interdisciplinary cooperation among the researchers.

The external conditions of the study were favored by circumstances prevailing at the time. For instance, with the consent of the subjects, it was possible to obtain a host of data from employment offices, statutory health insurance plans, local authorities, schools, etc. Considering the importance now given to the confidentiality of personal data, this might well be considerably more difficult today. More particularly, it was possible to induce the subjects of the control group (who were not in prison) to spend the time and effort involved in the extensive investigations. At the request of the subjects, many investigations took place during weekends. The subjects' basic willingness to contribute to scientific research tended to increase during the course of the study; this may well be due in part to the efforts of the researchers. They dealt very intensively with each individual subject and did not concern themselves exclusively with aspects relevant to the study, but also assisted with personal or welfare problems.

The findings presented here result from the cooperation of many representatives of law, medicine, psychology, and sociology, as well as that of social workers, students, and technical staff, whose contributions at all levels of the research project were considerable, from the conception of the study to the collection and evaluation of data to the preparation of this volume. Owing to circumstances at the university, various changes in the composition of the research team - with the exception of the head of the team and a few collaborators - were inevitable during the long phase of data collection and evaluation. Generally, these changes took place smoothly, particularly since the nucleus of the team remained the same during the data-collection phase. However, after this phase, which was marked by continuity, unity, and solidarity, a crisis developed at the beginning of the evaluation phase. The trends of the early 1970s, characterized by methodological (statistical) purism on the one hand and programmatic (criminopolitical) rigorism on the other, influenced team discussions of the research design agreed upon. The actual progress of evaluation was checked, yet the consistency and continuity of the study were not jeopardized in the end.

The broad, open-ended conception of the study yielded such a wealth of results and findings that they cannot be presented in concise form [see my *Kriminologie* (GÖPPINGER 1980) and the various monographs on specific areas of the Tübingen Comparative Study of Young Offenders listed in the bibliography]. For this reason, the present volume disregards aspects of secondary importance and concentrates on the essentials.

A group of 20- to 30-year-old male prisoners serving a sentence of at least 6 months and a control group from the general population were investigated. The heart of the study consisted of individual case studies, for which wide-ranging data on medical, psychiatric, and psychological aspects and the social spheres of each subject were collected by means of interviews with the subjects and other persons, the analysis of records, psychological tests, and medical and psychiatric examinations. While the medical, psychiatric, and psychological examinations of the subjects yielded practically no relevant distinctions, fundamental differences between the offender and the control group (from the general population) became apparent in the social spheres. The offender subjects differed less from the control subjects in their external circumstances than in their *behavior* in routine, daily affairs, their self-chosen relationships, and their entire life-style.

At the statistical level of the evaluation (Part II), within each separate sphere, we combined the most important *findings on social behavior* and picked out syndromes. These syndromes were of considerable criminological relevance - with respect to the early recognition of a life-style ultimately tending toward criminality - as they were found almost exclusively in the offender group.

On another level, we tried to arrive at a *complex, overall view* (Part III). We abandoned the statistical level and attempted to obtain a comprehensive view of the offender in the context of his social relationships by creating ideal types on the basis of criteria spanning the social spheres. The fruits of these efforts were *specifically criminological* criteria: criminorelevant constellations in the cross section of life, positions of the offense in the longitudinal section of life, and patterns of relevance and value orientation, which, taken together, form the *Criminological Triad*. This opens the way for the formulation of an *autonomous*, integrated criminology which is independent of its related disciplines, with its distinctive, consistent object of study, taking on definite shape in the concept of the *offender in the context of his social relationships*. At the same time, these criteria constitute the foundation of a *practice-oriented Applied Criminology* and a specifically criminological assessment of individual cases (Part IV). The comparative analysis of individual cases based on the ideal types that we have elaborated is the first practice-oriented criminological method - even at the international level - which allows a differential assessment of the individual offender in the context of his social relationships. The method does not rely on legal categories; taking into account social conspicuousness preceding and accompanying criminality, the method enables a specifically *criminological diagnosis*, which again leads to *conclusions for a prognosis*. It also shows criminologically relevant strengths and weaknesses of the subject. In this way, it provides a theoretical foundation for interventions according to (criminal) law relating to *prevention* and *prophylaxis* and to the treatment of offenders.

The aspects relevant to the assessment concentrate on the subjects' general social behavior in everyday life, which is easily accessible to people who deal with the subjects in practice (such as members of the legal profession, social workers, teachers, etc.) and who have no special psychological or psychiatric training. The method is also a valuable supplement to specialized knowledge in the fields of forensic psychiatry and psychology.

To show the criteria and procedures used in this method of comparative analysis of individual cases based on ideal types, a specific case is presented (Case A, Appendix). This example can show only some of the possible applications, not the entire spectrum.

It is true that the Tübingen Comparative Study of Young Offenders is marked by the circumstances prevailing at the time it was carried out. Yet, it was possible to detect definite formal criteria abstracted from specific behavior patterns caused by the prevailing circumstances, for example, in the sphere of leisure. Moreover, the validity of the findings beyond the specific historical moment became apparent in a comparison of these findings with those of other international studies, which - despite the different periods during which they were carried out and the differences in life circumstances - arrived at similar results concerning the behavior patterns of offenders. This is another reason why we are presenting our findings to an international public.

The first three parts of this American version largely correspond to the German edition: "*Der Täter in seinen sozialen Bezügen*" (GÖPPINGER 1983). In a few places, usually where knowledge of German circumstances (e.g., the German school system) is necessary, additional explanatory notes have been provided for non-German readers. The fourth part is a summary of the German book "*Angewandte Kriminologie*" (GÖPPINGER 1985), which describes the fundamentals of criminological individual case analysis on the basis of previously presented results.

First and foremost, I would like to thank Springer-Verlag for its cooperation in the preparation of the American edition, as well as I. KRAAN, certified conference interpreter, who translated the book with dedication and care, in close cooperation with us. My genuine thanks also go to Prof. em. Dr. P. P. LEJINS for his willingness to write a foreword to this edition and for the advice and encouragement he gave us. Furthermore, I am indebted to Dr. B. HARDIN for his expert advice in problems of language, as well as to my collaborators R. MISCHKOWITZ, M.A., and A. GREULICH, certified translator, for their critical review of the English text. Finally, I would like to mention in particular my former and current collaborators Prof. Dr. Dr. M. BOCK, Dr. J.-M. JEHLE and Dr. W. MASCHKE, who not only made important contributions to the German edition but also assisted in this translation.

Tübingen, April 1987 HANS GÖPPINGER

Contents

Appendix - The Criminological Assessment of a Case

Detailed Table of Contents

III Complex, Overall View

IV Applied Criminology - The Method and Criteria of Criminological Diagnosis and Prognosis

Appendix - The Criminological Assessment of a Case

I Object and Methods

1 Starting Point and Aim

An empirical[1] study aimed at the broadest possible understanding of how the persons studied actually live, rather than at achieving quick results in specific areas by applying standardized investigations, is a difficult and tedious enterprise. This was demonstrated once again - as in other comparable studies - in the "Tübingen Comparative Study of Young Offenders." The actual study, which began in 1965, was preceded by a prolonged period of specific planning and design and by a pilot study. After the (retrospective) investigations were completed, a lengthy phase of intensive evaluation began, the results of which are dealt with in the present report. Meanwhile, the further development of the subjects is being observed (prospectively) within the framework of a follow-up study.

The planning and design of the **Tübingen Comparative Study of Young Offenders** took place at a time when the research situation in the Federal Republic of Germany, contrary to that in the United States, was marked by a complete lack of comprehensive criminological studies; there were no comparative studies going beyond the simple collection of data from records and carried out *directly* with a large number of adult offenders. Therefore, a central aim of the present study was to develop basic criminological knowledge of how offenders actually live. Particularly in the field of criminology, this seemed all the more necessary as there are numerous theories claiming entirely different causes and concomitant circumstances of criminality: Theories related to personality predominated in the past, while today, theories which make social circumstances responsible for criminality (still) prevail. Criminality is regarded either as an effect of certain social structures or as a consequence of social reaction.

The present study complies with the traditional multifactorial approach insofar as such one-sided perspectives are rejected. It is marked by the self-evident, yet often neglected insight "that every offense is committed by an offender (or offenders), who is not, as it were, standing free in space as an entirely independent individual, isolated from any ties, but is always part of certain social fields, whose determining forces have an effect which is merely relativized by the individuality of each personality" (GÖPPINGER 1980, pp. 76ff.; translated by Ina Kraan). This view is closely related to the concept of the offender in the context of his social relationships, which took increasingly definite shape in the course of the study

[1] The term "empirical" as used hereafter is not only associated with a purely hypothesis-testing research design and standardized or quantifying methods of social research (see Sect. 4.1 below and Part III, Sect. 1.1). It also includes epistemological modes focusing on other kinds of rules and generalizations from experience which are gained by developing ideal-typical concepts and methods. Therefore, in the German text, the term *Erfahrungswissenschaft* (and *erfahrungswissenschaftlich)* in the tradition of M. WEBER, was used instead of *empirische Wissenschaft* (and *empirisch).*

(see Part III). It is not a theoretical model starting out from fixed hypotheses concerning the relevance of individual factors and certain causal relationships; rather, it should be understood heuristically in the sense that the *actual* complex of conditions and the real importance of individual factors are left open to discovery in the individual case.

Consequently, a research design based on one-sided theories was out of the question. Exclusive commitment of the study to any hypotheses was deliberately avoided so that it would remain open to unanticipated or unexpected circumstances and relationships. Thus, initially, we considered some seemingly simple and naive-sounding questions, which, however, demanded extremely complex answers: What are the offenders to be studied like in comparison with the rest of the population? Do they differ at all from the "general" population in terms of their life histories, in somatic, psychiatric/psychological, and social aspects, or in their behavior patterns?

These extremely broad and open initial question had methodological implications for the design of a **comparative study:** Only against the background of what is usual in the "general" population can the significance and weight of individual characteristics, behavior patterns, and circumstances for (recidivist) criminality be assessed.

The group of *offenders* (O-subjects) was selected from 20- to 30-year-old male prisoners (regarding the method, see Sect. 2.2 below) serving sentences of at least 6 months. This *selection criterion* was based on the reasonable assumption that these offenders would generally have already had what might be called a "criminal career." This was important, since offenders characterized by marked criminality, not by chance or peripheral manifestations of delinquency, were to be studied. For various reasons, 20-30 years seemed a suitable age range: It is particularly "prone" to criminality, and the selection of younger subjects would have meant that the large number of offenders who did not receive repeated convictions until adulthood would have been disregarded (see Part II, Sect. 1.3). The latter group of offenders in particular had not been taken into account at all in previous criminological studies, which concentrated mainly on juvenile (age 14-17) and adolescent (age 18-21) offenders.

The offender sample was therefore expected to cover a *definite,* yet practically and theoretically important, *subgroup of offenders,* i.e., offenders demonstrating serious or recidivist criminality (see Part II, Sect. 4.3.1) and not "criminality" as such. A minimum sentence of 6 months was stipulated because it could be assumed that this would exclude offenders convicted for petty offenses and also for the important practical reason that the duration of the sentence, i.e., the time during which the subject would be available, had to be sufficient to carry out in-depth investigations.

In contrast, the *control group* (G-subjects), was intended to represent a cross section of the corresponding age group of the general male population. A group that would be "normal" in every respect was to be selected, meaning that there would be not only hidden delinquency, but also a certain percentage of previously convicted subjects in the group (see Sects. 2.1.2 and 2.3 below and Part II, Sect. 4.7).

The *size* of the groups was limited to 200 subjects each. Thus, the groups were small enough to enable the Institute to conduct comprehensive and in-depth investigations over a reasonable period and still large enough to guarantee statistically significant results (see Sect. 4.2 below).

Designing the research project as an initially retrospective comparative study (see Sect. 2.1 below) inevitably implied certain methodological decisions; it was decided, however, that the investigations should remain largely unimpeded by anticipated theoretical definitions.

This does not mean that there were absolutely no preconditions in the present study. Selection of some of a practically unlimited number of observable phenomena is always unavoidable, not only for the practical reasons of limited staff and resources, but also as a matter of principle. The selection was thus *influenced* by hypotheses and results in individual areas of previous research work. Nevertheless, these hypotheses and results *did not determine the study to the same degree* as they would have determined hypothetical-deductive studies, since we were aware that they had been gained mostly from the limited perspective of specific disciplines related to criminology, which do not do justice to the complex of conditions and consequences in criminality.

Even more decisive for the justification of the open procedure was the assumption - confirmed in the course of the study - that surprising, unanticipated facts and circumstances might play an important role. Therefore, **in-depth individual case investigations** of the social spheres and somatic, psychiatric, and psychological aspects of the subjects selected (for the systematic and not only exploratory significance of individual case investigations, see Part III, Sect. 1) were of central importance. This was not an expedition into unknown territory, as there were the first impressions and experience of extensive pilot studies to go on. Yet the subjects were not simply to be "questioned" as to whether they showed certain predetermined factors; rather, *the development and life pattern of every individual* as a whole were to be covered in as much depth and from as many angles as possible. First, therefore, it was essential to collect as wide-ranging information from as many spheres as possible on each subject's "personality in the context of its social relationships." This implied a *complex, multidimensional perspective.*

A research project focusing on such a complex object could be mastered adequately only with an **interdisciplinary approach.** Consequently, the Tübingen Comparative Study of Young Offenders was conducted by a research team composed of members of the legal and medical professions, psychologists, sociologists, and social workers. Interdisciplinary research did not mean that the team was simply a formal grouping of individual researchers solely responsible for their own special disciplines, but that the group as a whole was entirely responsible for the planning and conducting of the study (see Göppinger 1980, pp. 78ff.; Kaiser 1967). The aim of this interdisciplinary research was to weight the individual facts - collected in the different areas by various methods - in an overall view from the angle of the *common research object, which was not specific to any one of the separate disciplines* (see Parts III and IV).

2 Design of the Study

2.1 Methodological Implications of a (Retrospective) Comparative Study

Any study design inevitably implies methodological decisions with far-reaching consequences for the validity and range of its results. This also applies to the present retrospective comparative study, which traces back the subjects' development through life, starting from the time of the study (and which - as a long-term study - will be supplemented by a prospective follow-up study). Yet the limitations for the value of the results can be kept within narrow bounds if the problems and restrictions of the individual research techniques are kept in mind.

2.1.1 General Problems

There is one objection that is leveled more frequently against *comparative* studies in criminological research than any other: It is claimed that such studies compare two extreme populations and disregard intermediate groups; this objection is directed particularly at studies comparing delinquent and nondelinquent subjects. Yet the control group of the present study is not a contrasting group in any respect; it represents the "general" population. Therefore, delinquency does occur in this group (see Part II, 4.7; for information on the problem of hidden criminality, see Sect. 2.1.2 below).

Retrospective studies of prisoners are decried on the grounds that it is impossible to estimate accurately the effects of the current prison situation and earlier social reactions and punishment of the subjects' behavior. Moreover, the conviction and social stigmatization of the subjects can lead parents and other reference persons to change their attitudes, which can affect what they say about the subjects. Finally, the investigation of events that took place long ago can be impaired by memory lapses or other tendencies toward distortion.

These limitations cannot be fully eliminated for the present study, though they are narrowed down considerably by the systematic form of retrospection. To a large extent, it was possible to check and correct the data: Various sources of information were available for each area of investigation, and many written records from each relevant period were collected (see Sect. 3.2 below).

The research design of the *prospective cohort study* (e.g., West 1969; Wolfgang et al. 1972), in contrast, is intended to avoid the aforementioned objections from the outset. Even so, it cannot completely avoid the basic problems of retrospection. The design of the study is prospective only insofar as a population which is not selected according to the characteristic of criminality is chosen, usually during childhood, and then observed as to its further development, with reference to later criminality, among other things. Otherwise, the data are necessarily collected retrospectively. This holds not only for the period preceding the time of the study, but also for the further development in later life: Generally, and also specifically for the occurrence of delinquency, a subject's development can be investigated retrospectively only at certain intervals for each stage of the study.

Moreover, prospective cohort studies are confronted with a number of serious practical problems. If one wants to make any statements on a period of time relevant to the occurrence and development of delinquency, investigations must be conducted continuously over at least 10-20 years, which constitutes an enormous research effort. At the same time, the long study period can lead to a significant drop-out quota: Subjects may are no longer willing to participate, may move away or may no longer be able to participate in the study for some other reason. A further risk of distortion is that the subjects become familiar with the research questions. Because they are investigated repeatedly, they are able to "see through" the questions. Another much more serious risk is that the study itself may have an (uncontrollable) influence on the attitudes and behavior patterns of the subjects. Finally, there is the decisive practical drawback that criminality, especially serious and persistent criminality, is only scantly represented in randomly selected populations. Detailed observation of the development of delinquency for a larger group, rather than in a few individual cases, would therefore require a considerable number of subjects. This number would have to be projected with reference to the prevalence of recidivist criminality according to the selection criteria applied to the O-group (see Sect. 2.2 below). This would mean a great deal of information on thousands of subjects, yet would also make it impossible to proceed beyond data that are easy to collect, and would therefore forestall any comprehensive statement on the specific reality of the subjects' lives.

2.1.2 The Problem of Hidden Criminality

A basic objection to all "offender-oriented" studies of "convicted persons" was made, particularly in connection with the discussion on the labeling approach (e.g., SACK 1969). It is claimed that convicted persons, and especially prisoners, constitute a group selected by criminal prosecution authorities, not according to criteria of delinquency, but according to other social and personal aspects. In other words, it is not criminality that distinguishes the convicted from the nonconvicted population, since criminality is really ubiquitous, i.e., distributed evenly throughout the entire population.

With a strict application of the premises underlying the labeling approach, according to which deviant or criminal behavior as such is (socially) nonexistent as long as it is not noticed or there is no official reaction, hidden criminality, i.e., nonrecognized or nonprosecuted criminality, should be in fact irrelevant. Yet, apart from this, the reference to hidden criminality could question the validity of a comparative study such as the present one only if the subjects' *actual* delinquency did *not* show the same striking differences between prisoners and the general population as their *officially recorded* delinquency, but were similarly or even equally distributed among convicted and nonconvicted persons. *Only then* could the somatic, psychological/psychiatric, or social differences between prisoners and the general population be interpreted as mere criteria of selection or "criminalization" by criminal prosecution authorities; *only then* would they have nothing to do with the kind and frequency of prosecuted and actual delinquency; and *only then* would a comparison between convicted persons and the general population be criminologically meaningless.

It is precisely the *premise of equal distribution* of criminality that is obviously *incorrect*; the investigated delinquency is also more serious and frequent among prisoners than in the general population. This was shown in a study of actual delinquency (SCHÖCH 1976) supplementing the present one (see Part II, Sect. 4.2.2). It has also been confirmed by numerous differentiating studies (see in particular the critical survey of HINDELANG et al. 1981).

Finally, it should be noted again that the above reservations do not affect the present study, especially as the G-group (control group from the general population; see Sect. 2.2 below) is *not* a group of "nondelinquents" (see Sect. 1 above and Sect. 2.3 below); there was no intention of correlating observed differences between O- and G-subjects with delinquency as such. The aim of the study was not to make any statement on *criminality in all its forms,* e.g., chance, single offense, petty, but to discover the concomitant social, somatic, and psychological/psychiatric circumstances lastly leading to (recidivist) criminality. Therefore, the comparison between O- and G-subjects is not obstructed by the fact that several subjects in the G-group had been previously convicted, and that practically all G-subjects indicated that they had committed offenses, albeit only few and minor ones, in the study by SCHÖCH (see Part II, Sect. 4.2.2).

2.2 Selection of the Groups in the Study

From 1965 to 1970, two sample groups were randomly selected for the Tübingen Comparative Study of Young Offenders: 200 prisoners and 200 persons from the "general" population. Only German citizens were selected because of the possibility of language difficulties and cultural differences in the case of foreigners and the impossibility of obtaining documents relating to the past life and social environment of foreigners corresponding to those available for German citizens.

The **offender group** was to be representative, at the time of the study, for all male inmates of the penal institution in Rottenburg who were between their 20th and 30th birthdays (average age 24.89 years) and had sentences of at least 6 months to serve. Only prisoners who had been sentenced by the district courts of Hechingen, Rottweil, Tübingen, and Stuttgart and committed by the corresponding departments of public prosecution were considered eligible for the study. Rottenburg is in the immediate vicinity of Tübingen, and at that time the penal institution in Rottenburg offered a cross section of the prisoner population, with the exception of persons convicted for capital crimes and those sentenced to prison under the Juvenile Court Act *(Jugendgerichtsgesetz).*

The samples were drawn as follows: Up to 1970, the Institute of Criminology in Tübingen was kept continuously informed of the commitment of any prisoners to the penal institution complying with the aforementioned criteria. Subjects were continuously selected from among these prisoners by means of tables of random numbers and interviewed as soon as possible after their committal. There should be no systematic distortions in this successive selection of subjects, as the time of committal to Rottenburg was not related to criteria which could have been relevant to the study; thus, for example, the distribution of the individual groups of offenses was approximately random throughout the year.

The **control group** from the "general" population also consisted of 200 subjects. It was matched to the offender sample for the criteria age (average age 26.03 years), sex, and, geographically, for the jurisdictions of the district courts concerned. There were no other selection criteria.

The selection procedure for the control group was more complicated than that for the offender group. As there was no overall population register for the four areas covered by the district courts of Hechingen, Rottweil, Stuttgart, and Tübingen, the following two-stage selection procedure was applied:

There were 869 municipalities in the four districts. The populations of several of these municipalities were selected to serve as subpopulations from which the control subjects were chosen. To reflect the various sizes of the municipalities, eight categories of municipalities were defined. According to the 1960-1961 census of the Baden-Württemberg Statistics Office, a total of 240924 men between 20 and 30 were living in the four jurisdictions of the district courts. Their distribution percentage among the categories of municipalities covered by the census was used to determine the number of subjects to be selected from each category.

Assuming, for instance, that 6% of the population lived in municipalities of 500-1000 residents, 12 of the total sample of 200 subjects would have to be selected from these municipalities. As three municipalities were chosen from this category, four subjects would have to be selected from each municipality. (Merely in Stuttgart, the only large city, were the subjects drawn from one municipality alone.)

The subjects were selected according to the principle of systematic random sampling: The necessary quotas of subjects were taken systematically and at regular intervals from the population registers or, in larger municipalities, from the registers maintained by the conscription service.

The subjects' addresses and the most important data in the registers were recorded on pre-prepared forms. Subsequently, the subjects were contacted.

The *drop-out rate* was minimal: In the offender group there were only four subjects who refused to participate and eight who could not participate because they were released prematurely or transferred to another institution. In the control group 16 of the initially selected subjects could not participate, mainly because the records in the population registers were obsolete or the subjects moved away from the area of the study; in four cases participation was precluded by mental or physical disability; four subjects refused to participate (see Sect. 2.3 below). In both groups, the subjects who dropped out were substituted by systematically selected new subjects.

Several subjects who had first refused to cooperate were persuaded to participate in the study after intensive discussions with the study's social workers.

2.3 Representativeness

The *offender sample* represented a cross section of all young adult inmates of the penal institution in Rottenburg during the study period who were serving sentences of at least 6 months. This resulted in the selection of a group which - insofar as any statement may be made on the basis of prison statistics *(Strafvollzugsstatistik)* - reflects the largest group in the overall prison population.

Table 1. Comparison between male prisoners in the Federal Republic of Germany and O-subjects

	Male prisoners 1965-1969[a] (n = 30489)	O-subjects (n = 200)
Age		
20 to under 30 years	53.5% (16313)	100%
Of whom 20 to under 24 years	28.0%	32.0%
24 years	13.2%	12.5%
25 to under 30 years	58.8%	55.5%
Length of sentence		
Over 5 months	64.2% (19569)	100%
Of which over 5 to 6 months	8.8%	11.5%[b]
over 6 to 9 months	14.7%	20.0%
over 9 to 12 months	18.2%	15.0%
over 1 to 2 years	32.4%	31.5%
over 2 to 5 years	24.4%	19.0%
over 5 years	1.0%	.5%
Indefinite	.3%	2.5%
Number of previous convictions		
1	17.4%	12.0%
2	15.7%	21.5%
3	12.4%	16.5%
4	9.2%	11.0%
5-10	23.4%	25.0%
11-20	7.1%	2.5%
21 and more	.9%	-
Total of previously convicted prisoners	86.1% (26225)	89.0%

[a] Source of basic figures: *Rechtspflegestatistik Fachserie A, Bevölkerung und Kultur, Reihe 9, III. Strafvollzug* (prison statistics for the Federal Republic of Germany), corresponding year; the average of 5 years each was taken

[b] Exactly 6 months

With respect to *age structure,* prisoners aged 20-30 made up an average of 53.5% of all male prison inmates, according to the fixed date counts of the 1965-1969 prison statistics. Prisoners serving a *sentence of more than 5 months* made up 64.2% of the entire prison population (see Table 1).

The selection of O-subjects excluded *persons sentenced for capital crimes,* who, however, represented only a relatively small percentage of the entire prison population. This meant that certain forms of serious criminality were excluded from the outset (for details, see Part II, Sect. 4.3.3).

The group of offenders serving *short sentences* was (and still is) also a large one, particularly if distortions resulting from fixed date counts are taken into account (see below). This subgroup of prisoners is suited neither for research aims such as the present one (see Sect. 1 above) nor for any research related to "classic criminality," in view of its heterogeneous composition (it includes many first and traffic offenders).

The data on the offender population are - from a purely methodological viewpoint - representative only for offenders corresponding to the criteria applied in the Tübingen study and committed by the departments of public prosecution of the district courts of Hechingen, Rottweil, Stuttgart, and Tübingen. However, as these district courts' sentencing policy does not differ substantially from that

Table 2. Social class of G-subjects in comparison

	KLEINING and MOORE[a] (n = 14375)	G-group (n = 200)	
		Class of family of orientation[b]	Subject's class
Upper class, upper middle and middle middle class	17%	15.0%	18.0%
Lower middle class	38%	38.0%	35.5%
Upper lower class	30%	29.5%	39.0%
Lower lower class and "socially despised"	15%	17.5%	7.5%

[a] See KLEINING and MOORE 1968, p. 547
[b] See Part II, Sect. 2.1.2.1

throughout the entire Federal Republic of Germany (see KESKE 1983), it is reasonable to assume that any statements concerning the prisoners included in the Tübingen Comparative Study of Young Offenders also apply, in principle, to all young adult offenders in the Federal Republic of Germany complying with the selection criteria. A comparison of the characteristics of prison inmates presented in prison statistics with those of the O-subjects supports this assumption, although the characteristics represent merely a few external variables.

One must consider that comparisons with data in official statistics are possible only within certain limits, as no data specifically on groups corresponding to the O-subjects in age and sentence length could be referred to either in criminal statistics relating to court proceedings *(Strafverfolgungsstatistik)* or in prison statistics. In interpreting prison statistics - which were used for the comparison since they contain the most information on prisoners - it must be taken into account that the data are collected on fixed dates and therefore refer only to inmates in prison on a specific day (March 31 of each year). Prisoners who serve a sentence falling between two fixed dates (not including either of them) are entirely disregarded. This leads to distortions, in particular to an underrepresentation of prisoners serving short sentences and to an overrepresentation of prisoners serving long sentences. This can also affect other characteristics, especially the extent of previous convictions.

The similarities between the O-subjects and male prison inmates in the Federal Republic of Germany with respect to distribution of *age groups, sentence length,* and *number of previous convictions* (see Table 1) must be viewed in the light of these reservations.

On the basis of its selection, the *G-group* was expected to be representative for the corresponding age group of the total male population of the same geographical region. In addition, we checked to what extent it was representative for the entire Federal Republic of Germany for certain external criteria.

With respect to *social stratification,* the subjects in the G-group were rated according to the social class of their families of orientation and their own social class on the basis of the index developed by KLEINING and MOORE (1968; for more details, see Part II, Sects. 2.1.2 and 2.3.4). Subsequently, they were compared with their population samples selected from the Federal Republic and from West Berlin (see Table 2).

For *social class of family of orientation,* the G-group was similar to the sample of KLEINING and MOORE, while for *subject's social class* there was a shift in the lower class to the upper lower class, i.e., a shift from temporary laborers and unskilled workers to skilled workers (on this marked upward mobility, see Part II, Sects. 2.1.2.3 and 2.3.4.2).

The G-group showed up more favorably for other criteria as well: The average intelligence quotient was somewhat higher (see Part II, Sect. 3.4.3.2) and the number of previously convicted subjects somewhat lower (see Part II, Sect. 4.7) than the corresponding figures for the population of the Federal Republic of Germany.

A *reason* why the values in the G-group differed for these criteria may be the *selection procedure* itself, besides the overrepresentation of students owing to the regional accumulation of universities in the area of Tübingen, Reutlingen, and Stuttgart. Generally speaking, samples drawn from population registers do not include persons who have no fixed abode or who change their place of residence without registering their new address. Precisely this group may well rank at the lower end of the social scale and include more persons with previous convictions. Moreover, four initially selected subjects with a considerable number of previous convictions refused to participate - one of them even ran away - presumably because they (mistakenly) expected criminal prosecution. These drop-outs (see Sect. 2.2 above) may be responsible for the absence of G-subjects corresponding to the criteria of the O-group with respect to offenses and penalties, though a proportion of approximately 1%-2% was to be expected.

3 Investigative Procedure

3.1 Conduct of the Examinations and Data Collection

In keeping with the research aim, i.e., the fullest possible comprehension of the subjects in the context of their social relationships, the following investigations were conducted: interviews, psychological tests, explorations, and laboratory tests carried out with *subjects* themselves; interviews with *other persons* for data collection on the *environment* of the subjects; and, in particular, data collection from *records.*

3.1.1 Contacting the Subjects

The O-subjects were contacted directly in the penal institution by the social workers, while the G-subjects first received a mimeographed note informing them of the aim of the study and the method of selection and notifying them of a visit by a social worker.

The object of the *first personal contact* with each of the selected subjects was to inform them of the aim of the study, the method of selection, and so on, and to persuade them to participate. A subject's consent to participate in the study was confirmed in a written statement, which also contained the permission to request records and information from authorities and the subject's contact persons. The subjects were informed of the team's obligation to maintain professional discretion and observe anonymity in publications.

The first interview with an *O-subject,* which lasted 2-3 hours, centered on his current situation, difficulties, and problems, and on his relatives, with the aim of creating the basis for a confidential relationship. These interviews were of no immediate use for the study itself and were not recorded.

The first interview with a *G-subject* was more problematic. The G-subjects were not always receptive to the study, and circumstances at home often made it impossible to hold a conversation in private. If any information was collected at all during these first interviews, it was limited to more or less superficial facts and formal data, which were at least useful as points of reference for requesting records from authorities and institutions.

3.1.2 Collection of Data and Examination of the Subjects

Subjects were invited to the Institute of Criminology as soon as possible after the first interviews, so that the external situation of the actual investigations would be practically the same for both groups. The direct investigations took 2-4 days, depending on the subject's life history, and the investigations in the Institute lasted an average of 20-25 hours per subject. The O-subjects were brought to the Institute by an employee of the penal institution, who was not present during the investigations. Due regard was paid to the daily routine of the penal institution, and there were practically no difficulties concerning appointments. Appointments with G-subjects were much more difficult. Because of their working hours and commitments during leisure time, the G-subjects could often come to the Institute only during weekends.

As a rule, the investigations in the Institute started with an extensive *interview* conducted by a social worker. Detailed data on each period of a subject's life were collected in unstructured interviews, following a guideline guaranteeing that nothing important was forgotten. The information was recorded and then set down in the form of a report. To avoid overtaxing the subjects, the individual phases of the interview were limited to a maximum of 3 hours.

After the data from the social environment of the subjects had been collected and the written information and documents received, further interviews usually took place. Gaps in information and any points which were unclear were corrected, and the subjects were confronted with any discrepancies between their own statements and information provided by other persons or derived from documents or the data collected in the subject's social environment. The total length of the interviews varied according to the life history of a subject; they generally lasted 10-15 hours.

After the interviews with the social workers, the psychologists conducted *psychological tests* and a supplementary *short psychological exploration.* A test battery, i.e., a combination of various tests, was administered, so that the individual test results would complement each other. The test battery included the tree test, the Rorschach test, the Wartegg design test, and, as a nonprojective test, the Wechsler Adult Intelligence Scale. The Rosenzweig Picture Frustration Test and/or the *Persönlichkeits- und Interessentest,* a test which measures personality traits and specific interests, were administered to a number of subjects in addition (for the individual tests and results, see Part II, Sect. 3.4.3).

The *medical examinations* included a psychiatric exploration (see Part II, Sects. 3.1.2 and 3.4.2), an electroencephalogram, and - for some of the subjects - an echoencephalogram, and/or chromosome examinations (see Part II, Sect. 3.3).

The direct data collection and the examinations of a subject were concluded by a discussion between the subject and the director of the Institute, who was also the head of the team.

As the direct data collection and examinations turned out to be much more intensive than the subjects had expected, several of them needed to be persuaded to come to the Institute for repeated visits. Moreover, the in-depth investigation of a subject and his life required a fair amount of cooperation, which was possible only on the basis of a confidential relationship between team member and subject.

As a whole, the O-subjects were more willing to give information, even if it was to their disadvantage or "negative." The G-subjects, in contrast, tended to hold back and gloss over or play down facts. Some G-subjects did not open up until several interviews had taken place and then approached the team member with their personal difficulties and problems, which occasionally meant a considerable additional expenditure of time. This was accepted for the sake of correctness of data.

3.1.3 Data Collected in the Social Environment of the Subjects

Other persons at the place of residence (or from the general environment) of a subject were interviewed to obtain further information. The social workers visited a subject's parents, relatives, and, if he was married, his wife and parents-in-law, and also his fellow employees, employers, friends, and acquaintances. Few subjects (mainly O-subjects) refused to give permission for this, despite all efforts to obtain it. The relatives of several subjects had died or could not be contacted because they were living in the German Democratic Republic or foreign countries. Nonetheless, the home and family environment could be investigated for 136 O- and 164 G-subjects. Relatives who lived far away or who could not be visited at home despite the subjects' permission were contacted by letter, which often resulted in additional information.

In many cases relatives could not be contacted during the first visit - whether because they were out or because they simply did not answer the door - so that more than one visit was necessary to obtain an interview. The interviews with relatives followed certain guidelines. They covered the same topics as the interviews with the subjects and were also recorded and summarized in a report. They took several hours; if necessary, more than one visit took place until the necessary data had been collected. This was particularly the case for the relatives of the G-subjects, who, like the subjects themselves, tended to hold back information and not open up for several visits. Subsequently, however, they often did not content themselves with their role as interviewees, but tried to contribute toward the aim of the study and the problems mentioned, countering questions with other questions and expressing their own ideas.

The relatives of the O-group, in contrast, were often familiar with the interview situation, usually because of previous experience with the police or other institutions. Nonetheless, the business of the study could often hardly be approached until some current crisis had been dealt with. Thus, often enough, the social workers had to help with welfare problems before they could begin their work as researchers.

At the same time, domiciliary visits provided an opportunity to conduct on-the-spot investigations of a subject's dwelling, and occasionally his place of work or leisure could also be viewed. Impressions were recorded in descriptive reports and sometimes in photographs. They covered the residential area, location, furnishings, arrangement, condition, and atmosphere of the dwelling and place of work or leisure.

Finally, in the investigations of the social environment additional, much clearer, and more extensive information than the often sparse written information (see Sect. 3.1.4 below) could be obtained in personal conversations at local authorities' offices, police stations, clergymen's offices, and schools, especially in small communities.

3.1.4 Data Collected from Records and Written Information

To check and supplement the information provided by the subjects and their relatives and that obtained from their social environment, any relevant authorities or institutions that the subject had been involved with were requested to provide all available records for consultation and to give general written information as well as answers to specific questions. The letters of request to the authorities and institutions referred to the permission of the subject and the decree of the Ministry of

Justice of Baden-Württemberg notifying all legal authorities of Baden-Württemberg of the Tübingen research project and requesting them to provide assistance.

Generally, 12-20 letters of request were written per subject; the number was substantially higher when a subject had frequently been convicted or committed to homes. Certain difficulties arose when a subject had often changed his place of residence - frequently without giving proper notice of his change of address - and when there were no records because a subject had stayed at a certain place for only a short time. Another problem was encountered with expellees and refugees, since comparable information from the authorities and institutions of their countries of origin could not be counted on. Any records in existence were requested from the head of the federal procedure for emergency acceptance *(Leiter des Bundesnotaufnahmeverfahrens)* in Giessen.

As a rule, an *extract from the register of convictions* was obtained for each O- and G-subject from the departments of public prosecution holding the records (at that time). If applicable, the extract was supplemented by information from the *juvenile records (gerichtliche Erziehungskartei)*. With this information, the corresponding *case records* could be requested from the court which had passed the sentence. If a sentence had already been served, the *records of execution of sentence (Vollstreckungshefte)* and *prison records* were requested from the corresponding authorities. In case of parole, probation, or an order for supervision of a probationer, the *probation service records* and written reports of the probation officers were obtained. In addition, the prison records of the term being served in the penal institution in Rottenburg were available for the O-subjects.

Additionally, information and records were requested from the *youth and social welfare offices* under whose supervision an O- or G-subject had spent at least part of his childhood. If it could be assumed that further youth or social welfare authorities, *homes*, or *reform schools* had any records, they were asked to lend them for a short time or to furnish a written report.

Furthermore, information and copies of certificates were obtained from *school authorities*, as were records from *local authorities* and *clergymen's offices* of the communities where a subject had grown up or lived for some time. Records pertaining to work and employment could be obtained from the various *statutory health insurance plans* and *employment offices*. Records and written information were also requested from the local police forces.

The data collected from records were extremely informative, particularly since the files usually contained more information and observations on the lives of the subjects than that what could have been expected considering the purpose of the records. This information - also used as a basis for further inquiries or checks with the subjects or other persons - contributed substantially to the completeness of data (see Sect. 3.2 below). In contrast, the additional written information requested, especially that provided by local authorities and institutions - when they provided more than formal data - was often very carefully worded and noncommittal, in some cases even biased in "favor" of the subject. The social workers' personal inquiries mostly showed that these institutions usually did not give any negative information on a person in the community as a matter of principle, but that they were able and - when guaranteed absolute discretion - willing to give corresponding verbal information.

3.2 The Problem of Completeness and Correctness of Data

The open procedure of the present study meant that the volume of relevant facts could not be determined in advance. Therefore, there were certain facts whose importance was not recognized until the study was well under way, but efforts to collect these data for all subjects were limited, partly for economic reasons. Consequently, despite the wealth of information, there was no overall *completeness* in the clarification of all details, especially as for some questions, contradictions between certain pieces of information remained unresolved despite all efforts. For this reason, "unclear" is occasionally found in the presentation of the results of the investigations (see also below Part II, Sect. 1.3).

Nonetheless, the *degree of truth* and the *correctness* of the data on the subjects' personalities and social spheres should be very high. The extensive and in-depth investigations conducted with the subjects by several researchers of different disciplines substantially reduced the subjects' opportunities for persisting in untrue statements. Records in particular (and partially the written information) were an effective corrective, as were the investigations of the social environment. Yet, although some of the information was very accurate, the contents of records could not be categorically assumed to be correct: Time and again it became apparent that the information relating to the immediate concern of the record was very reliable, while the information which was of marginal importance for the purpose of the records, and had thus been only incidentally collected, was often incorrect (regarding the degree of truth of information in records, see GÖPPINGER 1980, pp. 114ff.).

4 Evaluation of the Data

4.1 Preliminary Remarks

In studies which follow the usual procedure of empirical social research, the manner of evaluation is normally predetermined by the investigations. The mode of investigation, the research instrument, and the methods of evaluation are a unity reaching all the way down to the technical details of data processing.

Apart from the psychological and medical examinations, which used standardized testing methods in part, the investigations in the present study were to remain open to avoid the shortcomings of strictly hypothesis-testing studies. Owing to their design, hypothesis-testing studies investigate from a limited perspective which cannot be avoided or corrected. The open procedure in the present study meant that methods of evaluation had to be applied in retrospect to the manifold and complex individual data, especially those in the social spheres. In no way did this entail a loss of objectivity. The multitude of different pieces of information from various investigations even enabled the correction of facts usually considered to be "hard" (e.g., number of siblings). Standardized methods of data collection simulate a higher degree of precision only in that reality is adapted to what data can be collected with the research instrument. This is particularly true in the "soft" processes of estimation and classification. Moreover, once the data have been collected, any information not included in the categorization is *irretrievably lost* in standardized procedures. By categorizing after the data are collected, as was done in the present study, the "*surplus*" which does not belong to any category remains. Thus, particularly in problematic estimations and classifications, it was possible to consult the entire contents of the complex individual case investigations. In this respect, the procedure in the present study is certainly no less objective, although it involves much greater efforts than that in standardized investigations.

4.2 Stages and Directions of the Individual Evaluations

4.2.1 Processing the Data

First, a data sheet was conceived on the basis of the experience from the pilot studies and the knowledge obtained from the relevant literature. The sheet served as a guideline for the collection of data by the social workers and as a reminder of the topics to be covered. New experiences were continuously incorporated in the initial stage of the study.

Specially instructed research assistants transferred the facts from the records and from the social workers' comprehensive interview protocols to the data sheets, at the same time checking the data for completeness. Any gaps in information or unclear aspects found were arranged in a catalog of specific questions, which the social workers used to collect further data. After the investigation of a subject had been preliminarily concluded, the case was discussed in two differently composed small committees of the researchers concerned. If anything remained unclear, further data were collected. Any other questions of a fundamental nature were discussed in the "large committee," where the entire research team discussed pending problems.

In the next stage of the evaluation, a separate form was developed for each main area of investigation, and the results of each sphere were arranged on these forms. Again, detailed commentaries were made. Each individual data sheet, and therefore each individual case, was again checked for accuracy of transfer and completeness of information before the data were transferred to a data carrier and submitted to a normal error-checking program.

4.2.2 Statistical Evaluation

As a rule, the statistical evaluation took place as follows: First, characteristics were compared with respect to frequency in both samples, and the correlations between the differences were checked in significance tests (chi square test). Correlations between variables were presented in multidimensional table analyses. The phi coefficient and Pearson's contingency coefficient ($\bar{C}$) in its corrected form according to LIENERT (1967, pp. 560ff.) were used in the calculations. However, the number of variables whose covariation can be presented in a table is limited, as tables with more than three dimensions become too intricate. Furthermore, the number of variables analyzed simultaneously in one table is strictly limited by the size of the sample. Subgroups of 200 subjects are often too small to ensure significant results in inferential statistics.

Classical multivariate methods such as analysis of variance or factor analysis were not used. The external conditions for these methods, such as interval scale (exceptionally, also ordinal scale), normal distribution, and linear relationships between variables, are given for only a small part of the data, and then not even for the most important part. Besides these rather technical considerations, we decided as a matter of principle not to show correlations spanning the various spheres by way of statistical models (for details, see Part III, Sect. 1.1).

4.3 Evaluation with Regard to a Complex, Overall View

Besides the essentially quantitative-statistical evaluation of the findings in the various spheres, we attempted to obtain a complex, overall view of the wealth of information from the individual case investigations (for the methodological justification of this procedure, see Part III, Sect. 1). This overall view took into account the specific complex of conditions in the individual case better than the foregoing steps of evaluation, without remaining on the level of purely illustrative descriptions of individual cases.

To begin with, parallel to the work on the first data sheets, *overview forms* were created (see Part III, Sect. 4.2). The individual pieces of information were abbreviated and combined in tabular surveys. These forms were supplemented by detailed *descriptions of daily routines* (see Part III, Sect. 3.2). In these descriptions, it became particularly obvious that the separate areas of investigation interlocked and differed in weight.

A further emphasis was on full utilization of the advantages of the *comparative* design of the study. By nature, statistical comparisons take into account merely variables which can be collected as individual data and for which comparable facts are available for a large proportion of the subjects. Yet there was some reason to assume that essential and characteristic differences between O- and G-subjects existed as well in circumstances prevailing for only a few (in extreme cases only two) subjects. Though such differences can be of some importance in a complex, overall view, they are not generally valid. This limitation was offset by the possibility of recognizing life circumstances which had occasionally not even been assumed to be of any relevance. The aim of these comparisons was a contrasting description of the (ideal-)typical behavior of the O- and the G-group in the various - particularly the social - spheres of the study (see Part III, Sect. 2).

The endeavor to match O- and G-subjects who were as identical as possible in all external, particularly decisive life circumstances as "*twin pairs*" and to compare them (see Part III, Sect. 4.3) pursued a similar aim. As there was no technical procedure for this kind of matching, the direct experience from the investigations had to be referred to once again. Had we attempted to avoid this problem by matching earlier on, we would have been limited to (theoretical) knowledge or (hypothetical) assumptions. In this way, the direct knowledge of a wealth of life circumstances, sometimes surprisingly relevant, could be included in the matching.

Further work at this level of evaluation was equally geared to obtaining a complex, overall view (of the offender in the context of his social relationships). Here, it was important to integrate both the individual findings elaborated in the separate spheres by means of the statistical evaluation and the foregoing steps of evaluation into *constellations in the cross section* (see Part III, Sect. 3.3) and *courses in the longitudinal section* (see Part III, Sect. 4.4). The impression gained from the individual case descriptions that the essential differences between the O- and the G-subjects can become visible only in an overall view of their life patterns had to be objectified, i. e., made accessible for verification and presentation. For this purpose, criteria spanning the various spheres had to be formed. Otherwise, a comparison of the subjects in an overall view would have been impossible. In a protracted process, these criteria were continuously refined and changed in meaning by continuously checking whether and how they really applied to the subjects. To some extent, the results of the statistical evaluation could be used to this end. As a rule, however, the fact that these criteria spanned the various spheres required being familiar with all life circumstances of a subject, which meant that all individual case descriptions had to be consulted constantly.

4.4 Summary

The evaluation of the data took place on two different levels, a statistical evaluation in the spheres on one level and a more qualitative elaboration of a complex, overall view on the other. Though there were two different levels where two different means of obtaining knowledge were applied, it should not be forgotten that these levels are interdependent and stimulate each other. One reason for this is that the individual case investigations, where factual truth was strongly emphasized, were a starting point *and* a constant corrective for the processing in the statistical evaluation and the efforts to find relationships spanning the various spheres (see Part III, Sect. 1.3). On the one hand, reciprocal stimulation became evident when typical manifestations gained on one level motivated the quantitative assessment of "variables" which went beyond the level of formal or external data on the other level. In this way alone, a substantial increase in knowledge was obtained. On the other hand, referring back to how frequently characteristics occurred was a constant corrective for the immediate experience from the direct contact with the subjects and their environment on the other level of evaluation.

That all this could be effective was guaranteed by the external form of cooperation, the small and large committees, the innumerable meetings, and constant informal communication among team members. Last but not least was the conviction that the team was working together on something important, the results of which were becoming discernible.

II Results in the Separate Areas

1 Preliminary Remarks

1.1 Division into Separate Areas

The following presentation of the various findings from the separate spheres offers no unified picture. This is a result of the - of necessity somewhat arbitrary - division into separate spheres introduced for the purpose of analysis.

A rough division into social, somatic, and psychological/psychiatric areas offered itself, considering the traditional division of objects among the disciplines related to criminology and the interdisciplinary composition of the research team. Yet the boundaries are fluid, depending on the conception of the discipline. Moreover, it was our aim to replace the model of an interdisciplinary criminology consisting of *completed* individual parts with an integrative criminology, where every individual contribution already has a *specifically criminological* perspective (see Part I, Sect. 1; in this connection, and regarding the assumed boundaries between the related disciplines, see GÖPPINGER 1980, pp. 7 ff. and 76 ff.). In this respect, there is a constant conflict in the efforts to appreciate individual results as such and yet see their interdependency with the whole.

In part, the interdependency was taken into account by referring to other spheres and to the complex, overall view (see Part III) or by summarizing from this specifically criminological angle. It should be noted, however, that the various results are not to be understood as parts of the disciplines related to criminology: They gain their real importance when seen as part of a (criminological) whole.

The division into areas and their share in the following presentation are to a certain degree themselves a result of the study. The heart of Part II is the presentation of the *social spheres* (see Sect. 2 below), as the findings in these spheres were of considerable importance. Here again, it should not be forgotten that the division into separate spheres, however logical it may seem, is artificial. It is certainly true that the family of orientation is in a certain sense an environment which initially surrounds a person entirely. Step by step, it is extended or succeeded by the subject's own material (spheres of performance, leisure) and personal (contacts, ties, family of procreation) relationships. The division between the spheres of performance and leisure seems obvious as well. Nevertheless, in the course of the study, it became apparent that difficult definitions were necessary or that overlapping occurred (e.g., in the sphere of abode, there is a transitional phase during which the subject is entirely oriented away from home but still sleeps there) and that criminologically essential knowledge could often not be gained until the spheres were examined in their reciprocity. For instance, the spheres of leisure and contacts are closely related in many respects. But even though the spheres of performance and leisure, for example, can be considered *complementary* in many respects, their direct relatedness becomes apparent in criteria such as the "expansion of leisure time at the expense of the sphere of performance." Thus, it is often the *interdependency* of the spheres which points out the specific differences between the O- and the G-subjects.

As always in statistical processing, a further simplification of a complex reality occurred insofar as, in the separate spheres as well, life circumstances had to be split into questions and variables. Consequently, details of individual cases were lost in the classification according to abstract criteria. It was attempted to compensate for this loss of reality by referring back to the *individual case studies,* using the impressions and knowledge gained there as illustrations and pointing out relationships which became apparent in the individual cases (concerning the further importance of individual case studies, see Part III, Sects. 1.2 and 1.3).

1.2 Comparisons with Other Studies

Each summary of a sphere in Part II contains a short overview of the pertinent results of the relevant studies. Generally, only studies conducted on the basis of the classical multifactorial approach in criminology were taken into consideration. In only a few exceptional cases were studies concerned with merely one specific aspect included.

Exemplary, and best comparable as a retrospective comparative study in terms of breadth of investigations and design, is the research of the GLUECKS (GLUECK and GLUECK 1957, 1974), though they left off at a point beyond which the Tübingen study particularly wanted to proceed (for details, see Part III, Sect. 1). The more recent study of WEST (1969, 1982; WEST and FARRINGTON 1973, 1977) is also worthy of notice. As a prospective cohort study, it is, in a certain sense, the touchstone for the factual soundness of the methodological objections to retrospective comparative studies (concerning methodology, see Part I, Sect. 2.1).

Yet a comparison of the results of the large multifactorial studies with those of the present study poses some difficulties. On the one hand, the samples of the studies differed, as they were always formed according to special points of view. On the other hand, the differences in their design and, even more pronouncedly, in the training of the researchers in different disciplines rendered their comparison difficult. It is very unlikely that concepts such as "conspicuous" or "antisocial behavior", "mental disorders", "neurotic", etc. were used in the same way. Additionally, in comparisons on an international level, the differing legal systems and criminal codes must be taken into consideration, as they may mean that "criminality" is defined differently from one country to another and therefore occurs to a differing extent. For example, in the United States, the concept of "delinquency" includes acts or behavior patterns which, in the Federal Republic of Germany, are mainly still considered "social conspicuousness." Finally, since the time of the early studies by HEALY and BRONNER (1926, 1936) or the later ones by the GLUECKS, changes have taken place in the social, moral, and cultural situation - again with different national colorings. These considerations compel one to use the utmost care when generalizing common results of the large multifactorial comparative studies.

Consequently, it is all the more surprising that the studies, providing they applied comparable criteria, led to similar results, in particular in what are called the social spheres in the present study. The interpretation or criminological importance given the individual findings varies considerably, yet the findings themselves, especially facts which are easy to determine, are not so heterogeneous as to make any comparison futile. In view of these findings, the present study can certainly be included in the tradition of multifactorial studies. In addition, however, it was attempted to go beyond this stage of knowledge to obtain a complex, overall view integrating the individual results (see Part III).

1.3 General Information on the Presentation

Considering the way the offender group was selected (see Part I, Sect. 1), it was expected that the offenders would already have gone through what can be called a "criminal career" and that they had usually committed an offense during their youth. It was all the more surprising, then, that a substantial percentage of them - 43% (86 subjects) - had *no* criminal record at juvenile age. In the course of the evaluation, it became increasingly apparent that these subjects, hereafter referred to as "late delinquents" (O_2), differed markedly from the other O-subjects, the "early delinquents" (O_1). In the following, the offender group is differentiated accordingly - in retrospect - for important characteristics. An early delinquent or *O_1-subject* is one who committed his first registered offense before his 18th birthday, while a subject who had no criminal record until after this date was a late delinquent or *O_2-subject*. One's 18th birthday is also an important date, since offenses committed before this date are merely sentenced according to the Juvenile Court Act *(Jugendgerichtsgesetz)*, whereas later offenses may be sentenced according to the Criminal Code *(Strafgesetzbuch)*.

With respect to the age of the subjects at the time of the study, the age variation resulting from the selection criterion was superimposed by the fact that the individual subjects were investigated one after another (see Part I, Sect. 2.2). Thus, the indications "at the time of the study" and "during the period of the study" do not represent a uniform date, but vary from subject to subject. Insofar as the data are concerned with the external circumstances and behavior of the subjects, the *time of the study* is the time of their last imprisonment for the O-subjects and the beginning of the individual investigations in the Institute for the G-subjects. In the following, statements beyond this period are made only in exceptional cases and are always indicated. Similarly, the *period of the study* is the period before their last imprisonment for the O-subjects and before the beginning of the individual investigations for the G-subjects.

The medical and psychological test data, in contrast, generally refer to the time when they were actually collected, thus, for the O-subjects, to some time during their last imprisonment.

Prior to the *presentation of the figures,* it should be noted that several subjects had to be disregarded for a series of criteria. In addition to several subjects for whom not all data were collected (see Part I, Sects. 3.1.2 and 3), several subjects were occasionally disregarded for reasons of contents or systematics. For the family of orientation, for example, four O-subjects who had grown up almost exclusively in homes were disregarded. This is mentioned wherever it occurs. It was generally possible, however, to keep the number of such unclear cases low because of the wealth of sources of information (see Part I, Sect. 3.2). Small deviations in the total populations because of unclear cases could not always be avoided. They are not explained individually in the following.

2 The Social Spheres

2.1 The Family of Orientation

2.1.1 Preliminary Remarks

The family of orientation is considered to be of special importance insofar as it is generally the "environment" per se of a person for a relatively long time. It should not be forgotten, however, that the family of orientation is an intricate complex of conditions, where not only the family and its environment form the child, but the child itself also exerts an influence. In this sense, it will presumably remain impossible to comprehend completely by empirical means the process of growing up, particularly the reciprocal relationship between parents and child, whether by retrospective investigations or participant observation.

Moreover, in the present study, the problems related to retrospection must be taken into consideration, particularly the subjects' selective faculties of memory, considering how far back in time their childhood was. Here in particular, the combination of various data collection techniques (see Part I, Sect. 3) proved essential. We did not assume a priori that information from records or interviews with other persons were more objective: By using all sources of information, we tried to obtain an accurate picture of the individual case. In order to rule out conscious and unconscious misrepresentations, a basic stock of "hard" data, for example, stays in camps and assistance by public institutions, was collected by means of criteria which were easy to objectify. The evaluation differentiated between external and internal circumstances; the internal circumstances were subdivided into structural and functional aspects.

As mentioned above (see Sect. 1.3 above), it was not always possible to consider each subject for all criteria. Especially for the family of orientation, where the facts to be collected had occurred some time earlier, there was a considerable quota of uncertain or entirely unclear information for several criteria. These cases are not mentioned in the tables; the figures in the tables and their interpretation relate to unequivocal positions only. Moreover, four subjects were completely disregarded since they had grown up almost exclusively in homes.

Additional information on the sphere of the family of orientation can be found in Dolde (1978), who, however, uses a partially different categorization.

2.1.2 External Circumstances of the Family of Orientation

2.1.2.1 Socioeconomic Status

The socioeconomic situation of the subjects was determined by means of the index of class self-rating developed by Kleining and Moore (1968), which rates according to the occupation of the main breadwinner (see Dolde 1978, pp. 166 ff.).

Table 3. Social class of family of orientation

	O-subj (n=196)	G-subj (n=200)	O_1-subj (n=113)	O_2-subj (n=83)	In comparison, the sample of KLEINING and MOORE[a] (n=14375)
Upper and middle middle class (UM+MM)	4.6%	15.0%	5.3%	3.6%	17%
Lower middle class (LM)	14.8%	38.0%	14.2%	15.7%	38%
Upper lower class (UL)	35.7%	29.5%	37.2%	33.7%	30%
Lower lower class (LL)	44.9%	17.5%	43.4%	47.0%	15%

Significance level: O-G: $p<.001$; O_1-O_2: *n.s.*, not significant

[a] KLEINING and MOORE 1968, p. 547. The sample covers the 16- to 65-year-old residential population of the Federal Republic of Germany and West Berlin in 1967 and 1968. The categories "industrial" and "nonindustrial" as well as "lower lower class" and "socially despised" were taken together

The data were complete and detailed enough for this criterion. The index was modified, however, in that the subjects were rated by us, not by themselves. Table 3 shows the social stratification of the subjects.

The O-subjects are clearly overrepresented in the lower class, especially in the lower lower class. Yet one should be cautious in interpreting this result. No less than 47% of the G-families also belonged to the lower class (for a differentiated discussion of the problem of social class, see Sect. 2.1.3.4 below; in connection with intergenerational mobility, see Sects. 2.1.2.3 and 2.3.4.2 below).

2.1.2.2 Other External Circumstances

The individual case investigations also allowed a detailed presentation of the "external circumstances" of the families of the O- and the G-subjects. As the *immediate "environment" of the subject,* these circumstances have a much stronger effect than social class alone. Thus, in some cases it was shown that a "bad reputation in the community," which does not necessarily have only socioeconomic causes, often made it difficult for a subject to find an apprenticeship, in particular in small communities, and could thus indirectly influence the post-school sphere of performance. "Physical disability of a parent or other person rearing the subject" often meant considerable difficulties and strains for the entire family far beyond mere socioeconomic aspects.

For a presentation of such additional facts leading to "problems of adaptation" see Table 4.

The strains mentioned occurred much more frequently in the O- than in the G-group, especially "bad reputation in the community" and "social conspicuousness or criminality" of a parent, other person rearing the subject, or sibling. For the present, it can be stated that considerably more O- than G-subjects grew up much longer in family circumstances marked by various "problems of adaptation" (on the relationship with social class, see Table 10). But not until the social workers' direct investigations of the environment did the actual extent of neglect in the family circumstances of many O-subjects become visible.

Table 4. Other strains in family of orientation

	O-subj ($n=196$)	G-subj ($n=200$)	Sig. O–G	O_1-subj ($n=113$)	O_2-subj ($n=83$)	Sig. O_1–O_2
Over 6 years in inadequate housing conditions[a]	29.1%	3.5%	++	31.7%	25.3%	n.s.
Living on "social welfare" for at least 1 year, except if caused by illness	9.2%	2.5%	+	11.5%	6.0%	n.s.
Bad reputation in the community (father and/or mother)	31.1%	4.0%	++	39.8%	19.3%	+
Physical impairment of a person rearing the subject	18.9%	8.0%	+	25.7%	9.6%	+
Social conspicuousness or criminality of a person rearing the subject[b]	49.0%	12.5%	++	54.9%	41.0%	n.s.
	($n=165$)	($n=176$)		($n=94$)	($n=71$)	
Social conspicuousness or criminality of siblings[c]	40.4%	7.9%	++	52.1%	25.4%	++

Significance level: +, $p<.05$; ++, $p<.001$; *n.s.*, not significant

[a] Primitive dwellings, hostels for the homeless, bunkers, huts, overcrowded dwellings without any private area for the subjects

[b] Promiscuity and other sexual conspicuousness, conspicuously high alcohol consumption, particularly aggressive behavior, being regarded as an outsider, or registered delinquency excluding traffic delinquency

[c] Siblings with whom the subject lived for at least 6 months, including step- and foster siblings

The difficulties related to *resettlement* after World War II, which occurred rather frequently in both groups, can also be considered external problems of adaptation; 43.5% of the O- and 29.5% of the G-families (i.e., at least one parent) were expellees, refugees, or immigrants. In both groups, these families had a lower socioeconomic status than the domestic families. Yet here again, observing social class alone is misleading for the specific importance of the family as the "environment" of the subject. The G-immigrants belonging to the lower lower class had mostly just moved down to this social class ($G=13$ of 19; $O=9$ of 42; $p<.001$). Before their resettlement, they had often been independent farmers or artisans.

Despite the frequent downward occupational mobility measured by class index, the main breadwinners of the G-immigrants were capable of procuring ordered housing circumstances earlier than those of the O-immigrants. Only 6.8% of the G-, as compared with 38.4% ($p<.001$) of the O-immigrant families, lived in inadequate housing conditions for more than 6 years (on these subjects, see Sect. 2.2.2.2 below). Furthermore, according to the *individual case studies,* they usually provided for a better education of the subjects. Once again, the difference between the O- and the G-group was the specific *reaction* to the *same* "objective" problems of adaptation.

2.1.2.3 Vertical Mobility of the Family of Orientation and Intergenerational Mobility

There were practically no differences in *vertical social mobility* of the family of orientation. It is merely striking, that, as mentioned above in relation to immigrants and resettlers, 19 of the 35 G-families of the lower lower class had just moved down to that social class, as opposed to only 20 of the 88 O-families (O_1: 13 of 49; O_2: 7 of 39; $p<.001$).

Obvious differences existed, however, in the comparison of the socioeconomic status of the families of orientation with that of the subjects, i.e., in *intergenerational mobility*. In a separate examination of the subjects of the upper lower class - for whom both upward and downward mobility is possible - it became apparent that 69.1% of the O- and only 11.3% of the G-subjects had moved down the scale. Here again, the rating of subjects according to a class index only unsatisfactorily expressed their actual social position. Nonetheless, the fact of a clearly divergent socioeconomic development for the O- and the G-subjects remained (for details, see Sect. 2.3.4.2 below).

2.1.3 Internal Circumstances of the Family of Orientation

The division into structural and functional aspects is artificial insofar as certain conditions can be viewed structurally if given circumstances are taken into consideration; if the reactions of those concerned are also taken into account, there is a transition toward a functional approach.

2.1.3.1 Structural Aspects

Table 5 shows the distribution of the most important structural variables.

It is revealing that *loss of parent(s),* which should be considered purely a matter of fate, occurred to the same extent in both groups. In only relatively few cases did the mother remarry after the death of a subject's father (O = 8; G = 3). The *individual case studies* showed that the previous "style" of the G-family remained practically unchanged or that corresponding compensations occurred, whether the mother remarried or not. The G-subjects developed other strong ties and accepted offers of such; the G-mothers, despite economic burdens or employment (for details, see below), saw to it that their children were adequately supervised and taken care of. In contrast, the attempts to find a substitute home for the O-subjects often failed because of the behavior of the O-subjects themselves, and mothers felt responsible to only a small degree. Thus, any already existing lack of ties and supervision was accentuated (see GÖPPINGER 1980, p. 262).

For structural incompleteness of family as well, there were no differences between the O- and the G-subjects providing the incompleteness was continuous, i.e., providing there were no *changes of parents or other persons rearing the subject.*

Such changes took place especially when the family was temporarily incomplete because a subject's parents were separated or divorced. A total of 19.4% of the O-subjects, but only 7% of the G-subjects had one or more stepfathers or their mothers had male companions. At least one change of parent or other person rearing the subject occurred for 15% of the G-group, as compared with 38.3% of the O-group ($p<.001$; see also DOLDE 1978, p. 238).

The reactions of the subjects and their families to a *"separation from the mother"* also differed. Before the subjects were 5, mostly going to stay with the father, rela-

Table 5. Structural family circumstances

	O-subj ($n=200$)	G-subj ($n=200$)	Sig. O-G	O_1-subj ($n=114$)	O_2-subj ($n=86$)	Sig. O_1-O_2
Orphans: Father dead	15.0%	14.5%	n.s.	14.0%	16.3%	n.s.
Mother dead	5.5%	2.5%	n.s.	4.4%	7.0%	n.s.
Both parents dead	1.5%	-	n.s.	0.9%	2.3%	n.s.
Grew up exclusively in homes (3 orphans)	(4)	(0)	-	(1)	(3)	-
	($n=196$)	($n=200$)		($n=113$)	($n=83$)	
Subject grew up in structurally incomplete family[a]						
Always	15.8%	15.5%	n.s.	12.4%	20.5%	n.s.
Over 1 year	33.2%	15.0%	++	31.0%	36.1%	n.s.
Under 1 year or not at all	50.0%	69.5%	++	56.6%	43.4%	n.s.
Subject is illegitimate	18.4%	3.5%	++	22.1%	13.3%	n.s.
Subject has 5 or more siblings	15.8%	8.5%	+	20.4%	3.6%	+
Subject is an only child	15.8%	12.0%	n.s.	16.8%	14.5%	n.s.
Subject was separated from mother[b]						
Age 0-2	9.2%	5.5%	n.s.	10.6%	7.2%	n.s.
Age 3-5	5.6%	2.5%	n.s.	4.4%	7.2%	n.s.
Age 6-13	21.9%	6.5%	++	23.9%	19.3%	n.s.

Significance level: +, $p<.05$; ++, $p<.001$; *n.s.*, not significant
[a] Separation and divorce of parents, being an orphan, illegitimacy
[b] For at least 3 months

tives or other persons served as substitutes for the mother. At school age, however, the O-subjects were more frequently committed to homes (G=3 of 13; O=22 of 43; $p<.001$; $O_1=18$ of 27; $O_2=4$ of 16; $p<.05$) while the earlier "substitutes" continued for most G-subjects. (On stays in homes, especially the reasons for committal to a home, which are revealing in this context, see Sect. 2.2.2.3 below).

The difference in *number of siblings* was shown to be dependent on social class and was therefore a spurious correlation (on social stratification and other variables, see Table 10; see also DOLDE 1978, pp. 230ff.). The number of only children was approximately equal in both groups. There was an obvious difference in the proportions of illegitimate O- and G-subjects (see GÖPPINGER 1980, pp. 260ff.).

That the structural and functional views necessarily interlock was also shown plainly by the *employment of the mother* (see Table 6). About the same number of mothers were employed in both groups, and the rate of employment generally increased with the age of the subjects. G-mothers always worked more often at home by the hour, and, if they were away, their children were supervised more frequently. This indicates that the G-mothers were more careful and attentive, which was also confirmed by the *individual case studies*. This is a particularly illustrative example of the fact that an external condition alone - which is often the result of a fateful emergency - is of no importance unless the specific reactions to this condition are taken into account.

Table 6. Employment of mother

	Subjects' age	O-subj ($n=196$)	G-subj ($n=200$)	Sig. O-G	O_1-subj ($n=113$)	O_2-subj ($n=83$)	Sig. O_1-O_2
a) Mother employed	0- 2	38.3%	38.0%	n.s.	37.2%	39.8%	n.s.
	3- 5	47.5%	43.5%	n.s.	46.0%	49.4%	n.s.
	6-13	59.7%	57.5%	n.s.	53.1%	68.7%	+
b) At home and only by the hour (% of a)	0- 2	14.7%	32.9%	+	14.3%	15.2%	n.s.
	3- 5	14.0%	27.6%	+	13.5%	14.6%	n.s.
	6-13	11.1%	22.6%	+	11.7%	10.5%	n.s.
c) Child was always supervised (% of a)	0- 2	61.3%	85.5%	++	64.3%	57.6%	n.s.
	3- 5	52.7%	81.6%	++	51.9%	53.7%	n.s.
	6-13	29.9%	63.5%	++	25.0%	35.1%	n.s.

Significance level: +, $p<.05$; ++, $p<.001$; *n.s.*, not significant

2.1.3.2 Functional Aspects

The characteristic differences between the life patterns of the O- and the G-subjects were shown particularly well by their specific adaptation or attitude to the same "objective" circumstances, be they immigration, death of the father, or employment of the mother. This indicates the importance of functional internal circumstances in the family. In this context, it usually became apparent whether and how external difficulties were "compensated for."

Table 7 shows that unfavorable situations occurred substantially more often for the O-subjects for all internal circumstances. These differences proved to be largely independent of social class (see Table 10). They ranged from disrupted relationships between a subject's parents over lack of supervision, conspicuousness of the subject including theft and fraud (see also Sect. 4.2.1 below) and lack of emotional ties, to inconsistent child rearing and excessive corporal punishment in the heat of passion. There was a particularly obvious difference between the groups regarding the extent of "consistency in the parents' child rearing".

There were essential relationships between various variables. For example, the subjects who were not adequately supervised by their parents mostly came from families with disrupted relationships between parents (see Table 8).

Among the O-subjects who were brought up very strictly by their fathers were only a few whose fathers regularly participated in child rearing (see Table 9). Furthermore, the behavior of O-parents or other persons rearing the subject was often unpredictable; according to the *individual case studies*, the O-subjects often turned this to their own advantage by clever tactics.

Problematic as a whole were the relationships between O-subjects and fathers, which is expressed in the extent of corporal punishment as well as in the special affections and conflictual contacts of these O-subjects. The O-fathers ranked only fourth in a list of parents, grandparents, brothers, sisters and other relevant persons rated according to the affection the subjects felt for them (see DOLDE 1978, pp. 278 ff.), the O_1-fathers only fifth (in contrast, G-fathers ranked second). In the list of conflictual relationships, fathers ranked first in all groups.

Important differences between the O- and the G-subjects also became apparent in the detailed examination of the variables *"parental supervision"* and *"active*

Table 7. Functional family circumstances

	O-subj	G-subj	Sig.	O_1-subj	O_2-subj	Sig.
	($n=165$)	($n=167$)		($n=99$)	($n=66$)	
Disruption of parents' relationship[a]	46.1%	14.4%	++	53.5%	34.9%	+
Supervision of subject[b]	($n=178$)	($n=197$)		($n=107$)	($n=71$)	
Subject is supervised	74.2%	95.9%	++	74.8%	73.2%	n.s.
(Of these): Subject avoids supervision	37.1%	5.3%	++	51.3%	15.4%	++
No supervision	25.8%	4.1%	++	25.2%	26.8%	n.s.
Conspicuousness of subject at home[c]	($n=196$)	($n=200$)		($n=113$)	($n=83$)	
Total	56.7%	9.0%	++	68.1%	41.0%	++
In connection with theft and fraud	27.6%	2.5%	++	32.7%	20.5%	++
Positive basic attitude of	($n=144$)	($n=164$)		($n=89$)	($n=55$)	
Father	55.6%	88.4%	++	49.4%	65.5%	n.s.
	($n=178$)	($n=196$)		($n=105$)	($n=73$)	
Mother	82.9%	96.4%	++	83.3%	82.2%	n.s.
Strictness of child rearing	($n=130$)	($n=159$)		($n=80$)	($n=50$)	
By father: Very strict	33.9%	21.4%		37.5%	28.0%	
Normal	37.7%	63.5%	++	35.0%	42.0%	n.s.
Lax	28.4%	15.1%		27.5%	30.0%	
	($n=168$)	($n=199$)		($n=100$)	($n=68$)	
By mother: Very strict	7.7%	7.5%		3.0%	14.7%	
Normal	29.2%	71.4%	++	31.0%	26.5%	+
Lax	63.1%	21.1%		66.0%	58.8%	
Regular participation in child rearing of:						
	($n=152$)	($n=166$)		($n=94$)	($n=58$)	
Father	36.8%	71.7%	++	33.0%	43.1%	n.s.
	($n=183$)	($n=199$)		($n=107$)	($n=76$)	
Mother	45.8%	73.9%	++	55.1%	68.4%	++
	($n=126$)	($n=160$)		($n=77$)	($n=49$)	
Agreement of both parents with respect to child rearing	14.3%	73.6%	++	10.4%	20.4%	n.s.
	($n=196$)	($n=200$)		($n=113$)	($n=83$)	
Frequent violent punishment in the heat of passion	36.2%	9.5%	++	42.5%	27.7%	+

Significance level: +, $p<.05$; + +, $p<.001$; *n.s.*, not significant
[a] Frequent verbal and violent arguments; temporary or final separation/divorce
[b] Knowledge of activity and company, and at least partial supervision of homework
[c] Insincerity, disobedience, quarrelsomeness, running away

Table 8. Disruption of parents' relationship and supervision

	Supervision by parents	Parents' relationship		Significance, correlation
		Disrupted	Intact	
O-subjects ($n=142$)	There is supervision	29.0% (20)	68.5% (50)	++
	Subject avoids it, and no supervision	71.0% (49)	31.5% (23)	phi=.45
G-subjects ($n=166$)	There is supervision	75.0% (18)	95.1% (135)	+
	Subject avoids it, and no supervision	25.0% (6)	4.9% (7)	phi=.38
Significance		++	++	
Correlation		phi=.54	phi=.48	
O_1-subjects ($n=89$)	There is supervision	21.3% (10)	61.9% (26)	++
	Subject avoids it and no supervision	78.7% (37)	38.1% (16)	phi=.55
O_2-subjects ($n=53$)	There is supervision	45.5% (10)	77.4% (24)	+
	Subject avoids it and no supervision	54.5% (12)	22.6% (7)	phi=.50
Significance		+	n.s.	
Correlation		phi=.45	phi=.26	

Significance level: +, $p<.05$; ++, $p<.001$; *n.s.*, not significant

Table 9. Relationship between strict child rearing and participation of father in child rearing

	Very strictly reared			
	O-subjects ($n=44$)	G-subjects ($n=34$)	O_1-subjects ($n=30$)	O_2-subjects ($n=14$)
Father participated in child rearing				
Regularly	36.4% (16)	76.5% (26)	33.3% (10)	42.9% (6)
Irregularly	63.6% (28)	23.5% (8)	66.7% (20)	57.1% (8)

Significance level: O-G: $p<.001$; O_1-O_2: not significant

avoidance" of supervision by some of the subjects (see Table 7). The *individual case studies* showed that the O-subjects tended to turn away from the sphere of the family, often at a very early age, and "roam about," without their parents knowing or wanting to know about this or about the subjects' whereabouts, contacts, and leisure activities. Later on, this active avoidance of any kind of supervision continued in the specific conspicuousness in the sphere of performance (see Sect. 2.3 below).

2.1.3.3 A Critical View

The present results do not allow the interpretation that unfavorable conditions of socialization are, as it were, the links by which a low socioeconomic status affects future criminality. That the variables which best differentiate the O- and the G-

Table 10. Influence of social class

	O-subjects ($n=196$)		G-subjects ($n=200$)		Comparison O-G of same class		Comparison L-M in same group	
	Lower class ($n=158$)	Middle class ($n=38$)	Lower class ($n=94$)	Middle class ($n=106$)	Lower class	Middle class	O-subj	G-subj
More than 6 years in inadequate housing conditions[a]	34.8% (55)	5.3% (2)	5.3% (5)	1.9% (2)	++	n.s.	++	n.s.
Living on welfare for at least 1 year, except if due to illness	10.8% (17)	2.6% (1)	5.3% (5)	.0% (0)	n.s.	n.s.	n.s.	n.s.
Bad reputation in the community (father and/or mother)	36.1% (57)	10.5% (4)	5.3% (5)	2.8% (3)	++	n.s.	+	n.s.
Social conspicuousness or criminality of a person rearing the subject[b]	53.8% (85)	29.0% (11)	16.0% (15)	9.4% (10)	++	+	+	n.s.
Social conspicuousness or criminality of siblings[c]	45.1% (64)	13.0% (3)	11.7% (11)	3.3% (3)	++	n.s.	+	+
Physical impairment of a person rearing the subject	20.9% (33)	10.5% (4)	12.8% (12)	3.8% (4)	n.s.	n.s.	n.s.	+
Subject had 5 or more siblings	19.0% (30)	2.6% (1)	11.7% (11)	5.7% (6)	n.s.	n.s.	+	n.s.
Subject grew up in structurally incomplete family[d]								
Always	16.4% (26)	13.2% (5)	23.4% (22)	8.5% (9)				
More than 1 year	33.5% (53)	31.6% (12)	12.8% (12)	17.0% (18)	+	n.s.	n.s.	+
Less than 1 year, never	50.0% (79)	55.3% (21)	63.8% (60)	74.5% (79)				
Subject is illegitimate	19.0% (30)	15.8% (6)	6.4% (6)	.9% (1)	+	+	n.s.	n.s.
Subject was separated from mother from the age of 6 to 13[e]	22.8% (36)	18.4% (7)	6.4% (6)	6.6% (7)	++	+	n.s.	n.s.
Disrupted relationship between parents[f]	($n=132$)	($n=33$)	($n=72$)	($n=95$)				
	48.9%	36.4%	15.3%	13.7%	++	+	n.s.	n.s.
Supervision of subject[f]	($n=143$)	($n=35$)	($n=92$)	($n=105$)				
Subject is supervised	69.9%	91.4%	92.4%	99.0%	++	n.s.	+	+
Of these: subject avoids supervision	36.0%	40.6%	4.7%	5.8%	++	++	n.s.	n.s.
No supervision	30.1%	8.6%	7.6%	1.0%				
Conspicuousness of subject at home[f]	($n=158$)	($n=38$)	($n=94$)	($n=106$)				
As a whole	57.0%	55.3%	10.6%	6.6%	++	++	n.s.	n.s.
Associated with theft and fraud	25.9%	34.2%	4.3%	.9%	++	++	n.s.	n.s.
Positive basic attitude of								
Father	($n=111$)	($n=33$)	($n=69$)	($n=95$)				
	50.5%	69.7%	91.3%	86.3%	++	n.s.	+	n.s.
Mother	($n=140$)	($n=38$)	($n=92$)	($n=104$)				
	80.7%	84.2%	97.8%	95.1%	++	n.s.	n.s.	n.s.
Strictness of father in child rearing	($n=102$)	($n=28$)	($n=66$)	($n=93$)				
Strict	32.4%	39.3%	21.2%	21.5%				
Usual	38.2%	35.7%	57.6%	67.7%	n.s.	n.s.	n.s.	n.s.
Lax	29.4%	25.0%	21.2%	10.8%				
Strictness of mother in child rearing	($n=134$)	($n=34$)	($n=93$)	($n=106$)				
Strict	8.2%	5.9%	8.6%	6.6%				
Usual	25.4%	44.1%	73.1%	69.8%	n.s.	n.s.	n.s.	n.s.
Lax	66.4%	50.0%	18.3%	23.6%				
Regular participation in child rearing								
Father	($n=121$)	($n=31$)	($n=70$)	($n=96$)				
	47.9%	58.1%	68.6%	74.0%	++	n.s.	+	n.s.
Mother	($n=148$)	($n=35$)	($n=93$)	($n=106$)				
	56.1%	80.0%	88.2%	91.5%	++	n.s.	+	n.s.

Table 10 (continued)

	O-subjects ($n=196$)		G-subjects ($n=200$)		Comparison O-G of same class		Comparison L-M in same group	
	Lower class ($n=158$)	Middle class ($n=38$)	Lower class ($n=94$)	Middle class ($n=106$)	Lower class	Middle class	O-subj	G-subj
Agreement of both parents with respect to child rearing[f]	($n=97$) 13.4%	($n=29$) 17.2%	($n=67$) 76.1%	($n=93$) 72.0%	++	++	n.s.	n.s.
Frequent/brutal punishment in the heat of passion[f]	($n=158$) 37.3%	($n=38$) 31.6%	($n=94$) 5.3%	($n=106$) 13.2%	++	+	n.s.	n.s.

Significance level: +, $p<.05$; ++, $p<.001$; *n.s.*, not significant
[a] Primitive dwellings, hostels for the homeless, bunkers, barracks, overcrowded apartments with no own sphere of living for the subject
[b] Sexual conspicuousness, considerable alcohol consumption, aggressive behavior, being an outsider, or registered criminality without traffic offenses
[c] With whom the subject lived together for at least 6 months: O (L=142; M=23); G (L=86; M=90)
[d] Parents separated or divorced
[e] For at least 3 months
[f] Populations and explanations, see Table 7

group are distributed irrespective of social class in the G-group clearly speaks against this (see Table 10; see also DOLDE 1978, p.300).

The differences in conditions of socialization, particularly functional internal circumstances, are more important than the mere fact of social class, since they express a great deal more of the specific reality of life in which a subject grew up. Nevertheless, here again, one should be careful with general causal interpretations, above all because of two findings: On the one hand, there are a considerable number of subjects, especially among the O_2-subjects, who grew up in ordered family circumstances and yet became seriously delinquent. Family circumstances possibly prevented as early an onset of criminality as for the O_1-subjects. On the other hand, there were enough G-subjects for whom criminality did not occur or remained a temporary episode despite unfavorable circumstances. Evidently, it depends on additional conditions whether "positive" or "negative" circumstances affect criminality at all. These various possibilities cannot, however, be expressed in general probability statements on the importance of the family of orientation for criminality.

The partially substantial tendencies of the G-subjects' to gloss over facts when presenting the circumstances in their families, which came to light in the intensive investigations, must be seen in this context. In statements on their parents, the G-subjects mainly expressed understanding for their parents' difficulties and justified their failure. The subjects regretted negative external circumstances such as a lack of educational opportunities but tried to compensate for this lack by their own efforts (see Sect. 2.3 below). In contrast, the O-subjects tended to put their family circumstances into an unfavorable light to relate their criminality more easily and plausibly to these circumstances, either for themselves or for others.

Furthermore, it was shown that only the persistence in the efforts to obtain correct information in the collection of data revealed the differences between the subjects' presentations and the additional findings based on the data collected from other sources (for the O- as well as for the G-subjects, though to a lesser extent and mostly in the opposite sense). Without these efforts, the presentations of the O- and the G-subjects could not have been compared; in this way, the presentations themselves became an essential material criterion.

Neither can any general statement be made on the direction of causal relationships. That the subjects were not only passively subjected to circumstances at home is shown by the findings on the subjects' own conspicuousness, such as their active avoidance of any parental supervision. In the *individual case studies,* it became evident that severe disruptions in the family of orientation occasionally developed only because of the behavior of the subject. It was reported, for example, that parents could not "cope with" a subject from the beginning or that he couldn't "get into line." Furthermore, "special affections" or "conflictual contacts," as well as all variables of style of child rearing always depend on the behavior of the child (subject) as well.

This does not call into question the importance of circumstances in the family of orientation for the development of a person. Yet their importance, at least with respect to recidivist criminality (for other possible disadvantages, see GÖPPINGER 1980, pp. 240 ff.), is not specific enough to allow any *general* theoretical statements. Whether such "deficits," perhaps only one of them, may or may not be of considerable importance *in the individual case* is in no way decided, but remains to be determined empirically.

2.1.3.4 Excursus: Social Class as a Factor

It is a common fact that approximately half of the population (47% of the G-group in the present study; 45% in KLEINING and MOORE) belongs to the lower class. This means that a categorization into social classes on the basis of socioeconomic circumstances describes other criteria of "inequality" than those separating the O- and the G-group. There are only very specific (and extremely few) members of the lower class who become recidivist offenders in the sense of the O-criteria. The percentage of O-subjects in the corresponding segment of the entire population amounts to approximately 1%–2% (see Part I, Sect. 2.3), while 15% of the population belonged to the lower lower class in the sample of KLEINING and MOORE (1968). A specific class behavior, as assumed by the older criminal sociology, as well as a class-specific policy of selective sentencing, as is occasionally currently assumed, would have had to become apparent in the lower lower class of the G-group, as it was not a contrast but a true control group (on the criminality of the G-group, see Sect. 4.7 below).

Furthermore, the correlation between social class and criminality cannot be interpreted as a one-way influence between dependent (criminality) and independent (social class) variables. On the basis of the present findings, there is no doubt whatsoever that a large number of O-subjects grew up in extremely problematic circumstances, including social conspicuousness and criminality of a parent or other person rearing the subject, but Table 10 shows that this is *no class*-specific correlation.

On the one hand, the differences between the O- and the G-subjects usually remained when only the lower class subjects were compared (Table 10, 4th column from the right). On the other hand, there was no relationship, with a few insignificant exceptions, between these variables and social class in the G-group (Table 10, 1st column from the right). The frequency of strains - also in the internal circumstances of the family - among the O-subjects of the lower class (Table 10, 1st column from the left), therefore, *cannot* be explained by social class. Moreover, considering in particular the considerable differences in intergenerational mobility, it seems to be equally plausible in many cases that only a subject's specific individual behavior led to a low socioeconomic status.

The *individual case studies* repeatedly confirmed that many subjects "felt attracted" by a different environment than that of their families of orientation or that they "just liked it there" (see GÖPPINGER 1980, p. 267). This sense of well-being, which is difficult to describe, was merely possible if a subject's entire life-style, including organization of time and external social manners, largely corresponded with this "other environment." However, these were always specific groups of reference, which in the case of the O-subjects again mostly belonged to the lower class according to the criteria of common indices. Yet they owed their attractiveness to characteristics which had nothing to do with social class (see Sects. 2.4.3.3 and 2.5.3 below).

This is shown very clearly in the results of the study of WEST (1969, 1982; WEST and FARRINGTON 1973, 1977), who selected a cohort in a London working class neighborhood and found differences between the delinquent and nondelinquent juveniles which are similar to those in the present study.

2.1.4 Summary

The findings on the family of orientation showed two general tendencies: The essential differences between the O- and the G-group relevant to (recidivist) criminality did not appear in external circumstances, for which data were easy to collect, but only in the detailed examination of the specific behavior of the subjects and their families. Problems of adaptation ensuing from the social conspicuousness of parents were more important than socioeconomic status as such. Immigrant or expellee G-parents reacted to "refugee" problems in a different way than O-parents did. Structural incompleteness of family and employment of mother as such were insignificant. However, frequent changes of parents or other persons rearing the subject or insufficient supervision of subjects during mothers' employment did have an effect. As the statistical frequencies and the *individual case studies* showed, *functional internal circumstances* had a more lasting effect than structural conditions, such as being an orphan or the number of siblings. But a disrupted relationship between parents, inconsistent and unpredictable child rearing, and disrupted emotional relationships between parents and subjects were *not* specific enough to be *causally related* with future delinquency in a *general* way.

This tendency corresponds largely to the *results of other multifactorial studies*. "Broken home", insofar as it means a merely external incompleteness of family, is also not considered to influence delinquency in any significant way by HEALY and BRONNER (1926, p. 123), OTTERSTRÖM (1946, pp. 142, 145), FERGUSON (1952, p. 145), McCORD and McCORD (1959, pp. 83 ff.), PONGRATZ and HÜBNER (1959, p. 55), Statens offentliga utredningar (1973 a, p. 210), and WEST and FARRINGTON (1973, pp. 69 ff.). While GLUECK and GLUECK (1974, p. 64) and McCORD and McCORD (1959, p. 83) do mention "broken home" and illegitimacy as deviance propitious, they also describe the influence of "internal" factors such as lack of cohesion in this connection. In contrast, the report of the Centro Nazionale di Prevenzione e Difesa Sociale (1969, pp. 77, 97, 352 ff.) states that a higher proportion of the delinquents, especially recidivists, had lost their fathers.

The remaining findings on *socioeconomic circumstances* lack uniformity. Similar to the present study, WOLFGANG et al. (1972, pp. 54 ff.), WEST and FARRINGTON (1973, p. 27), and GLUECK and GLUECK (1974, pp. 60, 67) found that the families of delinquents were overrepresented in the lower classes. On the other hand, HEALY and BRONNER (1926, p.121), POWERS and WITMER (1951, p.230, 234), and Statens offentliga utredningar (1972, p. 108) saw no relationship between standard of living and delinquency.

Increased *social conspicuousness and criminality of the parents* of delinquents is also reported by MCCORD and MCCORD (1960, pp.104ff.), WEST and FARRINGTON (1973, p.33), and GLUECK and GLUECK (1974, pp.51ff.). The (socio)psychological interpretations of these findings lack uniformity. HEALY and BRONNER (1926, p.129), OTTERSTRÖM (1946, pp.156, 179ff.), and Statens offentliga utredningar (1972, p.108) state that conspicuousness and delinquency of parents are not decisive. The same holds for conspicuousness of siblings of delinquents. While indications on the influence of number of siblings and position in sibling order (necessarily) depend on differing psychological interpretations, the findings of a large number of siblings (WEST and FARRINGTON 1973, pp.31ff.) and of stronger social conspicuousness and criminality of the siblings of delinquents (GLUECK and GLUECK 1974, p.53; WEST and FARRINGTON 1973, p.37; 1977, pp.109ff.) seem to have been determined directly.

As regards *functional internal circumstances,* MCCORD and MCCORD (1959, p.83), ROSENQUIST and MEGARGEE (1969, p.305), FERRACUTI et al. (1975, pp.61ff.), and GLUECK and GLUECK (1974, pp.67ff.) present comparable indications on inner conflicts in the family and weaker family ties for delinquents. The negative influence of marital disharmony on children is regarded as more important than the mere fact of a missing person of reference by HEALY and BRONNER (1926, p.123; 1936, pp.29ff.), PONGRATZ and HÜBNER (1959, p.56), MCCORD and MCCORD (1960, p.101), ROSENQUIST and MEGARGEE (1969, p.169), and GLUECK and GLUECK (1974, p.67).

With respect to the results on *child rearing behavior* of parents, there is almost complete accordance with the facts described in the relevant literature. MCCORD and MCCORD (1959, p.77), PONGRATZ and HÜBNER (1959, p.39), Statens offentliga utredningar (1973a, p.212), and GLUECK and GLUECK (1974, pp.65, 68, 155) regard inconsistent, erratic and contradictory child rearing behavior as a particularly negative influence. For the indifferent, too lax, or too strict attitudes of the parents of many O-subjects, there were also comparable findings of other authors, such as POWERS and WITMER (1951, p.254), MCCORD and MCCORD (1959, p.83), WEST and FARRINGTON (1973, pp.49ff.), and GLUECK and GLUECK (1974, pp.67, 155). Furthermore, a feeling of rejection was described by MCCORD and MCCORD (1960, pp.109ff.), ROSENQUIST and MEGARGEE (1969, p.332), the report of the Centro Nazionale di Prevenzione e Difesa Sociale (1969, pp.37ff.), GLUECK and GLUECK (1974, p.155), and WEST and FARRINGTON (1973, pp.57ff.). On *corporal punishment,* especially by fathers, there are similar indications in MCCORD and MCCORD (1959, p.77; 1960, pp.115ff.), Statens offentliga utredningar (1971, p.155; 1973a, p.211), WEST and FARRINGTON (1973, p.51), and GLUECK and GLUECK (1974, p. 155). *Employment* and *absence* of the mother as such is also seen as not having any influence (PONGRATZ and HÜBNER 1959, p.39; FERGUSON 1952, p.145). The kind of supervision during the mother's absence is practically not covered by the other literature; however, GLUECK and GLUECK (1974, p.63) determined an *insufficient supervision of delinquents,* partially due to employment as well as to alcoholism or prostitution.

A second general trend resulting from the Tübingen Comparative Study of Young Offenders was that the presence of one or several characteristics alone, even functional internal circumstances, does not necessarily have any bearing on future delinquency. Thus, there was the large group of the late delinquents, who, despite better circumstances than the early delinquents, became seriously delinquent. In contrast, a number of G-subjects did not become delinquent at all or became delinquent only temporarily and usually not seriously despite extremely unfavorable circumstances. Therefore, it depends on additional factors, which can also be somatic or psychological/psychiatric, whether the circumstances in the family of orientation have any (positive or negative) influence at all on the subject's further development.

This fact should remind us to be extremely careful in making *general* causal statements, for example on relationships among social class, socialization, and criminality where these *opposite possibilities* are evened out. It is in no way possible

Table 11. Syndrome of family strains

	O-subj ($n=196$)	G-subj ($n=200$)	O_1-subj ($n=113$)	O_2-subj ($n=83$)
1. Lower lower class and/or living in inadequate housing conditions for more than 6 years and/or living on welfare for more than 1 year through one's own fault.	54.6% (107)	20.0% (40)	53.1% (60)	56.6% (47)
2. Social conspicuousness and/or criminality of a person rearing the subject[a]	49.0% (96)	12.5% (25)	54.9% (62)	41.0% (34)
3. The subject is not adequately supervised and/or actively avoids supervision[b]	46.9% (92)	8.5% (17)	57.5% (65)	20.5% (17)
4. (1+2+3) Syndrome of family strains	20.9% (41)	1.0% (2)	28.3% (32)	10.8% (9)

[a] See Table 4
[b] See Table 8

to treat socioeconomic status or internal circumstances of the family simply as given facts and examine their (one-sided) influence on the subject. The results on intergenerational mobility and the indications on early conspicuous behavior of the subjects show that disruption and problems of adaptation in the family of orientation may well be the result of the conspicuousness of the subject.

A *concurrence of certain factors,* however, can be particularly important for the cases concerned. This was shown in the *syndrome of family strains,* consisting of criteria which are easy to objectify, selective in the statistical sense, and of special factual importance, as they take into account a *subject's own behavior as well as that of his parents.* These are: belonging to the lower lower class plus the additional variables of external circumstances which express a reinforcement of a lifestyle at the lower end of the social ladder and are not a matter of *fate.* Moreover, there are the criteria "social conspicuousness or criminality of parents" as well as "lack of supervision of subject", which was traced back in part to the subject's "active avoidance of supervision." These aspects make up a syndrome (see Table 11) which, though it applied to only one-fifth of the O-subjects (20.9%), occurred for no more than two G-subjects (1%).

These figures do not permit speaking of a typical concurrence for the entire O-group. Yet the small number of two G-subjects (1%), one of whom became seriously delinquent (see Sect. 4.7 below), allows the conclusion that if the syndrome occurs, the absence of criminality must be regarded as an exception. This reinforces the rather drastic impression from the *individual case studies* that there is a relatively clearly definable group of families (among the O_1-subjects no less than 28.3%) which should be regarded as a marginal group in the sense of the colloquial expression "asocial".

Thus, with due care, the circumstances of the family of orientation can be said to have a certain predisposing effect (concerning equal opportunities, see GÖPPINGER 1980, pp. 240ff.). However, they rarely have a determinative effect on the development of a person, since it is very well possible that their "positive" or "negative" effects are superimposed by a subject's own behavior or compensated for by opposite developments in other spheres, whether concurrently or later on, in particular in the spheres of self-chosen contacts and ties and those of leisure and performance.

2.2 The Sphere of Abode

2.2.1 Preliminary Remarks

The sphere of abode is the external framework of a person's life. Yet it influences him not only with respect to space in its broadest sense (what kind of place of residence, neighborhood, dwelling), but also by its specific atmosphere (character of neighborhood, neighbors, nature, etc.). Thus, the sphere of abode is important in more than a merely formal way for a person's entire life. Furthermore, it is in no way an unchanging, given quantity: In many respects, a change of abode or the organization of the sphere of abode is to some extent a decision of the person concerned. Thus, the sphere of abode, together with other criteria, mainly from the other social spheres, certainly offers some access to the personality in the context of its social relationships (see Göppinger 1980, pp. 274ff.).

In the following, the sphere of abode is the actual place of residence and abode (not the official place of residence according to registration rules) with its environment, i.e., the area where the subject's everyday life with his family, at work, and during leisure time (including the corresponding contacts and friendships) usually takes place. It is important what kinds of places of abode there were during a subject's life (parents' home, homes, correctional institutions or military barracks, his own dwelling and marital home, possibly also roaming about without a fixed abode), as well as when and in particular how frequently a subject changed his place of abode.

Special (only short-term) places of abode which were either included in the actual place of abode in its broader sense or from which the subjects came back to their permanent places of residence or abode (e.g., place of work or the various places where the subject spent his leisure time, such as taverns, sports grounds and holiday places) are included in the discussion of the corresponding spheres (see also Sect. 2.4.4 below).

2.2.2 Places of Abode and Committal

2.2.2.1 Overview

Even an overview of the life history of the subjects from the point of view of their *main* places of abode at different ages shows differences between the O- and the G-group (see Table 12).

The majority of the subjects in both groups grew up in their parents' home, with one or both parents (see Sect. 2.2.2.2 below). Staying with persons other than their parents played a greater role for the O- than for the G-subjects. Obvious differences between the two groups appeared mainly for committals to homes (see Sect. 2.2.2.3 below). The sudden increase in the number of committals to homes from the age of 7 and especially from the age of 14 on is striking: After beginning

Table 12. (Main) Place of abode at different age levels

	Age 0–3		Age 4–6		Age 7–11		Age 12–13		Age 14–17		Age 18–19		Age 20 to time of study		Immediately before time of study	
	O (n=200)	G (n=200)	O (n=199)	G (n=200)	O (n=200)	G (n=200)	O (n=200)	G (n=199)	O (n=200)	G (n=200)	O (n=199)	G (n=199)	O (n=200)	G (n=199)	O (n=200)	G (n=199)
With parent(s)	93.0%	98.0%	90.4%	95.5%	86.0%	96.5%	88.0%	97.4%	69.0%	90.5%	52.0%	81.4%	26.0%	38.2%	29.5%	31.1%
With other person rearing the subject	5.5%	2.0%	9.0%	4.0%	7.5%	3.0%	5.5%	2.0%	5.0%	2.0%	3.0%	.5%	.5%	.5%	.5%	1.0%
In home	1.5%	-	.5%	.5%	6.5%	.5%	6.5%	.5%	12.5%	1.0%	7.0%	-	1.0%	-	1.0%	-
With master/employer (contact with the family)	-	-	-	-	-	-	-	-	8.0%	5.0%	5.0%	4.5%	-	.5%	1.5%	-
(Alone) as subtenant/company housing	-	-	-	-	-	-	-	-	4.0%	1.0%	13.6%	9.5%	21.0%	14.1%	20.5%	12.6%
In barracks/Foreign Legion	-	-	-	-	-	-	-	-	-	-	3.0%	3.5%	3.0%	8.5%	2.0%	4.5%
In own/marital dwelling	-	-	-	-	-	-	-	-	-	-	-	-	12.5%	37.7%	13.5%	50.7%
In sanatorium/nursing home	-	-	-	-	-	-	-	-	-	-	-	-	-	-	.5%	-
In penal institution	-	-	-	-	-	-	-	-	1.5%	-	14.6%	-	32.5%	-	3.5%[a]	-
Without fixed abode/roaming about	-	-	-	-	-	-	-	-	-	.5%	2.0%	.5%	3.5%	.5%	27.5%	-

[a] Subjects who had been released from prison immediately before their last imprisonment

to go to school or work, the subjects were not only additionally and more extensively supervised than before (by the school or employer) but also confronted with higher requirements in the sphere of performance. This meant that conspicuousness or negligence had different consequences than during previous periods (see also Sects. 2.3.2 and 2.3.3 below).

The subjects' further development in the sphere of abode differed as well: A large section of the O-group left their parents' home (see Sect. 2.2.2.6 below) between the ages of 14 and 17, many G-subjects only from the age of 19 on. The O-subjects' families of orientation were replaced by committals to homes and, later on, increasingly by committals to prison (see Sect. 2.2.2.4 below), besides by their own dwellings (particularly at the place of an apprentice's master or in company housing). From the age of 19 up to the time of the study, one-third of the O-subjects spent most of the time in prison. Immediately before their last imprisonment, almost one-third of the O-subjects had no fixed abode; many of them were "roaming about" (see Sect. 2.2.3 below). A G-subject's parents' home, in contrast, was normally succeeded - besides by his own dwelling (e.g., in connection with occupational training) or barracks in the course of military service (see Sect. 2.2.2.5 below) - by his own (marital) home (see Sect. 2.2.2.7 below).

2.2.2.2 *Parents' Home*

During the subjects' childhood, many families temporarily lived in inadequate housing conditions, not least as a consequence of World War II and the postwar period. Exclusively because of World War II - either as a direct consequence of war or as refugees or expellees - almost as many subjects of both groups, namely, 36 O- (25 O_1-, 11 O_2-) and 32 G-subjects, had lived in inadequate housing conditions for at least 3 months up to the age of 13. Regardless of this, overcrowded dwellings where the subjects had no space to themselves were of some importance in both groups: Up to the age of 13, 35 O_1-, 27 O_2-, and 20 G-subjects lived in such housing conditions for some time together with their parents; 21 O_1-, 3 O_2-, and 3 G-subjects lived in primitive dwellings and 17 O_1-, 8 O_2-, and 8 G-subjects in hostels for the homeless, huts, and former bunkers (multiple answers).

There were marked differences between the two groups, however, in view of *how long* the subjects lived in such housing conditions: While 17% of the O- and 11% of the G-subjects grew up in such conditions for 1 to less than 6 years, only 3.5% of the G-subjects, as compared with 29% of the O-subjects, lived in such conditions for more than 6 years (see also Sect. 2.1.2.2 above).

Particularly revealing were the differences between the subgroups of 65 O- and 44 G-subjects who were particularly affected by the consequences of war with respect to place of abode and committal because the subjects, together with their families of orientation, had emigrated to the Federal Republic of Germany after the war as *refugees, expellees, or resettlers* before the age of 13 (subjects born to refugee parents in the Federal Republic of Germany were disregarded). Not only did the O-subjects stay in refugee camps and emergency housing temporarily (more than 6 months) more frequently than the G-subjects (O: 48%; G: 30%); they also remained in such conditions for longer periods of time (6 years or more) more often (O: 40%; G: 5%).

The *reasons* why O-families lived in inadequate housing conditions for more than 1 year were mostly: too low family income as a consequence of unemployment, irregular employment or low-paid work of the main breadwinner, and a large number of children. As far as is known, most of these O-families later continued living in such inadequate housing conditions. Of the six G-families who had lived in poor housing mainly because of flight, expulsion, or late repatriation, four saved money for their own home during this period and then immediately moved to their new home, and one rented a house after living in inadequate housing conditions for 7 years and thus provided for an adequate dwelling. The sixth subject was also able to improve his situation by going to live with the (procreation) family of his sister, which was well off, after his *Abitur* (high-school graduation; see Sect. 2.3.2.1 below).

The *individual case studies* also repeatedly showed that these differences were not due so much to external difficulties, such as the availability of adequate housing, as they were to the differing willingness or ability of parents to improve their housing situation by their own efforts. The parents of the G-subjects, furthermore, tried to provide their children with some space to themselves, even in very crowded housing conditions, and they provided for ordered circumstances in the household even in unfavorable conditions. The O-subjects often had no space to themselves, in some cases not even beds to themselves in the parents' dwellings, which were frequently underfurnished and occasionally neglected or extremely dirty. On the other hand, however, a number of O-subjects did not take advantage of extraordinarily favorable conditions at home, whereas some G-subjects were able to overcome unfavorable housing conditions in their families of orientation by establishing close ties with the family of a schoolmate or friend.

2.2.2.3 Stays in Homes

Almost half (43%) of the O-subject but only 6% of the G-subjects had been committed to homes before the age of 21 (at least for a short time). Stays lasted no more than a few weeks or months for the majority of the subjects. Especially during childhood, only a few subjects lived in homes for longer periods of time (see Table 12). Committals to homes gained in importance when the subjects were older: 7% of the school-age O-subjects (up to and including the age of 13) and 13% of the O-subjects at the age of occupational training (between the ages of 14 and 17) stayed *predominantly* in homes. Four O-subjects grew up almost exclusively in homes at school age and at the age of occupational training, while only one G-subject spent the majority of his youth in a home.

Short (minimum 3 months) stays in homes were also taken into account in Table 13, on the *reasons* for committals to homes. This did not affect the basic differences between the O- and the G-group with respect to the importance of stays in homes.

Although there were often several reasons for a committal to a home, unequivocal trends became evident in the essential reasons: During all three intervals of the study (for the definition of the intervals, see Sects. 1.3 above and 2.4.1 below), the O-subjects, especially the O_1-subjects, were committed to homes in particular because they, and often their parents or other persons rearing them, were socially conspicuous. The G-subjects, in contrast, were almost exclusively committed to homes because of external circumstances, such as loss of a parent or other person rearing the subject, or education and training away from home. The O_2-subjects were between the O_1- and the G-subjects: During the second and third intervals they were clearly underrepresented for stays in homes as compared with the O_1-group.

Table 13. Stays in homes of at least 3 months and reasons for stays

	Before the age of 14				Age 14–17				Age 18–20			
	O-subj ($n=200$)	G-subj ($n=200$)	O_1-subj ($n=114$)	O_2-subj ($n=86$)	O-subj ($n=200$)	G-subj ($n=200$)	O_1-subj ($n=114$)	O_2-subj ($n=86$)	O-subj ($n=200$)	G-subj ($n=200$)	O_1-subj ($n=114$)	O_2-subj ($n=86$)
Stays in homes	18.0%	3.0%	19.3%	16.3%	32.5%[a]	1.5%	43.0%	18.6%	17.0%[b]	0.5%	21.0%	11.6%
Main reasons (multiple entries)												
Social conspicuousness of subject (and "offenses")	20	1	16	4	49	–	41	8	33	–	24	10
Neglect by/social conspicuousness of a person rearing the subject	19	–	12	7	16	–	11	5	–	–	–	–
Other circumstances/exigencies (e.g. death of a person rearing the subject)	14	5	6	8	6	–	4	2	5	–	–	–
School/training away from home	–	1	–	–	10	3	4	6	–	1	–	–

[a] For 58 O-subjects, committal according to Juvenile Court Act *(Jugendgerichtsgesetz)*
[b] For all O-subjects, committal according to Juvenile Court Act

Corresponding to the reasons for committals, practically all (58) of the O-subjects concerned from between the ages of 14 and 17 had been committed to *reform schools;* of these 28 O_1- and four O_2-subjects had been sent to strictly run or closed wards or to reform schools. From 18 to 20 years, 15 O_1- and three O_2-subjects had been committed to such wards or reform schools. The remaining O-subjects and all the G-subjects concerned had lived exclusively in (open) *hostels for pupils or apprentices.*

Long-term *committals to detoxification centers or sanatoria,* on the other hand, were of no importance in either group. Only a few subjects had been temporarily committed to tuberculosis sanatoria during childhood; one G-subject and five O-subjects had been temporarily committed to detoxification centers or psychiatric hospitals as adults because of alcoholism.

2.2.2.4 Imprisonment

Besides committals to homes, imprisonment played an important role for the O-subjects from their youth on: 78.5% (157) of the O-subjects had been imprisoned (including pretrial detention) at least once before the term during which they were selected for the Tübingen study, 57% of them (64% of the O_1-, 48% of the O_2-subjects) for a period of at least 1 month (see also Table 14). In contrast, only four subjects of the G-group had ever been imprisoned up to the time of the study, two for 2 and two for 4 weeks (concerning the delinquency of the G-subjects, see Sect. 4.7 below).

In accordance with the definition of the O_2-subjects (first conviction after 18th birthday), stays in prison from 15 to 18 years of age concerned (almost) only the O_1-subjects: About 40% of them had been in prison temporarily, one-third of these for more than 6 months. Between the ages of 18 and 20 and after the age of 20, somewhat more than half of the O_1-subjects were temporarily imprisoned (the term during which they were selected for the Tübingen study was not included), long-term sentences increasing disproportionately. This may be partially due to the summation of several short prison sentences (see Sect. 4.3.1 below).

The distribution and development of imprisonment among the O_2-subjects was different: The proportion of temporarily imprisoned subjects rose from only 19%

Table 14. O-subjects' stays in prison according to age-groups[a]

	Age 14–17		Age 18–20		Age 21 and over	
	O_1-subj ($n=114$)	O_2-subj ($n=86$)	O_1-subj ($n=114$)	O_2-subj ($n=86$)	O_1-subj ($n=114$)	O_2-subj ($n=86$)
Up to 6 months	26.3%	1.2%[b]	19.3%	15.1%	23.7%	39.5%
Over 6 months up to 1 year	9.7%	-	7.0%	1.2%	7.9%	4.7%
Over 1 year to 2 years	3.5%	-	14.9%	2.3%	13.2%	10.5%
Over 2 years	.0%	-	12.3%	.0%	10.5%	5.8%
Not in prison	60.5%	98.8%	46.5%	81.4%	44.7%	39.5%

[a] Total duration of all stays in prison within each age-group, excepting the imprisonment leading to a subject's selection for the study
[b] Pretrial detention without subsequent sentencing

between the age of 18 and 20 to over 60% after 20. Long-term spans between terms in prison also increased, yet the emphasis remained on short prison terms of up to 6 months.

2.2.2.5 Military Service

In contrast to the O-subjects' committals to prison or homes, another kind of institutionalized stay, although a much less limiting one, was of great importance for the G-subjects: staying in a barracks during military service. Almost twice as many G-subjects (40%) as O-subjects (24%) were enlisted for military service (some as volunteers). In the O-group, the O_2-subjects, with 32.5% (as compared with 17.5% of the O_1-subjects), were drafted disproportionately more often for military service. This, as well as the high proportion of G-subjects, was probably due to the administration policy of not drafting anyone with a certain number of previous convictions.

There were further differences: The majority of the drafted G-subjects completed military service or engaged themselves for further service (only five subjects were prematurely exempted, two of whom because of physical impairments). Only about half of the drafted O-subjects, in contrast, completed military service: Besides one subject who was exempted in retrospect, 12 O_1- and nine O_2-subjects were prematurely dishonorably discharged from military service. The divergent behavior of the O- and the G-subjects in the sphere of performance deserves mention in this connection (see Sect. 2.3 below), as completing military service poses several performance requirements which are quite comparable to those in working life in general.

2.2.2.6 Age of Separation from Parents' Home

The subjects' age when they left home (parents, foster parents, etc.; i.e., the environment the subjects grew up in) "for good" turned out to distinguish clearly between the two groups. (For the four O-subjects who grew up almost exclusively in homes, leaving home was defined as being released from the home.) Leaving home "for good" meant that a subject had no longer mainly slept "at home" for more than 1 year (see Table 15).

Table 15. Age of subjects when they left parents' home "for good"

	O-subjects ($n=198$)	G-subjects ($n=200$)	O_1-subjects ($n=114$)	O_2-subjects ($n=84$)
Under 16	15.2%	4.0%	12.3%	19.1%
Up to the age of 17	42.9%	14.5%	47.4%	36.9%
Up to the age of 20	76.3%	51.5%	79.8%	71.4%
After the age of 20	95.0%	83.0%	94.7%	95.2%
Not yet	5.0%	17.0%	5.3%	4.8%
Median age	19.6 years	21.9 years	19.2 years	20.1 years

Significance level: O–G: $p<.001$; O_1–O_2: not significant

A total of 43% of the O-subjects had already left their parents' home at the age of 18, compared with only 15% of the G-subjects. Almost half of the G-subjects still lived at their parents' home at the age of 21 (compared with only one-fourth of the O-subjects). Thus, the median age of the O- and the G-subjects varied by more than 2 years.

Although the O_2-subjects were positioned between the G- and the O_1-subjects in this respect as well, the high percentage of O_2-subjects who left home before the age of 15 is striking; the figures are even higher for the O_2-group than for the O_1-group.

The *reasons* the subjects gave for leaving home are rather impressive (see Table 16): For most (90%) of the G-subjects who had left home, the following reasons - in chronological order - were decisive: occupational training or employment away from home, military service, or marriage. One-third of the O-subjects (even half of the O_1-subjects) left home because they were committed to a home or prison, one-third of them because they had quarreled with their parents or for no specific reason. Again, the differentiation of the O-group presented no uniform picture: The O_2-subjects were more similar to the G-group in mentioning "occupational training" and "military service," while efforts to become independent accounted for a higher percentage than in the O_1-group.

A detailed look at the O-subjects who left home because of stays in homes or prison showed that this was the immediate, yet, seen as a whole, only superficial reason for the separation for a considerable number of the subjects: Only barely half of the O-subjects (see Sect. 2.2.2.3 above) committed to homes between the ages of 14 and 17 and only four of the O-subjects (see Sect. 2.2.2.4 above) committed to prison stayed in a home or prison for more than 1 year during this period (all committals taken together). For the majority of these subjects, in contrast, this reason alone meant no minimum absence of 1 year, and therefore no separation from home. In these cases, it was decisive that a subject had chiefly no longer stayed at home before his committal or had used his home only as a place to sleep. After being released from a home or prison, the O-subjects often took advantage of the opportunity to become "independent" by not going back home and finding other dwellings or even only temporary places to sleep.

Table 16. Reasons for leaving parents' home "for good"[a]

	O-subj ($n=198$)	G-subj ($n=200$)	O_1-subj ($n=114$)	O_2-subj ($n=84$)
No special reason (striving toward independence)	15.2%	2.5%	13.2%	17.9%
Quarreling with parents	17.7%	2.0%	18.4%	16.7%
Negative circumstances at parents' home	4.5%	2.0%	4.4%	4.8%
Committal to a home/imprisonment	34.3%	.0%	50.0%	13.1%
Training/occupation	18.7%	25.0%	12.3%	27.4%
Military service	13.1%	30.0%	8.8%	19.1%
Marriage/own household	6.6%	24.5%	5.3%	8.3%
Subject had not yet left parents' home	5.1%	17.0%	5.3%	4.8%

[a] Multiple answers

Disregarding the inevitable separation from home due to long-term stays in homes or prison (i.e., for more than 1 year), the following reasons for leaving the parents' home - besides military service - clearly distinguished the O- from the G-group: for the O-subjects, efforts to become independent and/or quarrels with parents; for the G-subjects, occupational training away from home or marriage.

The *individual case studies* showed that quarrels with parents or leaving home "for no specific reason" were often due to the subjects' pronounced efforts to become independent, which also became apparent in the other social spheres, and to the desire to avoid supervision - if there was any at all (see Sect. 2.1.3.2 above). But precisely those O-subjects who emphasized their early independence and freedom were not capable of obtaining and creating their own sphere of living. They often stayed with socially conspicuous acquaintances, partially prostitutes, or roamed about aimlessly.

Some G-subjects indicated reasons for leaving home which were similar in a formal respect. Yet these efforts toward independence, which were almost characteristic of some of the subjects, were never connected with the desire to avoid all supervision. This became evident in the various social commitments which the G-subjects undertook at their new places of abode. Moreover, most of these considerations were subordinated to other reasons, so that the separation desired by the subjects took place almost of necessity through changes in the sphere of performance or contacts and led to a new, usually ordered place to live.

2.2.2.7 Own Sphere of Living

At the time of the study, half (51%) of the G-subjects had their *own* (marital) *dwellings;* one-third (31%) of them still lived with their families of orientation, and the remaining subjects lived alone, usually as subtenants, in company housing, student accommodations, etc. (see Table 12). Despite leaving home substantially earlier, only a few O-subjects had their own sphere of living. With interruptions due to imprisonment, about one-fourth of the O-subjects after the age of 20 still or again lived with their parents, one-fourth lived chiefly as subtenants (usually for a short time and with frequent changes) or in company housing or had only a more or less disordered temporary place to sleep. Including the married O-subjects, only 13% of the O-subjects mainly lived in their own or marital dwellings after 20 years of age, while one-third of them (with variations in length from subject to subject; see Sect. 1.3 above) spent this period mostly in prison (their "last" imprisonment was disregarded).

That 67% of the O-subjects (compared with only 3.5% of the G-subjects) were at least temporarily without official places of residence, 32% longer than 1 month and 12% longer than 6 months, showed the differing importance of one's own sphere of living. Also immediately before the time of the study, almost one-third (28%) of the O-subjects (and no G-subject) had no own, more or less stable sphere of living. A number of these subjects (who were often on the run after committing an offense) were "roaming about" without a fixed abode (see Table 12 and Sect. 2.2.3 below).

The *individual case studies* in particular showed that these behavior patterns were in no way temporary and exclusively connected with a previous offense, flight, or release from prison, but rather a generally noticeable, fundamentally different attitude of the majority of the O-subjects. Thus, in the past as well, the majority of the O-subjects had chosen their dwellings rather indiscriminately and taken whatever was available. The G-subjects, in contrast, had selected their dwellings carefully not only with respect to how far away they were from their work, but also with respect to various other (social) aspects (e.g., general neighborhood, vicinity to nature, opportunities for their children to play).

Considerable differences also occurred in *organization* and *atmosphere of the dwelling*. Among those subjects who had a permanent place of residence (see Sect. 2.2.3 below), 12% of the O-subjects, but only 4% of the G-subjects, had lived in inadequate housing conditions in terms of number of inhabitants and furnishings immediately before the time of the study. It became apparent that the G-subjects usually thought about how they were going to furnish their own dwellings or rooms and tried to give their dwellings an individual character - even if it was furnished very simply and modestly - by decorating it with personal objects. Any purchases were in relation to the subjects' current financial means. In contrast, the O-subjects usually spent much less time furnishing their dwellings. Apartments were often scantily furnished, uncomfortable, or even dirty. This gave rise to the impression that an O-subject did not consider his own dwelling a "home," all the more so as he often used even his marital home only as a place to sleep (see also Sects. 2.4.4.2 and 2.5.4 below). On the other hand, it was evident that some O-subjects, especially the married ones, attempted to furnish their apartments completely but not always expediently from the outset, which almost always led to financial difficulties.

2.2.3 Changes of Places of Abode

Besides the foregoing material aspects on different kinds of places of abode, it was attempted to determine the mobility (in space) of the subjects as well, by observing how frequently they changed their places of abode (see Table 17). A change was assumed only if a subject remained at the new place for some time (at least 6 months), which commonly meant that most previous social ties (acquaintances, memberships in clubs, etc.) were broken. Consequently, short-term changes such as vacations or stays in hospitals were not taken into account.

During childhood, the O-subjects and their families of orientation changed their places of abode more frequently than the G-subjects and their families did. However, a markedly higher mobility did not occur until the O-subjects were 14–19 years old, i.e., when they could increasingly change their places of residence and abode regardless of their families (of orientation). The sudden increase for the O-subjects between 13 and 14 years of age was particularly striking; a similar development did not occur for the G-subjects until after the age of 20. The mobility of the O_2-subjects between the ages of 12 and 19 was between that of the O_1- and the G-subjects; their behavior, however, corresponded more to that of the O_1-group with respect to the time of sudden increase and to the frequency of changes of places of abode. The O_2-group even surpassed the O_1-group after the age of 20.

Table 17. Changes of place of abode

	O-subj ($n=200$)	G-subj ($n=200$)	Sig. O–G	O_1-subj ($n=114$)	O_2-subj ($n=86$)	Sig. O_1–O_2
Up to the age of 11	67.0%	55.0%	+	71.1%	61.6%	n.s.
Age 12 to 13	23.0%	10.0%	++	28.9%	15.1%	+
Age 14 to 17	63.0%	15.0%	++	77.2%	46.5%	++
Age 18 to 19	71.5%	18.0%	++	81.6%	58.1%	++
Age 20 and over	91.5%	76.0%	++	88.6%	95.3%	n.s.
During the last month before the time of the study	46.0%	1.5%	++	39.5%	54.7%	+

Significance level: *+*, $p<.05$; *+ +*, $p<.001$; *n.s.*, not significant

Similar to the reasons for leaving home (see Sect. 2.2.2.6 above), the *reasons* why the G-subjects increasingly changed their places of abode after the age of 20 were essentially military service, occupational training away from home, and especially the establishment of their own household after marriage. For the O-subjects, however, stays in homes or prison were only partly responsible for the frequent changes (see Sect. 2.2.2.6 above). Founding their own household in connection with marriage and military service were not decisive either, because of the smaller number of O-subjects as compared with G-subjects. Thus, the O-subjects changed their places of abode substantially more often than the G-subjects, regardless of these reasons.

The *individual case studies* showed that the O-subjects only exceptionally developed strong social ties at their places of abode, whether with people, to a job, or to a club. For them, a change simply meant a change of personal and material contacts which were interchangeable anyway. On the other hand, particularly O-subjects living in *"Asozialensiedlungen"* (a kind of social ghetto, i. e., buildings or blocks where, for example, people on social welfare live) were often strongly attached to their environment. The G-subjects exhibited a continuity similar to that in the other spheres. This continuity was regularly connected with a complex social integration expressed not only in their work and (usually small) circle of friends, but often also in club memberships and volunteer activities, and was opposed to a change of abode if it was at all desirable for other reasons.

Considering the numerous places of abode of the O-subjects, it did not seem useful - and was often impossible - to count them, as the O-subjects themselves often could not remember all the places they had stayed in the course of their lives. Instead, the period immediately preceding the period of the study - a period still fresh in the memory of the O-subjects - was analyzed in detail (see Table 18).

Apart from the fact that practically no G-subjects, but almost one-half of the O-subjects, changed their places of abode at least once during this period (see Table 17), there were differences between the O- and the G-group with respect to a discrepancy between last *(main) place of residence* registered with the police and *actual place of abode* of a subject. Including the roughly 15% of the O-subjects registered as being "without fixed abode," more than 40% of the O-subjects, but only 12% of the G-subjects were not chiefly at their (main) official places of residence immediately before the time of the study.

Table 18. Last place of residence and last place of abode (immediately before time of study)

	Last (main) place of residence					
	In municipalities of up to 20000 inhabitants		In municipalities of over 20000 inhabitants		No fixed abode	
	O-subj ($n=91$)	G-subj ($n=99$)	O-subj ($n=80$)	G-subj ($n=101$)	O-subj ($n=29$)	G-subj ($n=0$)
Last place of abode:						
At place of residence	70.3%	90.9%	68.8%	86.1%	-	-
In other municipalities of						
- up to 20000 inhabitants	7.7%	3.0%	7.5%	4.0%	3.4%	.0%
- over 20000 inhabitants	13.2%	6.1%	18.8%	9.9%	51.7%	.0%
Constantly changing	8.8%	.0%	5.0%	.0%	44.8%	.0%

More informative than numerical differences are the *reasons* for the discrepancy between official place of residence and place of abode: Apart from one G-subject who had moved in with his girlfriend after a quarrel with his wife, all the G-subjects were staying at places other than their main official places of residence because of their studies, military service, a job away from home, or stationary hospital treatment. If necessary, they were also officially registered at their second places of residence.

These kinds of reasons applied for merely one-fourth of the 81 O-subjects who were not at their official places of residence immediately before the time of the study. About half of these O-subjects were on the run because of a previous offense or a warrant for arrest (21 subjects), or were roaming about for no specific reason or had gone on a "spin", in some cases abroad (20 subjects). Another 17 subjects were on the road in connection with temporary jobs, often as magazine salesmen, "sales representatives," or showmen's helpers.

The *direction of mobility* in view of how places of residence or abode were distributed - large, medium, or small towns or countryside - showed, with certain reservations, a tendency toward (large) cities, especially for recidivist offenders. No less than half of the subjects who were not at their official places of residence immediately before the time of the study were staying in cities with a population of over 20000. In comparison with the place of residence, (large) cities were preferred as the place of abode by more O- than G-subjects. This holds especially for the O-subjects who had no fixed abode in the end or who, because of frequent changes, could not be assigned to any definite place and stayed almost exclusively in urban areas.

These tendencies proved even more differentiated in the *individual case studies*. The O-subjects felt especially attracted by the "milieu" of large cities as *places of leisure* (see Sects. 2.4.3.3 and 2.5.3 below), without transferring their places of abode or residence to the large city. On the other hand, it was a kind of refuge for the subjects who had no place to stay, or other difficulties. According to the subjects, it was a place where further opportunities and alternatives opened up. Although such areas are located mainly in large and industrial cities, it was impressive how an O-subject, for example in a small town which was unknown to him and whose inhabitants denied in good faith that such a "milieu" existed, would find the street or tavern corresponding to or at least similar to the "milieu" of the large city in a few hours. Thus, it is certainly not only the large city which offers such opportunities to those who are familiar with this sphere.

2.2.4 Summary

In essence, the following were the important points for the behavior of the subjects in the sphere of abode: After separating from their parents' home comparatively early, the O-subjects changed their places of abode significantly more often than the G-subjects during the following years, especially between the ages of 14 and 19. These changes were not exclusively due to stays in homes or imprisonment, which was shown in the detailed study of places of abode immediately before the time of the study: About two-fifths (81) of the O-subjects were not staying at their last registered places of residence. Half of them were roaming about without a fixed abode or were on the run because of a previous offense. These subjects in particular felt to a certain extent attracted by large cities. The G-subjects, in contrast, rarely changed their places of abode. They showed an extreme continuity, accompanied by various social commitments in a certain area. A differentiation of the O-group as to O_1- and O_2-subjects did not reveal any uniform tendencies.

The specific characteristics and behavior patterns of recidivist offenders with respect to place of abode are not - as is often assumed in the relevant literature - limited to inadequate housing conditions in the family of orientation, stays in homes (later prison), and lack of place of residence. These facts merely express particularly succinct aspects of an organization of life differing fundamentally from that of the "general" population, all the more so as the sphere of abode is the framework for the other social spheres.

As opposed to the sphere of performance, for example, the sphere of abode has scarcely been focused on as an independent sphere in empirical criminological research and the corresponding *literature*. Even the large multifactorial studies limited themselves to certain individual aspects, whose weight, also with respect to the other social spheres, was difficult to estimate. GLUECK and GLUECK (1950, p.157) and PONGRATZ and HÜBNER (1959, pp.71ff.) indicate that children who live in homes are more jeopardized (with respect to criminality). Yet PONGRATZ and HÜBNER only examined subjects who had stayed in homes and thus had no possibility of comparison. The high mobility of delinquent subjects together with the lack of a permanent residence is also emphasized by WOLFGANG et al. (1972, p.58) and GLUECK and GLUECK (1974, p.101). In other studies as well, more negative, often neglected housing conditions were found for the (delinquent) subjects (GLUECK and GLUECK 1950, p.81) as was overcrowding (Statens offentliga utredningar 1972, p.108); these circumstances are, in agreement with the results presented here, not considered decisive for delinquency.

2.3 The Sphere of Performance

2.3.1 Preliminary Remarks

All aspects pertaining to the development of the subjects at school, in occupational training, and during employment belong to the sphere of performance. As opposed to other spheres where performance is also required, for example in the framework of social obligations to one's own family, requirements concerning performance and behavior at school and work are governed by strict, formal rules.

Compulsory school education brings the first clear distinction between "work" and leisure, which marks later employment. Conspicuous behavior in particular becomes immediately socially visible. Therefore, one emphasis of the following presentation is conspicuousness at school (see Sect. 2.3.2 below).

Employment is of central importance for the sphere of performance, as working is usually the only possibility of earning one's living. This applies to the subjects of the present study as well, with the exception of the few who were still in occupational training or pursuing higher education. Considerable difficulties ensue if one disregards the necessity of working most of the days of the week or if one does not fulfill even a small part of the requirements. These aspects of behavior at work were taken into account in particular in the following presentation of the occupational sphere of performance (see Sects. 2.3.3 and 2.3.4 below).

As mentioned above (see Sect. 1.3 above), statements cannot be made for every one of the criteria for all subjects. Though there were practically no unclear cases for the sphere of performance in particular - due to the manifold objective sources of information and "hard" data (see also Part I, Sect. 3.1) - a certain (small) number of subjects could not be taken into account for certain criteria for reasons of content. The 23 students of the G-group in particular were ruled out in the discussion of employment and occupational training - with the exception of seven subjects who had completed occupational training before their studies. One O-subject who had stayed almost continuously in homes or prison was ruled out on questions of employment and one O-subject who was still an apprentice was excluded on occupational training and occupational position. Figures varied, furthermore, in relationships with characteristics from other spheres; the variations are indicated in the corresponding spheres. Thus, the tables present differing parent populations.

In addition to the present results, KOFLER (1980) and SCHMEHL (1980) give further information and details. They will be referred to occasionally in the following.

2.3.2 School

2.3.2.1 *Level of Education*

With respect to the kind of school attended and educational success, the O-subjects plainly did not reach the same level as the G-subjects (see Table 19).

The terms used in the following correspond to the currently valid definitions of the Education Act of Baden-Württemberg. The *Hauptschule (Volksschule* during the period of the study), as the regular school, follows the compulsory 4 years of *Grundschule* (primary school) and lasts until one's 15th birthday (one's 14th birthday during the period of the study). The subjects who had to repeat one or more grades and did not extend their school education voluntarily received a school certificate *(Abgangszeugnis)*. They were classified under non-completed *Hauptschule*. The subjects who finished the *Hauptschule* with a certificate of successful completion *(Abschlußzeugnis)* were classified under completed *Hauptschule*. During the 1950s and early 1960s, when most of the subjects went to school, the *Hilfsschulen* and *Sonderschulen*, special schools for educationally subnormal or maladjusted children, were of minor importance, as their capacity was rather small at that time. Today, *Sonderschulen* may well play a more important role.

Weiterführende Schulen (secondary schools) lead to higher diplomas which permit one to complete higher-qualified occupational training (diploma: *Mittlere Reife*) or to go to a university

Table 19. Achieved level of education[a]

		O-subjects (*n* = 200)		G-subjects (*n* = 200)	
Hilfs-/Sonderschule	unsuccessful	8.5%	53.0%	1.5%	9.0%
Hauptschule (regular school)					
- not completed		44.5%		7.5%	
- completed	successful	43.5%	47.0%	58.5%	91.0%
Weiterführende Schule (secondary school)					
- without *mittlere Reife*		2.5%		5.5%	
- *mittlere Reife*		1.0%		13.0%	
- *mittlere Reife* before *Abitur*		-		2.0%	
- *Abitur*		-		12.0%	

Significance level: $p < .001$

[a] See Schmehl 1980, p. 29

(diploma: *Abitur*). The subjects who successfully completed the 6th grade of a *weiterführende Schule* achieved the *mittlere Reife*; the subjects who completed the 9th grade of a *weiterführende Schule*, the *Abitur*.

The figures were particularly striking when only the subjects who attended *weiterführende Schulen* were taken into consideration: Seven of the 14 O-subjects stopped and went back to the *Hauptschule*, as compared with only five of the 70 G-subjects. The differences between the O- and the G-group became particularly evident when the subjects were divided into two groups according to *educational success* (the subjects who completed the *Hauptschule* or a *weiterführende Schule*) and *no educational success* (the subjects who went to a *Sonderschule* or did not complete the *Hauptschule*).

As the average *intelligence* (see Sect. 3.4.3.2 below) of the O- and the G-subjects differed, it seemed likely that intelligence was responsible for the differences in educational success. As expected, there was a relationship between IQ and educational success in both groups: More subjects with above-average intelligence completed school more often than did subjects with average or below-average intelligence. When intelligence was held constant, however, i.e., when the O- and the G-subjects from the same intelligence group were compared, it became apparent that the relationship between belonging to the O-group and (no) educational success does not disappear but remains for average and below-average intelligence - though it is somewhat less obvious (see Table 20). Intelligence, therefore, *cannot* explain the marked differences in educational success between the O- and the G-group; additional circumstances must pertain.

Table 20. Educational success in relation to intelligence, social class, and conspicuousness in social environment

	Educational success	O-subjects ($n=200$)	G-subjects ($n=200$)	Sig.
IQ according to WAIS				
up to 90	yes	23.2% (19)	73.9% (17)	++
	no	76.8% (63)	26.1% (6)	
91-109	yes	57.8% (59)	89.9% (98)	++
	no	42.2% (43)	10.1% (11)	
110 and over	yes	(16)	98.5% (67)	
	no	(0)	1.5% (1)	
Class of family of orientation[a]				
Lower lower class and socially despised	yes	31.8% (28)	82.9% (29)	++
	no	68.2% (60)	17.1% (6)	
Upper lower class	yes	55.7% (39)	91.5% (54)	++
	no	44.3% (31)	8.5% (5)	
Lower, middle, upper middle class	yes	68.4% (26)	93.4% (99)	++
	no	31.6% (12)	6.6% (7)	
Conspicuousness in the social environment				
Yes	yes	38.6% (44)	79.5% (35)	++
	no	61.4% (70)	20.5% (9)	
No	yes	58.1% (50)	94.2% (147)	++
	no	41.9% (36)	5.8% (9)	

Significance level: ++, $p<.001$

[a] According to KLEINING and MOORE (1968), see Sect. 2.1.2.1 above; four children who grew up in homes (O-subjects) were disregarded (see Sect. 2.1.1 above)

When the relationship between *social class* and educational success was examined, it became evident that in *both* groups, the lower the social class, the higher the proportion of failures. When the O- and the G-subjects of the same social class were compared, however, the marked differences remained for all three social class groups - decreasing slightly, the higher the social class (see Table 20).

A similar picture emerged when the influence of *conspicuousness and strains in the immediate social environment* of the subjects was examined. This category included: growing up in camps, in *Asozialensiedlungen* (a kind of social ghetto, i.e., buildings or blocks where, for example, people on social welfare live) or in neglected housing conditions for at least 1 year, and serious social conspicuousness of family members (alcoholism, serious criminality, etc.). Here again, the proportion of failures was higher in both groups if this conspicuousness occurred; when it was held constant, however, the differences between the O- and the G-group remained (see Table 20).

The O-group's relatively low degree of educational success can therefore *not* be explained solely by the greater extent of characteristics influencing educational success, such as low IQ, low social class of family of orientation, and social strains. However, these characteristics were examined only individually. Yet even if they coincide, the differences between the O- and the G-group remain, though the absolute figures are too small for a statistical significance test.

2.3.2.2 Conspicuousness at School

Behavior patterns at school are more important than the external fact of educational success. Pupils become conspicuous in two principal ways, either by not meeting performance requirements or by not meeting behavior requirements (not complying with school regulations).

The most stringent criterion for inadequate performance is having to *repeat a year*. The reasons for this measure may well differ considerably, especially when repeating a year in the *Hauptschule* and in a *weiterführende Schule* is compared.

When the subjects who attended a *weiterführende Schule* were disregarded, i.e., only the subjects who had repeated a year in the *Hauptschule* examined - which usually meant that they had not completed the *Hauptschule* - the difference was rather obvious: 53% of the O-group and only 13% of the G-group repeated a year ($p < .001$). The difference became even more pronounced when the subjects who had repeated 2 or more years were contrasted (O = 44; G = 3). As explained above for the relationship between educational success and intelligence (see Sect. 2.3.2.1 above), differences in intelligence cannot be the only explanation for the differing proportion of subjects who repeated one or more years.

Moreover, the *reasons* why subjects had to repeat a year in the *Hauptschule* were plainly divergent. For the (few) G-subjects (17), there were mostly exigencies (15), such as flight (after World War II) or illness, as well as reasons which the subjects themselves could not influence, such as not being mature enough to attend school. Negative behavior patterns, such as laziness, dawdling, or truancy were mentioned for the two remaining G-subjects. Precisely the latter behavior patterns were the reasons given for almost half (46) of the (96) O-subjects having to repeat a year.

That repeating a year cannot be considered apart from the kind of school the subjects attended is shown by the differences in *weiterführende Schulen*. A total of 12 of the 14 O-subjects did not advance to a higher class, yet 33 of the 70 G-subjects (almost half) did not either; thus, repeating a year in a *weiterführende Schule* can be termed "normal".

Of the behavior patterns opposing compliance with school regulations, *truancy* expresses most obviously that a pupil is trying to avoid constraints at school -

temporarily. As skipping a lesson occasionally may well be common, truancy was examined only in its serious form, i.e., *an unexcused absence from school of at least 1 day*. *Persistent truancy* meant that a subject frequently, i.e., more than once a month, and continuously, i.e., over a prolonged period of time, stayed away from school unexcused. *Occasional truancy* covered all other forms of truancy except for one-time exceptions. In order to have a period valid for all of the subjects, truancy was studied only during the period of compulsory school education, i.e., up to and including the age of 14 (see Sect. 2.3.2.1 above).

The varying distribution in the O- and the G-group is shown in Table 23 (see Sect. 2.3.2.5 below). Here again, it became apparent that the O-subjects were an extreme group. Somewhat more than half of the O-subjects at least occasionally skipped school for a day, most of them frequently and for long periods of time. In the G-group, these serious forms of truancy occurred for barely more than one-tenth of the subjects.

Truancy is only *one* form of maladaptation at school. There are many other *behavior patterns which disrupt lessons or the class or go against school regulations.*

These other modes of behavior, however, are not "hard" facts such as truancy or repeating a year, but depend on whether the behavior is taxed negative or "disruptive" at all - especially by the teacher. The possibility that the teacher's judgment might have changed in retrospect played only a minor role, as the information in school records was usually taken down immediately after the behavior occurred. The further difficulty that not all conspicuous behavior is shown in school records was compensated for by investigating such behavior patterns in detail, not only on the basis of school records and information provided by teachers, but also on the basis of the information given by the subjects and their parents (see Part I, Sect. 3). The conspicuous behavior found in this way ranged from laziness and total disinterest to annoying (such as silly or swaggering) and disruptive behavior (such as aggressiveness and constant unrest), to rebelling against school regulations (such as impertinence toward teachers, walking away repeatedly, lying and deceitfulness).

To obtain a better overall view, conspicuousness at school is divided into two categories in the following: *particularly conspicuous behavior at school,* including serious conspicuousness, especially aggressiveness toward fellow pupils or teachers and behavior expressing a serious rebellion against school regulations or an offense (such as theft) at school, and *conspicuous behavior at school,* covering any other conspicuousness insofar as it was not petty and did not occur only temporarily.

There were obvious differences, similar to those for truancy, between the O- and the G-subjects (see Sect. 2.3.2.5 below and Table 23). They became even more evident when ages at which the subjects first became conspicuous were compared. While 28% of the O-subjects concerned became conspicuous before the age of 7 and 49% before the age of 9, (only) 15.5% of the corresponding G-subjects became conspicuous before the age of 9. Conspicuousness in the form of *offenses* at school should be particularly emphasized. While offenses at school were known for only two G-subjects, 22 O-subjects committed offenses at school, 15 of them offenses against property (see Sect. 4.2.1 below).

Considering the reasons why the majority of the O-subjects were conspicuous at school, it should be mentioned that their relationship to school was marked by listlessness and that their parents were less interested in school matters than the

Table 21. Supervision by persons rearing O-subjects and O-subjects' behavior at school

	Actual supervision ($n=83$)	No supervision or subject avoids it ($n=92$)
Behavior at school of O-subjects		
Inconspicuous	63.9%	20.7%
Conspicuous	26.5%	40.2%
Particularly conspicuous	9.6%	39.1%

Significance level: $p<.001$; relationship: $\overline{C}=.59$

Table 22. Measures taken by schools against conspicuous behavior at school

Behavior at school:	Conspicuous			Particularly conspicuous	
	O-subjects ($n=66$)	G-subjects ($n=31$)	Sig.	O-subjects ($n=48$)	G-subjects ($n=6$)
External measures taken by schools					
No external measures known	72.7% (48)	67.7% (21)		27.1% (13)	(0)
Notification of parents	19.7% (13)	29.1% (9)	n.s.	16.7% (8)	(4)
Notification of police or youth welfare office, or expulsion	7.6% (5)	3.2% (1)		56.2% (27)	(2)

Significance level: *n.s.*, not significant

G-parents were. Even more important, especially with respect to serious violations of school regulations and persistent truancy, was the fact that the majority of the O-subjects lacked adequate supervision by the persons rearing them or actively avoided this supervision (see Sect. 2.1.3.2 above). There is a strong relationship between behavior at school and supervision (see Table 21).

The O-subjects who were not adequately supervised by the persons rearing them were chiefly unable to adapt to school inconspicuously. This became most obvious when the 49 subjects who *actively* avoided supervision at home were considered separately: Only four of them remained inconspicuous at school.

2.3.2.3 The Socioscholastic Syndrome

Truancy and other conspicuousness at school, even in serious forms, were of no great importance when regarded in isolation, as they occurred for both the O- and the G-subjects, though plainly less frequently and seriously for the latter. Much more important was the concurrence of certain kinds of conspicuousness, which can be called a *socioscholastic syndrome: Only* O-subjects demonstrated this syndrome.

Typical of the syndrome was – as the *individual case studies* showed in particular – a *close relationship* between conspicuousness *at* and *outside of* school: A subject tried to conceal his *persistent truancy* by *deceit*, e.g., forged excuses; during the

Table 23. School characteristics of O- and G-subjects and early and late delinquents

	O-subj ($n=200$)	G-subj ($n=200$)	Sig. O-G	O_1-subj ($n=114$)	O_2-subj ($n=86$)	Sig. O_1-O_2
1. *Educational Success*						
Yes	53.0%	9.0%	++	59.7%	44.2%	+
No	47.0%	91.0%		40.3%	55.8%	
2. *Truancy*						
No[a] truancy	48.0%	88.5%		38.6%	60.5%	
Occasional truancy	21.5%	8.5%	++	22.8%	18.5%	+
Persistent truancy	30.5%	3.0%		38.6%	21.0%	
3. *Conspicuous behavior at school*						
No[a] conspicuous behavior	43.0%	81.5%		28.9%	62.8%	
Conspicuous behavior	33.0%	15.5%	++	36.0%	27.9%	++
Particularly conspicuous behavior	24.0%	3.0%		35.1%	9.3%	
4. *Socioscholastic syndrome*[b]	15.0%	.0%	++	20.2%	8.1%	+
5. *Measures taken by schools against negative behavior at school*	($n=114$)	($n=37$)		($n=81$)	($n=33$)	
No external measures	53.5%	56.8%		50.6%	57.6%	
Notification of parents	18.7%	35.1%	+	18.5%	18.2%	n.s.
Notification of police, youth welfare office; expulsion	28.1%	8.1%		30.9%	24.2%	

Significance level: +, $p<.05$; ++, $p<.001$; *n.s.*, not significant
[a] Or only minimal
[b] See Sect. 2.3.2.3 above

resulting unsupervised time he usually *roamed about* and occasionally committed "offenses," such as minor damage to property and theft (regarding "offenses" during childhood in general, see Sect. 4.2.1 below).

The proportion of persistent truants was 30.5% for the O-group and 3% for the G-group. The proportion of persistent truants who additionally tried to conceal their truancy by forging excuses or other methods of deceit, used this time to roam about and committed an "offense" at least once, i.e., exhibited the socioscholastic syndrome, was 15% for the O-group and 0% for the G-group (see Sect. 2.3.2.5 below and Table 23). The syndrome was thus *in no way typical* of the O-subjects, as it concerned only a small proportion of them; however, it was *specific* to the O-group insofar as no G-subject demonstrated it. This leads to the conclusion that later (recidivist) criminality is only infrequently preceded by a marked socioscholastic syndrome. Nevertheless, if the syndrome occurs, it should be a strong indicator of later criminality.

2.3.2.4 Measures Taken by Schools

Schools have a great deal of room for discretion with respect to how they can react to conspicuous behavior: They can react school internally with school punishments, or they can inform parents or even the competent public institutions, for instance the youth welfare office, which naturally leads to certain consequences. While school-internal punishments such as extra written work occur for every pupil at some time, *measures which include notifying external institutions* are normally taken only rarely and in serious cases.

This was confirmed in our study. No external measures were known for somewhat more than half of the (considerably) conspicuous subjects (see Sect. 2.3.2.2 above), i.e., for 61 of the 114 O-subjects and 21 of the 37 G-subjects. This picture of a relatively consistent reaction to the O- and the G-subjects changed, however, when external measures were differentiated into notifying parents, notifying authorities, or dismissal from school. Such a differentiation into "hard" and "soft" measures is of use only if the measures are related to kind and seriousness of conspicuousness (see Table 22).

Despite the very small number of G-subjects, certain tendencies became apparent: Although the school reacted more severely to *serious forms of conspicuousness* in both groups, it more frequently made do with notifying parents in the case of the G-subjects. Apparently this was more frequently sufficient to make the parents of the G-subjects solve the behavior difficulties of their children. It was not sufficient for the parents of the O-subjects; they did not react or were not able to influence their children.

Particularly interesting was the reaction of schools to children who committed *offenses at school.* For 15 of the 22 O-subjects and for one of the two G-subjects, the school reacted severely, i.e., the police or youth welfare office were notified, or the subject was dismissed from school (for reactions to childhood delinquency in general, see Sect. 4.2.1 below).

2.3.2.5 Early and Late Delinquents

Although compared with the G-group, the O-group was extreme with respect to all aspects of school which were investigated, it was not consistent or homogeneous in itself. In the context of school it became evident - as in the sphere of the family - that the late delinquents (O_2-subjects, see Sect. 1.3 above), who did not commit any registered offense until after their 18th birthdays, i.e., normally some years after completing school, differed in a positive sense from the early delinquents (O_1-subjects, see Sect. 1.3 above), who were convicted for the first time immediately after leaving, or even during school (see Table 23).

The differentiation into early and late delinquents led to essential differences (which - as an examination showed - could not be explained by differences in social class or intelligence). While the picture of difficulties at school, and especially of conspicuous behavior, became so obvious as to seem typical of early delinquents, the late delinquents showed a greater extent of conspicuousness than the G-group, but differed just as clearly from the early delinquents: The majority of the O_2-subjects completed school successfully, and their behavior was mainly inconspicuous; those who did become conspicuous were considerably less seriously so.

2.3.3 Occupational Training

2.3.3.1 Start and Completion of Occupational Training

In the following, occupational training is defined as training in an occupation requiring an apprenticeship or training in a comparable or higher-qualified occupational career outside school providing it ends with a formalized, officially recognized examination and entitles one to use an occupational title. Thus, workers which the literature terms "unskilled", including workers termed "semiskilled", i.e., workers with a certain occupational qualification setting them off from unskilled labor, are not included here (as opposed to SCHMEHL 1980, pp. 149 ff.; see also Sect. 2.3.4.1 below).

According to this definition, the distribution in the groups plainly differed: There were only very few subjects without any occupational training in the G-group, while they accounted for almost one-fourth of the O-group. More than 40% of the O-subjects had failed to complete occupational training, as opposed to only 6% of the G-subjects (see Table 24).

It is obvious that educational success played a role in the decision to start and the ability to complete occupational training: Finding an apprenticeship may well have been more difficult for the subjects who did not complete the *Hauptschule* (see Sect. 2.3.2.1 above). It may have been more difficult for them to meet the theoretical requirements of occupational training as well. Correspondingly, there is a strong *relationship* ($\overline{C} = 0.53$) *between educational success and occupational training* in the O-group (the number of G-subjects was too small to guarantee statistically significant results). The subjects who did not complete the *Hauptschule* started occupational training or completed it substantially less frequently than the subjects who completed school successfully. When the O- and the G-subjects who did or did not complete the *Hauptschule* were compared however, the following picture emerged (see Table 25):

Although, of the subjects who completed the *Hauptschule*, almost as large a percentage of O- as of G-subjects started occupational training, the O-subjects failed to complete their training much more often than the G-subjects did. For the O- and the G-subjects who did not complete the *Hauptschule*, there was also an obvious trend: While only about 18% of the O-subjects successfully completed occupational training, 11 of the 18 G-subjects did so. Clearly, the G-subjects were able to compensate for their lack of complete school education, while this lack continued and grew worse for the O-subjects in occupational training.

The common assumption that *occupational status of the father* is to a large degree decisive for an occupational career must also be modified. For the O-subjects (a statistical analysis is useless for the small number of G-subjects), there was a relationship ($\overline{C} = 0.35$) between social class of family of orientation or occupational status of the father and the subject's occupational training.

Table 24. Occupational training

	O-subjects ($n = 199$)[a]	G-subjects ($n = 186$)[a]
Did not start occupational training	24.6%	7.5%
Did not complete occupational training	40.7%	5.9%
Successfully completed occupational training	34.7%	86.6%

Significance level: $p < .001$
[a] On the dropouts, see Sect. 2.3.1 above

Table 25. Occupational training in relation with educational success and social class of family of orientation

		Did not start training	Did not complete training	Completed training	Sig.
Educational success					
Yes	O-subj ($n=$ 93)	10.8% (10)	35.5% (33)	53.8% (50)	++
	G-subj ($n=168$)	5.4% (9)	5.4% (9)	89.3% (150)	
No	O-subj ($n=106$)	36.8% (39)	45.3% (48)	17.9% (19)	-
	G-subj ($n=$ 18)	(5)	(2)	(11)	
Social class					
Lower lower class	O-subj ($n=$ 88)	37.5% (33)	36.4% (32)	26.1% (23)	++
	G-subj ($n=$ 32)	18.7% (6)	9.4% (3)	71.9% (23)	
Upper lower class and above	O-subj ($n=108$)	14.8% (16)	45.4% (49)	39.8% (43)	++
	G-subj ($n=154$)	5.2% (8)	5.2% (8)	89.6% (138)	

Significance level: ++, $p<.001$

Yet, when the O- and the G-subjects whose parents came from the *same* social class were compared, the differences between the O- and the G-subjects remained (see Table 25).

Thus, the differences were largely independent of social class. For the subjects who did not come from the lower lower class, i.e., whose fathers were at least skilled workers, the O-group showed a severe lack of training, as opposed to the G-group. An equally evident trend appeared for the subjects from the lower lower class, i.e., those whose fathers were unskilled: More than 70% of the G-subjects, yet only somewhat more than one-fourth of the O-subjects completed occupational training.

Thus, there are two contrary trends: A large number (about 60%) of the O-subjects did not reach the level of occupational training of their *skilled* fathers, i.e., did not complete occupational training, and only a small number (26%) of them were able to do better than the occupational status of their *unskilled* fathers by completing occupational training. In contrast, the G-subjects from the lower lower class showed a distinct trend toward occupational qualification, and practically all (i.e., 90%) of the remaining G-subjects reached at least the level of occupational training of their fathers (on intergenerational mobility, see Sect. 2.3.4.2 below).

2.3.3.2 Subjects with No Occupational Training

The reasons why several subjects never started occupational training merit separate consideration.

As was shown above (Sect. 2.3.3.1), the seemingly pertinent reasons, i.e., *no educational success* and *low social class of family of orientation*, were not solely decisive. Though the subjects who left school without completing the *Hauptschule* were overrepresented (39 of 49) among the O-subjects who did not start occupational training, the mere fact of no educational success was no more an obstacle for occupational training for the O- than for the G-subjects: 67 of the 106 subjects who left school without completing the *Hauptschule* aimed at an occupational qualification.

The situation is similar with respect to occupational status of the father. Two-thirds of the fathers of O-subjects without occupational training had no occupational training themselves; yet the subjects with *unskilled* fathers did not always simply become unskilled workers: The majority of them (55 of the 88 O-subjects and even 26 of the 32 G-subjects) at least started occupational training.

A certain influence of the subjects' parents appeared, however, in the *reasons* the subjects and their parents gave for their lack of occupational training. For more than half of the 14 G-subjects and almost one-fourth (11) of the 49 O-subjects it was maintained that the parents' poor economic situation had prevented the subjects from starting occupational training, as they had to help support their families as early as possible.

Of greater importance than this external constraint to earn money immediately after leaving school was the subjects' own need to have some money of their own quickly. One-third of the O-subjects did not "feel like" spending a few years in occupational training with an initially lower pay. This was also often the reason for breaking off occupational training (see Sect. 2.3.3.3 below). Other circumstances, such as no aptitude and inability to find an apprenticeship, were mentioned for only one-third (17) of the subjects.

On the other hand, several unskilled workers achieved a certain degree of occupational qualification in the course of their work by assuming functions which were more qualified than those of unskilled workers after spending many years at the same job or after completing a short training in a semiskilled occupation, for example as a welder (see Sect. 2.3.4.1 below). Only 9 of the 49 O-subjects, yet 11 of the 14 G-subjects achieved this upward occupational mobility.

2.3.3.3 External Course of Occupational Training

In order to throw light on the reasons why subjects failed to complete occupational training, it was examined which circumstances went together with the success or failure of occupational training.

Continuity of training played an important role, i.e., whether the subjects stayed at the same place during their apprenticeship or whether and how often they changed or even chose a different occupation (see Table 26).

The majority of the successful subjects (88% of the G-, 62% of the O-subjects) completed their entire occupational training at one place. But 20 of the 24 G-sub-

Table 26. Changes and success of occupational training

	O-subjects ($n=150$)		G-subjects ($n=172$)	
Did not complete occupational training	54%		6.4%	
Of these:				
At first apprenticeship		46.9% (38)		(7)
After change of apprenticeship (same occupation)		24.7% (20)		(1)
After change of apprenticeship (different occupation)		28.4% (23)		(3)
Completed occupational training	46%		93.6%	
Of these:				
At first apprenticeship		62.3% (43)		87.6% (141)
After change of apprenticeship (same occupation)		18.8% (13)		5.6% (9)
After change of apprenticeship (different occupation)		18.8% (13)		6.8% (11)

jects who did change also completed occupational training, as compared with only 26 of the 69 O-subjects. Thus, not only did the O-subjects change much more often during training; they were also less successful after a change.

The *reasons* why G-subjects (17 of the 31) prematurely terminated their first occupational training - whether it meant a change or breaking off training altogether - were chiefly objective difficulties such as illness or moving or reasons connected with the occupation, whereas difficulties with instructors and fellow workers were rarely mentioned. In contrast, the O-subjects' main reasons could be traced back to their own negative conspicuous behavior, whether at work or otherwise.

At their first apprenticeship alone, almost one-third of the O-subjects (31 of the 107) were fired because they did not fulfill their tasks or repeatedly stayed away from work unexcused for one or even several days. A number of O-subjects were fired because they committed offenses at their places of work (11); for some, the contracts were terminated because of imprisonment (4). Besides difficulties with instructors and fellow employees (11), important reasons for the subjects to terminate their contracts were that they did not "feel like" completing their training (10) or wanted to earn more money (7). In contrast, objective reasons which the subjects were not responsible for or which were connected with the occupation played a role for less than one-third of them (together 33 of 107).

In the face of these reasons, it is not surprising that the O-subjects, after the termination of a contract, usually did not immediately begin occupational training again at another place or start to work, but simply did not work at all for some time: 70 of the 107 O-subjects exhibited such *intervals of nonemployment,* 45 of them more than once, as opposed to only 4 of the 31 G-subjects. That subjects who were fired because of delinquency or poor work performance needed a certain amount of time to find a new place of training or work even in a period of full employment (as at the time of the Tübingen study) is obvious. However, the subjects concerned mainly did not spend their time of nonemployment looking for a new job intensively, but rather - often as a continuation of behavior which had begun during their apprenticeship - loafing around and bumming. If the O-subjects terminated their contracts themselves because they did not "feel like" working anymore or wanted to earn more money, this usually led to a period of nonemployment as well; the subjects mainly terminated a contract without any specific prospects of a new job (regarding general behavior during nonemployment, see Sect. 2.3.4.4 below).

2.3.3.4 Behavior During Occupational Training

Behavior during occupational training was estimated on the basis of the information provided by the subjects and by other persons, especially employers, but also youth welfare offices, and on the basis of the information in the reports of the juvenile court assistance and probation officers (on the problem of data collected and estimations made in retrospect, see Part I, Sect. 2.1).

Behavior during occupational training was regarded as negative if it consistently did not correspond to minimum requirements at work - whether with respect to a subject's relationship with his instructors and fellow employees or to his work performance itself. If such behavior occurred only intermittently, behavior during occupational training was termed "varying". Indicators of this were: insufficient work performance, unreliability, belligerence, excessive alcohol consumption, and temporary, unexcused absence. Such behavior, if it occurs seriously, causes employers to

Table 27. Behavior during occupational training in relation to behavior at school and success of occupational training

		Behavior during training negative or varying	Behavior during training inconspicuous or positive	Sig.
Behavior at school				
Negative	O-subj (80)	73.7% (59)	26.3% (21)	++
	G-subj (31)	25.8% (8)	74.2% (23)	
Inconspicuous	O-subj (70)	40.0% (28)	60.0% (42)	++
	G-subj (141)	5.0% (7)	95.0% (134)	
Training				
Not completed	O-subj (80)	76.3% (61)	23.7% (19)	-
	G-subj (11)	(4)	(7)	
Completed	O-subj (70)	37.1% (26)	62.9% (44)	++
	G-subj (161)	6.8% (11)	93.2% (150)	

Significance level: $++$, $p<.001$

fire an employee (see Sect. 2.3.3.3 above). Any behavior which did not fall into the categories of negative or varying behavior during occupational training, was considered inconspicuous or positive.

Here again, there were pronounced differences: Of the 150 O-apprentices, 87 (58%) entered the categories of negative or varying behavior during occupational training, whereas only 15 (9%) of the 172 G-apprentices manifested such behavior.

As such serious negative behavior patterns during occupational training often led to the subject being fired and therefore to a change, if not an end of occupational training, behavior during occupational training also affected *success in occupational training*. In both groups there is a correlation between behavior during and success in occupational training (O: phi = .38; G: phi = .21). The subjects with negative behavior thus tended to break off occupational training. Yet there were considerable differences in the number of subjects who completed occupational training when the O- and the G-subjects with negative and inconspicuous behavior were compared (see Table 27).

Of the inconspicuous apprentices, the G-subjects were clearly more successful, yet almost two-thirds of these O-subjects completed occupational training. Of the subjects with negative behavior during occupational training, the O-subjects tended to stop and the G-subjects to complete occupational training. Here, the *individual case studies* showed that negative behavior during occupational training tended to occur more intermittently and less seriously for the G-subjects.

Negative behavior during occupational training was often preceded by *negative behavior patterns at school:* In the O- (phi = .34) and in the G-group (phi = .28), there was an obvious correlation between behavior during occupational training and behavior at school. Yet there were considerable differences when the subjects with and without conspicuous behavior at school were compared (see Table 27). Of the O-subjects with negative behavior at school, three-fourths showed negative behavior during occupational training, of the G-subjects only one-fourth. Obviously, most G-subjects were able to adapt to occupational life even if they had manifested negative behavior at school. Furthermore, it was noted that their behavior at school had been of a temporary nature and less seriously negative (see Sect. 2.3.2.2 above). In contrast, the O-subjects normally continued their negative behavior from school at their work. On the other hand, almost all of the G- and most of the O-subjects who exhibited inconspicuous behavior at school continued this behavior during occupational training. Yet 40% of the O-subjects who had completed school without any behavior problems did not comply with behavior requirements during occupational training.

2.3.4 Employment

2.3.4.1 Occupational Position (at the Time of the Study)

A rating according to formal descriptions of vocations alone generally does not say a great deal about a person's actual occupational situation, and it can even be misleading: On the one hand, the occupation a person underwent training for is not necessarily the occupation he practices; on the other hand, his actual occupational activities can differ considerably from those generally associated with a certain occupation. The category "*occupational position*" was to determine the *actual* occupational situation of the subjects both in the stricter context of the firm and in the broader context of the social system. Following sociological studies of occupation, a subject's occupational position was determined by means of "occupational status," "degree of responsibility," and "income."

As 108 O- and 9 G-subjects had no longer worked immediately before their last imprisonment or the time of the study, their last relevant activity was taken. Only subjects who had not worked for more than one year in freedom before the time of the study were defined as "not employed": two subjects who were roaming about as vagrants, one subject who lived by procuring, and one subject who had almost exclusively been in correctional education or prison. Determining the exact actual occupation of a subject was difficult, as the information the subjects gave on their occupation often turned out to be incorrect or misleading on closer examination. (This may explain why studies based exclusively on criminal records partially obtained different results than those here.)

To determine a subject's *occupational status*, his occupation was rated according to the index of Kleining and Moore (1968; see Sect. 2.1.2.1 above) for 70 precisely defined occupations. The index, which discerns seven classes, could be applied only in modified form, as it does not differentiate sufficiently at the lower end of the index, where the O-subjects are strongly represented: Unskilled labor was divided according to nonemployed persons (e.g., vagrants), temporary laborers, unskilled workers, and semiskilled workers (see Table 28).

There is an obvious difference in distribution in the two samples. Exactly 75% of the O-subjects remained below the status of a skilled worker (trained worker, journeyman); only 14% of the G-subjects were unskilled or semiskilled workers.

In order to obtain a more accurate picture of a subject's actual occupational situation, *income* and *degree of responsibility* were also taken into consideration to determine his occupational position. Both for income and degree of responsibility, a rating was made which typically corresponds to a certain occupational status.

Table 28. Occupational status of subjects[a]

	O-subjects ($n=200$)	G-subjects ($n=200$)
Nonemployed	2.0%	-
Temporary laborers	4.0%	-
Unskilled	49.5%	4.0%
Semiskilled	19.5%	10.0%
Skilled	21.0%	34.0%
Qualified	4.0%	30.5%
Highly qualified	-	10.0%
Students	-	11.5%

[a] See Kofler 1980, p. 31

(As this study covers a period of several years, an index taking into account general income increases had to be formed so that the answers would be uniform; see KOFLER 1980, p.38.) If a subject demonstrated a positive difference with respect to income and degree of responsibility, his occupational position was raised by one degree (see Table 29).

The correction with the supplementary criteria income and responsibility caused almost exclusively a shift from unskilled to semiskilled workers. The pronounced differences between the O- and the G-subjects remained in essence.

2.3.4.2 *Occupational Mobility*

Occupational position is the result of an occupational development. This can be illustrated particularly clearly by relating a subject's present occupational position to his initial occupational position *(intragenerational mobility)* and to the occupational (social) status of his father or "breadwinner" *(intergenerational mobility).*

Certain difficulties arose in determining upward or downward occupational mobility, as some of the 20- to 30-year-old subjects had not yet completed their upward mobility. Since the status of skilled worker is usually reached at the age of 20, the problem concerned only the rise from a skilled to a qualified position such as master craftsman. Had this possible upward mobility been taken into account, the differences between the O- and the G-subjects would have become even more pronounced.

Table 29. Occupational position - under consideration of income and responsibility[a]

	O-subjects ($n=195$)	G-subjects ($n=177$)
1. Very low position (unskilled)	35.9%	2.8%
2. Low position (semiskilled)	39.0%	13.0%
3. Medium position (skilled)	24.1%	52.9%
4. High position (qualified)	1.0%	32.2%

Significance level: $p<.001$
[a] See KOFLER 1980, p.41

Table 30. Intergenerational social mobility

	Total group		Middle class		Upper lower class		Lower lower class	
	O-subj ($n=194$)	G-subj ($n=177$)	O-subj ($n=38$)	G-subj ($n=87$)	O-subj ($n=69$)	G-subj ($n=58$)	O-subj ($n=87$)	G-subj ($n=32$)
Downward	39.2%	23.7%	89.5%	39.1%	60.9%	13.8%	-	-
Same	50.0%	50.3%	10.5%	60.9%	30.4%	46.6%	82.8%	28.1%
Upward	10.8%	26.0%	-	-	8.7%	39.7%	17.2%	71.9%

Significance level: O-G: $p<.001$

Considering the social status or class of the family of orientation measured by the index of KLEINING and MOORE (1968; see also Sect. 2.1.2.1 above), i.e., occupational status of "breadwinner," 35.7% of the O-subjects came from the upper lower and 44.9% from the lower lower class (i.e., from families of unskilled workers). There was a relationship between present occupational position (which is often lower than the one aimed at after leaving school; see Sect. 2.3.3.3 above) and social class of the family of orientation in both groups (O: $\overline{C}=.28$; G: $\overline{C}=.44$; see KOFLER 1980, pp. 51 ff.). Yet this general relationship expressed entirely different movements in *occupational intergenerational mobility,* which became apparent when class of family of orientation was held constant (see Table 30).

Consequently, social origin was not the only factor determining later occupational position; in both groups, only half of the subjects had an occupational position corresponding to the social class of their families of orientation. As a whole, there were two clearly opposite trends in intergenerational mobility: While a downward trend largely independent of social class of family of orientation was recognizable in the O-group, the G-subjects tended to maintain or improve the position reached by their families of orientation.

The development of a subject's *own occupational career* could be shown by comparing his present occupational position with his initial occupational position, i.e., by examining *intragenerational mobility.*

The starting point for this comparison was a subject's occupational position after he completed his first occupational training. If a subject had not started or completed occupational training, his initial occupational position was defined as the one he had during the first year he worked. "Low initial position" meant "unskilled" or "semiskilled worker," "high initial position" at least "skilled worker" (see Table 31).

Both groups predominantly maintained their initial positions. In the O-group, however, this was due to the fact that most subjects remained unskilled and thus could not move down by definition. (The 7.5% of the O-subjects who did move down from a low initial position were "semiskilled workers" who became "unskilled workers.") In contrast, one-third of the O-subjects with higher initial positions had moved down.

Consequently, in addition to the usually low initial position of the O-subjects, there was an obvious tendency to downward mobility. This is not typical of unskilled workers in general; the upward trend of the unskilled G-subjects was marked (61%).

Table 31. Intragenerational social mobility

	Total group		Low original level		High original level	
	O-subj ($n=198$)	G-subj ($n=177$)	O-subj ($n=135$)	G-subj ($n=28$)	O-subj ($n=63$)	G-subj ($n=149$)
Downward	15.2%	5.1%	7.5%	3.5%	32.0%	4.7%
Same	74.2%	58.7%	78.5%	35.7%	65.0%	63.1%
Upward	10.6%	36.2%	14.0%	60.7%	3.0%	32.2%

Significance level: O–G: $p<.001$

While *intergenerational* and *intragenerational mobility* were marked by an upward trend in the G-group, downward occupational mobility was predominant in the O-group: 44.9% of the O-subjects came from families with a very low occupational and social status ("breadwinner" unskilled); 68.1% of the O-subjects started their occupational careers as unskilled workers; 74.9% of the O-subjects were unskilled workers at the time of the study.

2.3.4.3 Job Changes

Continuity of employment was measured by the number of job changes. Yet the frequency of changes alone is not sufficient: For a meaningful statement, the number of jobs must be related to the total number of months a subject was employed. This shows the average duration of one job. Table 32 presents the extremely varying distribution.

Marked differences also occurred in the *reasons why the subjects changed jobs:* While two-thirds of the G-subjects mentioned occupational or family reasons, two-thirds of the O-subjects gave the following reasons:

They were fired because of purported offenses at work or in communal lodgings or because of unsatisfactory work performance; they left their jobs because of arguments with their bosses and/or fellow employees they themselves had caused; they wanted to avoid garnishment of wages; they feared arrest and took to flight; they did not feel like doing this type of work anymore - without having any prospects of another job; they did not want to work at all for some time.

Most job changes of the O-subjects were not planned, but spontaneous and based on their momentary mood - or "ill humor." The reason they gave for a change was often their feeling that working conditions and circumstances were adverse and unbearable, not the prospect of a new, more promising job. This became apparent in statements such as "I was sick of it," "I couldn't stand that place anymore," or simply "I just didn't feel like it anymore."

In contrast, job changes of G-subjects usually took place smoothly, i.e., a G-subject was already sure of his new job before he gave notice at his old job.

2.3.4.4 Regularity of Employment

Frequent job changes do not say anything about regularity of employment. Regularity of employment is a question of whether a new job immediately succeeds the former one or whether there are *periods without employment* in between. The sub-

Table 32. Duration of employment per job[a]

		O-subjects ($n=199$)		G-subjects ($n=177$)	
Frequent job changes	up to 3 months	77.9%	20.6%	2.3%	-
	up to 6 months		27.1%		-
	up to 9 months		20.1%		.6%
	up to 12 months		10.1%		1.7%
Job continuity	up to 24 months	22.1%	16.6%	97.7%	25.4%
	up to 36 months		5.0%		26.5%
	more than 36 months		.5%		45.8%

Significance level: $p<.001$

[a] See KOFLER 1980, p. 94

Table 33. Nonemployment[a]

	O-subjects (n=199)	G-subjects (n=177)
Continuously employed	14.1%	92.1%
Nonemployment		
up to 3 months	18.6%	5.7%
up to 6 months	14.1%	1.7%
up to 9 months	12.6%	-
up to 12 months	9.5%	-
up to 24 months	23.6%	.6%
up to 36 months	4.0%	-
more than 36 months	3.5%	-

Significance level: $p<.001$
[a] Since first employment; see KOFLER 1980, p. 108

jects who were dismissed because of an economic recession and were entitled to unemployment pay (this occurred only rarely, considering the economic situation at the relevant time) must be distinguished from the subjects who simply gave up their jobs for no compelling reason or who provoked their own dismissal. Accordingly, only periods of unemployment which *a subject had caused himself* were defined as "*nonemployment.*" Not caused by the subject himself (in case of doubt) meant that the subject received unemployment pay [see § 119, Unemployment Benefit and Support Act *(Arbeitsförderungsgesetz)*].

While 92% of the G-subjects never demonstrated nonemployment (through their own fault), 53% of the O-subjects exhibited periods of nonemployment totaling more than 6 months (see Table 33).

To show how regularly a subject had worked, the duration of nonemployment was related to the time the subject had or could have worked.

For this purpose, the number of months a subject had worked (including occupational training) was divided by the number of months the subject could have worked. Thus, the time of military service, illness, imprisonment, and unemployment through no fault of the subject was subtracted. Regular employment meant that a subject had worked at least 95% of the time he could have worked.

Almost all of the G-subjects (98.3%), but only 37.5% of the O-subjects had been *regularly employed.* The remaining O-subjects fell into two approximately equally large groups, those who had always worked irregularly (32%) and those who had first worked regularly, but toward the end only irregularly (30.5%). Thus, a large number of O-subjects "idled away" a considerable part of their occupational lives.

This was also shown in the frequency of *temporary labor,* i.e., short-term, usually hourly work (such as unloading trucks at the market) to earn some money, usually without the subjects' having to show any working papers. Almost half of the O-subjects (46%) had earned their living doing odd jobs at some time. Nevertheless, for 16% of these subjects, temporary labor had been more of an exception in their entire occupational development, and only 17% of the O-subjects often earned their living with odd jobs. In the G-group, only three subjects had ever done temporary labor, and then only on a short-term basis.

Only a small group of O-subjects used the time of nonemployment for meaningful activities or undertakings. Half (51%) of the O-subjects concerned mainly spent

Table 34. Behavior at work[a]

	O-subjects ($n=199$)	G-subjects ($n=177$)
Predominantly negative, constantly fluctuating	54.8%	1.1%
Predominantly inconspicuous, adequate	34.2%	48.0%
Predominantly satisfactory	8.0%	50.9%
Unclear, contradictory	3.1%	-

Significance level: $p<.001$
[a] See KOFLER 1980, p. 29

their time at home, "loitering," "gadding about," and "loafing around"; 22% simply roamed about without any destination, going from town to town, hoping for something to happen without being able to say what (see also Sect. 2.4.3.3 below).

Only 14% of these O-subjects did not commit any offenses during such periods; 24% of the subjects committed sporadic *offenses,* which were more the exception than the rule, while the majority of them (61%) committed offenses frequently or even "in series" (see also Sect. 4.6 below).

2.3.4.5 Behavior at Work

Here, *behavior at work* is understood in the strict sense of how the subjects performed their work. This estimation was based on the information provided by the subjects, other persons (such as employers), youth welfare offices, and by the reports of the juvenile court assistance or probation officers (see also Sect. 2.3.3.4 above).

The following indicators were decisive for mainly *negative behavior at work:* The subject was lazy, unreliable, irresponsible; he shirked work, worked reluctantly, had to be told to work, often stayed away from work unexcused, did slipshod work, drank more alcohol than usual in his occupation. The following aspects were decisive for mainly *satisfactory behavior at work:* The subject was diligent, aspiring, reliable, made an effort, was a help, considered himself "indispensable," had a sense of responsibility, took his work seriously, was a good worker. If the subject had made no particularly negative or positive impression or if he was fairly integrated, behavior at work was assessed as *inconspicuous* or adequate. *Fluctuating behavior at work,* finally, meant a frequent change between negative and inconspicuous behavior at work (see Table 34).

As the distribution shows, the negative conspicuousness of the O-subjects continued in their internal behavior at work. Thus, it was fair to assume that there were relationships between the individual occupational criteria.

2.3.4.6 The Syndrome of Lacking Occupational Adaptation

There was a strong relationship between job changes and regularity of employment for the O-subjects ($\overline{C}=0.68$; see KOFLER 1980, p. 118): The more frequently subjects changed their jobs, the more irregularly they worked. For the O-subjects who changed jobs frequently and stayed at one job for only a short time, jobs did not succeed each other immediately, but were interrupted by periods of non-employment. This corresponds to a generally negative behavior at work, which was closely related with frequent job changes ($\overline{C}=.51$) and irregular employment ($\overline{C}=.75$) (see KOFLER 1980, p. 130).

Table 35. Syndrome of lacking occupational adaptation (performance syndrome)

	O-subjects (n=199)	G-subjects (n=177)
1. Frequent job changes	77.9% (155)	2.3% (4)
2. Irregular employment	62.3% (124)	1.7% (3)
3. Negative or fluctuating behavior at work	54.8% (109)	1.1% (2)
(1+2+3) Syndrome of lacking occupational adaptation	42.7% (85)	.6% (1)

Significance level: O-G: $p<.001$

These three negative occupational aspects - frequent job changes, irregular employment, and negative or fluctuating behavior at work - can be understood as the manifestation of a *syndrome of a comprehensive inability to adapt to performance requirements in occupational life* - a syndrome which occurred fully for 43% and partially (two of the three criteria of lacking occupational adaptation) for 64% of the O-subjects (see Table 35).

This lacking occupational adaptation cannot be explained by the low occupational position predominant in the O-group, as it is not characteristic of unskilled workers: Only one (unskilled) G-subject demonstrated the syndrome.

Obviously, the O-subjects are an extreme group with respect to their inability to adapt to occupational requirements. Though the skilled workers of the O-group were as a whole less marked by negative forms than the unskilled workers, it would be incorrect to interpret this as a *consequence* of occupational position. The *opposite reasoning* seems correct: The occupational position of a skilled worker can be achieved and maintained in the long run only if at least minimal occupational requirements are met. Accordingly, particularly the subjects who moved down in occupation (see Sect. 2.3.4.2 above) demonstrate the characteristics of lacking occupational adaptation very clearly.

2.3.4.7 Employment, Imprisonment, and Special Situations in Life

In view of the question to what extent the occupational conspicuousness of the O-subjects could have been influenced by imprisonment, a strong relationship ($\overline{C}=.31$; see Kofler 1980, p. 62) appeared between occupational position and imprisonment (for details, see Sect. 4.3.1 below): There was a larger proportion of semiskilled and skilled workers among the subjects who had never been in prison before the study than among the subjects who had already been imprisoned. However, this does not clarify whether the subjects who had already served a term in prison had a low occupational position *because of* their imprisonment or whether the subjects with fewer convictions showed more commitment and endurance in the sphere of performance.

To answer this question, it was examined whether there were any changes in the sphere of occupational performance - possibly with a certain delay - after the subjects' first terms of imprisonment of at least one week. It was assumed that one's first imprisonment has far-reaching consequences with respect to its effects on one's psyche and on one's relationships with the environment. The examination was limited to phenomena which could be observed unequivocally from outside. Changes in the sphere of occupational performance could be observed for only 18 O-subjects, 17 of whom at least maintained their occupational position. As a rule, only the frequency of job changes increased.

When, additionally, the O-group was differentiated according to length of imprisonment before the time of the study to examine whether there were any differences in job changes, nonemployment, and behavior at work, the following relationships emerged: The longer (which often also means the more frequently) subjects were imprisoned, the more often did they change jobs ($\bar{C}=.45$), the more irregularly did they work ($\bar{C}=.44$) and the more negative was their behavior at work ($\bar{C}=.32$; see KOFLER 1980, pp. 100ff.; 116ff.; 132ff.). Yet these relationships cannot be interpreted as relationships of cause and effect. More frequent terms in prison certainly do lead to a number of job changes, and it may also be important that many subjects needed several days to find a job after they were released (although, in reality, the job market in the 1960s would usually have allowed the penal institution to arrange for a job). Yet it should be considered that frequent job changes had mostly already occurred *before* imprisonment and that remarkably many O-subjects, before they were arrested for an offense, had *not* worked for weeks or months already, i.e., that often only offenses committed during periods of nonemployment led to imprisonment (see Sect. 2.3.4.4 above). The comprehensive occupational instability of the O-subjects is therefore *not simply a consequence* of imprisonment but often developed before. Nevertheless, imprisonment may have an intensifying effect.

Finally, it should be noted that even the O-subjects who had *not been imprisoned* before their present term had been much more conspicuous in regard to their behavior at work (frequent job changes 51%; irregular employment 32%; negative behavior at work 35%) than the most predisposed G-subjects, i.e., the (28) unskilled G-subjects, of whom only one was concerned for each criteria.

On the other hand, other *special situations in life* and events were more frequently related (at least in time) to downward occupational mobility (33 O-subjects).

Such situations were in particular: Serious strains in the relationships with persons who were close to a subject and had given him support, discharge from military service, or fleeing from the German Democratic Republic. Other reasons to change jobs were the influence of a friend or acquaintance and - usually only imaginary - better pay at another job.

In conclusion, the O-subjects' lack of occupational success cannot be explained by imprisonment. Many subjects had either always been on the lowest occupational level or had already reached it *before* their first imprisonment.

2.3.4.8 Special Conspicuousness

Despite their usually negative experiences in occupational life, the O-subjects often did not adequately *estimate their occupational possibilities*. Many of them were out of touch with the reality of occupational life in their occupational plans, aims, and aspirations. This was an impression gained from the *individual case studies*. Practically no O-subject said that he mainly wanted to gain a firm foothold in his former occupation and achieve recognition and even promotion by constant performance at one place for several years, despite all difficulties involved.

Much more frequently, the O-subjects wanted to have a "dream job" with higher prestige and higher pay, such as being a "sales representative" or "self-employed." The subjects frequently took up ideas they had picked up from anywhere without any critical distance, and they rarely had a clear idea of the requirements and risks of the desired occupation. They usually failed to realize that it is necessary to possess a considerable amount of endurance, often for several years, and the ability to digest occasional failures to achieve occupational success.

This lack of sense of reality practically foretold the failure of any such plans. Even if the subjects had already had similar occupational aspirations and had failed to realize them, they did not learn from earlier setbacks. Thus, difficulties almost necessarily arose in the realization of any new plans. The subjects resigned quickly, "chucked it all," and were soon back in the same old rut as unskilled or temporary laborers, changing from job to job and soon committing offenses again. The subjects did not blame their own unrealistic estimation of their possibilities but circumstances, envious fellow employees, unfair superiors, traps, and the intrigues of probation officers.

In order to verify these impressions in the entire group, it was examined whether the subjects tended to overestimate their occupational possibilities and abilities according to the occupational plans and wishes they had mentioned - measured against the chance they stood to realize them. This did *not* exclusively mean the *actual* failure of new occupational developments, as other factors may have played a role too. It was attempted to determine whether a failure was already unmistakably apparent for outside observers in the stage of planning and whether this should have been recognized by the subjects as well had they applied some criticism. In this way, an *overestimation of occupational possibilities* was unequivocally determined for 53 O-subjects but only five G-subjects (see KOFLER 1980, pp. 144ff.).

A number of O-subjects, not only those whose occupational plans failed, often gave up working, "chucked it all," and only "gadded about." It was typical that, in contrast to the situation after the failure of occupational plans, there was frequently no external reason for giving up a job or work in general. The impression was that the subjects "shrugged of" the obligations of working, which they felt to be a burden, and "*broke away from the sphere of occupational performance.*"

Asked about their reasons for giving up work and not working for weeks or even months, the subjects often answered: "The idea just struck me," "I was fed up with everything," "I had enough," etc. These expressions were not directly aimed at employment, but expressed a general listlessness and discontent. The subjects did not know what to do with themselves, they felt dejected, at a loss, and wanted to "get out." Obligations at home and family ties were felt to be a burden, a constraint to be avoided; their occupation was often their last resort - but also a last constraint, a last pressure to evade. Often, the subjects simply shrugged off any "*musts.*"

These phenomena cannot be measured exactly or operationalized precisely. Their determination requires the estimation of moods and ill humor on the basis of a large quantity of information, including the self-estimation of the subject. Therefore, it is difficult to give exact figures. Nonetheless, members of the research team who judged entirely independently estimated that 77 O-subjects, as opposed to only three G-subjects, had "broken away from the sphere of occupational performance" frequently or occasionally for no discernible reason (see KOFLER 1980, pp. 151 ff.).

As the *individual case studies* showed, it was not so that many subjects suddenly stopped working, committed offenses at some time, and were arrested in the end: Usually, there was a slowly increasing *neglect of the sphere of occupational performance which went together with the commission of offenses* (see also Sect. 4.6 below).

Indicators of neglect were heavy drinking and frequent unexcused absences from work, "loafing around," frequent job changes - often accompanied first by sporadic offenses which were more the exception than the rule - until, finally, the subjects no longer worked at all and merely "hung around." The subjects often spent their time in the company of "buddies" in a similar situation. They sat together, drank, gambled, went from bar to bar to "pick up" girls, etc. When a subject (or the whole group) ran out of money, an offense was committed to obtain some. This sometimes led to whole series of theft or fraud, which did not stop until the subject was arrested.

It was attempted to determine this phenomenon in a quantitative respect. In this context, it was determined whether there was an interdependency between an increasing neglect of work and the onset of offenses. Only if this interdependency was apparent was the phenomenon considered to be present. This was the case for more than half (54%) of the O-subjects, for more than 20% of them even repeatedly, but for only one G-subject. Thus, it can be assumed that neglecting occupational obligations *and* committing offenses expresses an extensive maladaptation to social rules and obligations (see KOFLER 1980, pp. 157 ff.).

2.3.4.9 Early and Late Delinquents

In accordance with the findings from the spheres of family and school, the late delinquents (O_2-subjects), i.e., the subjects who were not convicted until after their 18th birthdays, and therefore, as a rule, after some years of employment or after completing occupational training, differed in a positive sense from the early delinquents (O_1-subjects), who had committed offenses shortly after they began working or started occupational training (see Table 36).

Approximately equally large proportions of early and late delinquents started occupational training, but the late delinquents tended to complete their occupational training, while two-thirds of the early delinquents failed to do so. This is also reflected in the differing numbers of subjects who last had the status of unskilled workers. There is only a small difference in job changes, and the major-

Table 36. Occupational training and employment of O- and G-subjects and early and late delinquents

	O-subj (n=199)	G-subj (n=186)	Sig. O-G	O_1-subj (n=113)	O_2-subj (n=86)	Sig. O_1-O_2
Occupational training						
1. Did not start training	24.6%	7.5%	++	23.0%	26.7%	n.s.
2. Started training	75.4%	92.5%	++	77.0%	73.3%	n.s.
Of these:						
a) Did not complete training	54.0%	6.4%	++	65.5%	38.1%	++
b) Negative behavior during training	58.0%	8.7%	++	74.7%	34.9%	++
3. Remained unskilled[a]	65.3%	13.4%	++	75.3%	54.6%	+
Employment as a whole	(n=199)	(n=177)		(n=113)	(n=86)	
4. Last occupational position unskilled[b]	74.9%	15.8%	++	82.3%	65.1%	+
5. Frequent job changes	77.9%	2.3%	++	82.3%	72.1%	n.s.
6. Irregular employment	62.5%	1.7%	++	67.3%	55.8%	n.s.
Of these:						
a) Exclusively irregular	51.2%	-	-	57.9%	39.6%	-
b) First regular, in the end irregular	48.8%	-	-	42.1%	60.4%	+
7. Predominantly negative or fluctuating behavior at work	56.8%	1.1%	++	77.9%	36.1%	++
8. Syndrome of lacking occupational adaptation (5+6+7)	42.7%	.6%	++	57.5%	31.4%	++

Significance level: *+*, $p<.05$; *++*, $p<.001$; *n.s.*, not significant
[a] Did not start or did not complete occupational training
[b] Had always been unskilled or moved down to the position of unskilled

ity (56%) of the late delinquents demonstrated irregular employment. In behavior at work, however, the late delinquents fared much better: 36% of the late, as compared with 78% of the early delinquents showed mainly negative or fluctuating behavior at work. Correspondingly, only a minority of the late delinquents fully demonstrated the syndrome of lacking occupational adaptation, as opposed to the majority of the early delinquents.

This - as compared with the O_1-subjects - relatively positive general impression of the O_2-subjects was based on categories describing occupational criteria as *static* characteristics, such as "mainly negative behavior at work." From this perspective, the *development* of the subjects in the *longitudinal section of life* was not evident, as, generally speaking, it cannot be adequately determined by statistical means. In contrast, the *individual case studies* showed in an impressive way that particularly the late delinquents increasingly neglected the sphere of performance before the time of the study and even more so before the offenses leading to their imprisonment (see also Sect. 4.6 below). This is also expressed here in the category of irregular employment. While most of the early delinquents worked irregularly during the entire period, the late delinquents usually worked regularly when they were first employed but worked more and more irregularly, particularly during the last period. These were signs that the O_2-subjects tended to approximate the extremely negative picture of the O_1-subjects' sphere of performance.

2.3.5 Summary

The results on the spheres of school and occupation fit into the relatively uniform picture provided by other multifactorial studies:

The studies reported that delinquents had to repeat a year at school more frequently or left school prematurely, played truant, or seriously violated school regulations and, partially, that the persons rearing the subject influenced development at school (see CONGER and MILLER 1966, pp. 66ff., 88ff.; GLUECK and GLUECK 1974, pp. 95ff., 154 ff.; FERGUSON 1952, p. 150; FERRACUTI et al. 1975, p. 74; HEALY and BRONNER 1936, pp. 61ff.; MCCORD and MCCORD 1959, pp. 77ff.; Statens offentliga utredningar 1971, p. 155; 1972, p. 109; 1973 a, p. 211; PONGRATZ and HÜBNER 1959, p. 40; POWERS and WITMER 1951, p. 272; ROBINS 1966, p. 215; ROSENQUIST and MEGARGEE 1969, p. 205; WEST and FARRINGTON 1973, pp. 98ff.; WOLFGANG et al. 1972, pp. 60ff.; Centro Nazionale di Prevenzione e Difesa Sociale 1969, pp. 380ff.).

The findings in the sphere of occupation were almost unanimous: Delinquents either do not start occupational training or break it off very soon; unskilled workers are overrepresented among delinquents, and their behavior at work is marked by frequent unplanned job changes, prolonged periods of unemployment, and unsatisfactory performance at work (FERGUSON 1952, p. 150; GLUECK and GLUECK 1974, pp. 160ff.; PONGRATZ and HÜBNER 1959, pp. 34ff.; ROBINS 1966, p. 54; ROSENQUIST and MEGARGEE 1969, pp. 201ff.; WEST and FARRINGTON 1977, pp. 64 ff.).

Compared with the G-subjects, the O-subjects had markedly less *school education*; more than half of the O-subjects had not even completed the *Hauptschule*. This negative picture of the O-subjects cannot be explained solely by the fact that they showed certain characteristics to a greater extent. As expected, these characteristics - namely, low IQ, low social class of family of orientation, and difficult social circumstances - influenced success at school. When these characteristics were held constant, however, the O-subjects still had significantly less school education than the G-subjects. Obviously, these relatively rough external or formal criteria do not suffice to describe or even explain the difference adequately.

The O-subjects were an extreme group, not only with respect to success at school but also with respect to *conspicuous behavior at school.* The majority of the O-subjects, but only 19% of the G-subjects exhibited the serious conspicuousness taken together in the categories of "conspicuous" and "particularly conspicuous behavior," which included persistent truancy. Concomitantly, conspicuous behavior was related with success at school ($\overline{C}=.32$), and failing at school was all the more frequent, the earlier the subjects' first conspicuousness occurred ($\overline{C}=.54$, see SCHMEHL 1980, pp. 69ff.). This means that the O-subjects who plainly did not comply with behavior requirements with respect to school regulations usually did not meet performance requirements either. There was also a strong relationship with circumstances at home; the subjects who were conspicuous at school were usually not supervised by the persons rearing them or avoided such supervision.

Problems at school and in particular negative conspicuous behavior were much more frequent and marked for the *early delinquents.* Thus, there is a certain probability that early delinquency is preceded by difficulties at school. School performance was mostly adequate or at least inconspicuous for the *late delinquents.*

It would be erroneous, however, to overestimate the importance of difficulties at school among the complex of conditions out of which criminality develops. On the one hand, about 30% of the early delinquents committed their first offenses shortly after leaving school, *despite inconspicuousness at school.* On the other hand, almost one-fifth of the G-subjects were conspicuous at school, just as were a considerable number of the late delinquents, who were not convicted until several years after leaving school.

The *socioscholastic syndrome,* which combines conspicuousness at and outside school, is a special aspect: Persistent truancy aided by deceit, roaming about, and committing petty offenses during the time gained. This combination of behavior did not occur frequently, but, since it concerned the O-subjects alone, it serves as a strong indicator of a danger of criminality.

Partly as a continuation of shortcomings and difficulties at school, partly as a consequence of downward occupational mobility, the O-subjects exhibited considerable *occupational shortcomings* as compared with the average population. A large percentage of the O-subjects did begin occupational training, but many of them stopped, often during the first year. While there was a tendency, in the G-group, toward upward occupational mobility or at least toward maintaining the position achieved, there was negative intragenerational occupational mobility in the O-group irrespective of social class: At the time of the study, 75% of the O-group held the position of unskilled workers.

This can be understood as an expression of a lack of stability throughout the entire sphere of performance. Lack of occupational success or downward occupational mobility were regularly accompanied by *frequent job changes, periods of nonemployment, and negative behavior at work or during occupational training,* which was usually preceded by conspicuous behavior at school. This occupational conspicuousness forms the *syndrome of lacking occupational adaptation,* which - as it concerned only the O-subjects, with the exception of one G-subject (who, however, also committed offenses) - can be considered specific to the O-subjects.

The results of the present study also show clearly that, although *external characteristics* such as social class of family of orientation and school education play a role in the occupational career of the subjects, they are not the decisive, determining factors for a development toward extremely conspicuous occupational behavior patterns. The striking differences between the O- and the G-group diminished only slightly when these characteristics were held constant, i.e., when their possible influence was eliminated. Previous *imprisonment* is equally not responsible for occupational shortcomings since downward occupational mobility had frequently already taken place or occupational conspicuousness occurred prior to it. Imprisonment was often preceded by times of nonemployment, during which the offenses were committed which led to the subjects' being imprisoned. Nevertheless, a development toward criminality and the imprisonment accompanying this development cannot be considered a simple consequence of occupational maladaptation. In most cases, there is an interdependency between the two developments: Occupational neglect goes hand in hand with the commission of offenses. An extreme conspicuousness in occupational career and a development toward recidivist criminality appear to be two symptoms of a general maladaptation (see Sect. 5 below).

In the differentiation according to *onset of delinquency,* the late delinquents presented a somewhat more positive picture: In the end, they had a higher occupational position and demonstrated fewer negative behavior patterns at work. However, it must be taken into account that the occupational development of the late delinquents - particularly during the period immediately before the study - tended toward an increasing neglect of the sphere of performance and therefore approached the negative picture of the sphere of performance of the early delinquents.

Finally, it should be mentioned that the simple facts of failing occupational training or remaining in the position of unskilled worker alone are of practically no importance. Much more decisive are criteria relating to a subject's behavior patterns at work and his attitude toward his occupation. These are: Job changes, regularity of employment, and behavior at work, whose negative variants form the criteria for the O-specific *syndrome of lacking occupational adaptation* (see above). As not all O-subjects - only 58% of the early and 31% of the late delinquents - demonstrated *all* three kinds of occupational conspicuousness, (recidivist) criminality (leading to a long term of imprisonment) is not necessarily accompanied by a lacking occupational adaptation *in the entire sphere of performance* (different for the last offenses, see Sect. 4.6 below, and for the "neglect of the sphere of performance" *at the time of the study,* see Part III, Sect. 3.3.3.1).

Conversely, however, the symptoms described in lacking occupational adaptation may well be a very strong indicator of a "development toward criminality" (see Part III, Sect. 4.4.2.1), as they practically did not occur in the general (G-)population.

It must be emphasized once again that this occupational behavior has nothing to do with - cyclical - "unemployment." Unemployed persons - if their unemployment was incurred through no fault of their own (under § 119, Unemployment Benefit and Support Act) - are entitled to unemployment benefits (initially) providing social security and also usually find work after a certain time or, even in case of long-term unemployment, remain socially integrated. The behavior shown to be relevant here is characterized by the facts that the subjects had caused their "nonemployment" themselves (they had either simply stopped working or had been fired because of their intolerable behavior), that they had not been registered with the employment office (and therefore had received no unemployment benefits or relief money), and that they had spent most of their free time "hanging around."

Lacking occupational adaptation or even a total neglect of the sphere of performance is of great importance in the complex of conditions out of which criminality develops - not least because irregular employment or nonemployment regularly meant that the subjects no longer had a secure living and that their lives became unstructured, which led to offenses more or less of necessity (see also Sect. 4.6 below).

2.4 The Sphere of Leisure

2.4.1 Preliminary Remarks

To *define* the concept of leisure and delimit the sphere of leisure from the other social spheres, a rather pragmatic-formal, yet easily and uniformly applicable formula was used, also under consideration of the impressions gained in the descriptions of daily routines (see Part III, Sect. 3.2): Leisure is the time which remains after deducting 8 hours of work a day (or the time spent at school), the time needed for the way to and from work (or school) for a 5-day week, and the time normally used for meals, sleep, and hygiene (see GÖPPINGER 1980, p. 290). Holidays and vacations were not taken into account, particularly since regular, planned vacations concerned almost exclusively the G-subjects and were unimportant for the O-subjects, if only because of their usually irregular employment (see Sect. 2.3.4.4 above).

The attempt to *systematize* the extensive data on leisure behavior rapidly showed, on the one hand, that the criteria commonly used to comprehend leisure inadequately reflect specific leisure behavior. These criteria are usually limited to an enumeration of leisure activities, such as how often the subjects went to the movies, to bars, or watched television, what hobbies they had, etc. On the other hand, these criteria were not able to distinguish clearly between the two groups. It became apparent that the leisure behavior and leisure structure of the two groups diverged to such an extent that even externally identical activities differed completely in content, that comparable undertakings took an entirely different course in time, and that attitudes toward leisure and planning and carrying out basically identical leisure activities varied considerably. The behavior patterns which were particularly characteristic of the O-group were especially problematic: The usual criteria did not allow satisfactory presentation of the irregularity and the constantly changing forms of these behavior patterns. Even examining the function of a certain organization of leisure led no further, as this in the end subjective point of view encompasses the entire scope of leisure behavior and does not permit a useful categorization. (One person finds distraction in a second job, another in the "milieu" of large cities.)

Criteria abstracting from the specific forms of leisure proved to be better suited to elaborate the characteristic structures of the behavior of the two groups and to guarantee a systematic understanding of the entire sphere of leisure. These criteria relate to the *extent in time* of leisure (availability of leisure, see Sect. 2.4.2 below), to *structure and course* of leisure activities (see Sect. 2.4.3 below) - again from an abstracting point of view, and to the *place* where leisure time is spent (place of leisure, see Sect. 2.4.4 below).

On the basis of these criteria, the leisure behavior of the subjects is analyzed for three unchanging intervals, irrespective of the individual duration of school or occupational training: Roughly, "school age" covers the period up to the age of 15 and "age of occupational training" that between the ages of 15 and 18. The third interval is the "period of the study" (see Sect. 1.3 above).

Four O-subjects were entirely disregarded for the "period of the study." They were barely over 20 at the time of the study, meaning that there was no prolonged interval for the "period of the study" after the "age of occupational training." Therefore, their behavior was taken into account only at "school age" and "age of occupational training."

2.4.2 Availability of Leisure Time

2.4.2.1 Limitation and Extension of Leisure Time According to Age-groups

According to the aforementioned definition of leisure, the time remaining between work and sleep only rarely coincides with the actual "spare" time which one can dispose of freely every day. Most people have manifold obligations due to their positions in the family, at work, in organizations, or in the local community, which they assumed voluntarily or came to assume through external circumstances. These obligations affect the way they dispose of their time. Overtime, spare-time work, or regular sports and hobbies (see also Sect. 2.4.3.1 below and Table 39), but also obligations and assistance in the family, among relatives or neighbors can lead to a considerable *limitation* of leisure time. While for some, only the weekend or perhaps merely part of it remains for "inactivity" or for specific plans, others can still freely dispose of a differing number of hours per day. However, a certain kind of leisure (and life) organization or certain leisure activities can also lead to an *extension* of the basically available "spare" time at the expense of the period of rest and sleep and the time intended for the sphere of performance (see also Sect. 2.4.3.3 below and Table 41).

The significance of the criterion "availability of leisure time" is in no way limited to the analysis of leisure behavior in the strict sense, but extends beyond, providing access to the understanding of a person's entire life-style. A life-style can be expressed, for example, in a "disorder" in the course of a day, which can be marked by an extension of leisure at the expense of sleep and the sphere of performance. A life-style can also be expressed in a subject's strict integration of many obligations (particularly during leisure time), and thus by a course of a day where each detail is organized (see also Part III, Sect. 3.2).

The two groups differed fundamentally with respect to availability of leisure time (see Table 37). Only few G-subjects exhibited a (predominant) extension of leisure time during the various intervals examined. A limitation of leisure time became increasingly important, especially in adulthood, when a heightened sense of responsibility and thus the fulfillment of manifold obligations are normally expected. Almost half of the G-subjects (41%) limited their leisure time by more than one activity (for the kinds of activities, see Table 39). Even the G-subjects who did not limit the main part of their leisure time showed a relatively balanced

Table 37. Availability of leisure time

	School age (up to age 14)		Age of occupational training (age 15-18)		Period of study	
	O-subj (n=177)	G-subj (n=196)	O-subj (n=189)	G-subj (n=193)	O-subj (n=189)	G-subj (n=198)
Predominantly limitation	13.0%	27.0%	7.9%	35.2%	4.8%	63.7%
No limitation or extension	40.7%	67.9%	33.3%	57.0%	10.0%	33.3%
Predominantly extension	46.3%	5.1%	58.7%	7.8%	85.2%	3.0%

Significance level: O-G: $p<.001$

Table 38. Direction of leisure time extension

	School age (up to age 14)			Age of occupational training (age 15-18)			Period of study		
	O-subj (n=177)	G-subj (n=196)	Sig.	O-subj (n=189)	G-subj (n=193)	Sig.	O-subj (n=189)	G-subj (n=198)	Sig.
Extension at the expense of									
Sphere of performance	50.8%	10.2%	++	57.1%	7.3%	++	82.0%	2.0%	++
Period of rest and sleep	41.8%	3.1%	++	62.4%	14.0%	++	89.4%	6.1%	++
Sphere of performance *and* period of rest and sleep	33.9%	2.0%	++	51.9%	4.2%	++	78.3%	.5%	++

Significance level: ++, $p<.001$

organization of leisure time, insofar as there were occasionally both extensions and limitations.

In contrast, a prolonged limitation of leisure time after school age occurred for only a few O-subjects. In spite of the usual increase of obligations in life, the O-subjects almost exclusively demonstrated considerable extensions of leisure time. Practically all the O-subjects had substantially extended the leisure time at their disposal by corresponding leisure activities (see Sect. 2.4.3.3 below and Table 41) for prolonged periods of time. These extensions took place at the expense of the period of rest and sleep or - usually additionally (see Table 38) - at the expense of normal employment, mostly in the form of serious tardiness, staying away from work (unexcused or on the pretext of being ill), or giving up working entirely in the sense of nonemployment (times of "real" unemployment - see also Sect. 2.3.4.4 above - were disregarded).

2.4.2.2 Direction of Leisure Time Extension

To examine in depth at the expense of which social spheres leisure time was extended, the G- and the O-subjects whose extension of leisure time at school age,

age of occupational training, and during the period of the study did not predominate, but had (temporarily) determined their leisure organization during a certain phase of the intervals (see Table 38) were also taken into consideration.

The essential difference between the two groups lay in the development of the *extension of leisure time at the expense of the sphere of performance:* The rather high proportion of such extensions at school age increased up to the period of the study for the O-subjects, while it decreased steadily for the G-subjects.

Less obvious was the difference between the two groups in the development of the *extension of leisure time at the expense of the period of rest and sleep:* Though there was a more marked increase during the intervals for the O-subjects - the proportion of these extensions more than doubled - the G-subjects' did not simply demonstrate an opposite development. For the G-subjects, this kind of extension of leisure time reached a certain high at the age of occupational training, but lost importance again during the period of the study.

A similar development occurred for the extension of leisure time *at the expense of the sphere of performance and the period of rest and sleep:* Here again, there was a continuous increase for the O-subjects and a certain high at the age of occupational training for the G-subjects. However, the extensions in *both* directions were much less significant for the G-group than for the O-group. This became particularly obvious for the period of the study, during which more than three-fourths of the O-subjects, as opposed to only one G-subject, extended leisure time in this extensive form. The extension in both directions usually went hand in hand with a total shift of the course of a day; for example, the subjects began their day in the afternoon and ended it late at night, which again affected the course of the following day.

In the framework of the *individual case studies,* two rather frequent developments became apparent for the O-subjects in this context: Especially the recidivist offenders who committed offenses against property had considerably extended their leisure time as early as at *school age,* particularly at the expense of the sphere of performance. The subjects played truant, roamed about all day, and came back home late. An extension (only) at the expense of sleep did not yet play a very important role during childhood, not least because there are practically no leisure activities at night for children and because parents or other persons (police, neighbors) would notice a child staying away at night. Insofar as there were any extensions at the expense of the period of rest and sleep, they normally occurred in connection with disordered (asocial) family circumstances, meaning that the subjects were unsupervised and could roam about "in the streets" until late at night.

Other O-subjects, in contrast, did not demonstrate any serious extensions of leisure time until the *age of occupational training.* In the beginning, leisure time was exclusively extended at the expense of sleep, but soon at the expense of the sphere of performance as well: The subjects caught up on their sleep the next morning and did not go to work. The initially sporadic, then more or less regular extension of leisure time at the expense of the sphere of performance and, consequently, a total shift of the course of a day always represented an important step toward social conspicuousness and a considerably greater danger of criminality.

Insofar as the G-subjects extended their leisure time at *school age* [especially in the higher grades of the *Hauptschule* (see Sect. 2.3.2 above)], they did so less frequently and stopped at the latest when they began working regularly.

At the *age of occupational training,* there were several G-subjects who temporarily demonstrated a conspicuous organization of leisure (cliques of hoodlums, "milieu" contacts) and also extended their leisure time during this period first at the expense of the period of rest and sleep, then sporadically at the expense of the sphere of performance. The latter, however, was usually limited to truancy at vocational school *(Berufsschule)* or staying away from work occasionally. There was no continuous extension of leisure time and, in particular, no shift in the course of a day. The subjects emphasized that even when they had "made a night of it," they had made a point of being at work on time the next day. Usually, this conspicuous way of life only lasted a short time, and a sudden change occurred very soon - frequently after the subjects came into conflict with the law for the first time: The subjects worked regularly again and returned to an inconspicuous life pattern (see also Sect. 4.7.2 below).

2.4.3 Structure and Course of Leisure

The simple presentation and enumeration of various leisure activities does not suffice for an analysis from material points of view, particularly since the activities as such occurred in both groups (see also Sect. 2.4.1 above). Informative, in contrast, was the examination of the *structures and courses* of the various leisure activities, which were divided according to three basic forms:

1. Planned, systematically pursued, and/or formally organized leisure activities with definite courses (Sect. 2.4.3.1)
2. Leisure activities with surveyable courses inside certain limits (Sect. 2.4.3.2)
3. Leisure activities with entirely open and unpredictable courses (Sect. 2.4.3.3)

In the following, certain activities are given as examples for each of the three forms. *As a rule,* these activities belong to that specific form. In the individual case, however, each activity - for example, reading, going to the movies, or going to a bar - must be examined as to whether the *course of the specific activity of the individual subject* corresponds to the criteria of the corresponding *form* or whether the individual leisure behavior demonstrates structures deviating from the norm. Here again, the necessity of detailed investigations became apparent, as they alone enabled recognition of the possibly entirely different organization of seemingly equal behavior patterns.

Going to the movies, for example, can normally be assumed to be a leisure activity with a surveyable course inside certain limits (e.g., when a subject occasionally or even frequently goes to see a certain movie to relax or to be entertained; the movie theater and the subject's return home are in essence determined in advance). Going to the movies, however, can also be entirely differently structured: Under certain circumstances, it can be the first stage of a nocturnal leisure behavior pattern with an entirely open and unpredictable course (e.g., when the movie theater is only a kind of meeting point for possible, individually indeterminable contacts and when, with respect to the further course of the evening, it is not sure whether the subject will watch the film at all or how long he will watch it and what the further course of the evening will look like). On the other hand, going to the movies can be a hobby for a movie fan or even a performance-oriented activity for a student working as a journalist. Then it would be regarded as a long-term, systematically pursued leisure activity with a definite course.

2.4.3.1 Leisure Activities with Definite Courses

Long-term, systematically pursued, and/or formally organized leisure activities with definite courses are largely purposeful and are pursued with some commitment. The usually voluntary forms of activity are often performance-oriented and generally limit the amount of leisure time at one's disposal to a considerable extent (for examples, see Table 39).

Table 39. Leisure activities with definite courses[a]

	School age (up to age 14)		Age of occupational training (age 15-18)		Period of study	
	O-subj ($n=200$)	G-subj ($n=200$)	O-subj ($n=200$)	G-subj ($n=200$)	O-subj ($n=196$)	G-subj ($n=200$)
Corresponding activities occurred for	65.0%	74.0%	64.0%	88.0%	25.5%	89.0%
In detail (multiple entries):[b]						
Prolonged occupational activity (particularly long way to school)	.0%	3.5%	4.0%	18.0%	4.1%	18.5%
Overtime (additional work for school)	.0%	1.5%	3.5%	1.5%	7.1%	25.0%
Additional job, "moon-lighting" (earning money)	12.0%	11.5%	4.0%	8.0%	4.1%	17.0%
Helping at home	28.0%	27.5%	11.0%	19.0%	5.1%	22.0%
Further education	-	-	1.5%	7.5%	1.0%	21.5%
Volunteer activities	2.0%	3.0%	.0%	8.0%	1.0%	14.0%
Hobby	15.0%	30.0%	21.0%	43.0%	11.2%	44.0%
Sports	39.0%	42.0%	49.0%	51.0%	9.2%	37.5%

[a] See GÖPPINGER 1980, p. 297
[b] Activities in parentheses for pupils

Such formally organized leisure activities became less and less important for the O-subjects. The G-subjects, in contrast, increasingly pursued such activities, usually several of them, particularly during the period of the study. During this period, the increase in particularly performance-oriented leisure activities was especially obvious for the G-subjects: About half of the G-subjects worked during leisure time, as opposed to less than 10% of the O-subjects.

As the *individual case studies* showed, the few O-subjects who pursued such leisure activities were generally not very interested in or dedicated to them. This holds both for work during leisure time and hobbies and sports. Such forms of activity took place only on a spontaneous and noncommittal basis. The subjects' enthusiasm and commitment did not last very long, and their (active) participation in corresponding clubs or groups ended at the latest toward the end of their youth. In many cases there were arguments, for example with a trainer or friends because of a subject's irregular attendance in a sports club or because of theft, which then lead to his exclusion. At the age of occupational training, 44% of the O-subjects were still members of sports or hobby clubs, during the period of the study, only 8%.

In contrast, once a G-subject had decided to pursue a certain leisure activity, he developed a considerable degree of commitment, and his activities demanded not only a large amount of time but also personal efforts. Even as adults, one-third of the G-subjects pursued hobbies and sports in clubs or informal groups. The G-subjects usually considered belonging to the group and regularly attending meetings and events an obligation, and not merely sporadic, noncommittal entertainment.

2.4.3.2 Leisure Activities with Courses Inside Certain Limits

Leisure activities with surveyable courses inside certain limits generally bring about a general mental and physical recuperation or to a certain extent easy enter-

Table 40. Leisure activities with surveyable courses inside certain limits (period of study)[a]

	O-subjects (n=196)	G-subjects (n=200)
Corresponding activities occurred for	81.2%	99.5%
In detail (multiple entries):		
Going to the movies	58.2%	35.0%
Watching television	47.7%	74.5%
Listening to music	47.7%	47.5%
Reading, making music, handicraft etc.	38.8%	74.5%
Going to bars, dances	32.7%	61.5%
Family	16.3%	67.5%
Rest, relaxation	14.3%	65.0%
Other events	12.2%	48.5%
Walks, hikes	11.2%	67.5%
Visiting relatives, friends, acquaintances	9.2%	58.0%
Visits from relatives, friends, acquaintances	2.0%	42.5%

[a] See GÖPPINGER 1980, p.299

tainment and relaxation. They offer the possibility of pursuing personal inclinations in an individually given (socially customary) framework and maintaining relationships with friends and relatives. These leisure activities do not entail obligations as the leisure activities with definite courses do, but they are still of a regular nature due to the external framework of time and place. This separates them from the leisure activities with entirely open and unpredictable courses. The main activities which usually belong to this form are presented in Table 40. For each classification, however, the specific course of the activities was verified for each individual subject.

Though everyone pursues such leisure activities, their importance for the individual and with regard to leisure in general differs considerably (see Sect. 2.4.3.4 below). The position of the individual activities in the two groups is also different: For example, during the period of the study, going to the movies came first (in percent) for the O- and last for the G-subjects, while activities which require a certain degree of "leisure," particularly those connected with maintaining relationships in a group, were favored by the G-subjects but not by the O-subjects (see also Sect. 2.5.3 below). The G-subjects mentioned such activities much more frequently, which - together with the greater importance of the aforementioned structured activities - indicates that their leisure time was more differentiated in its organization than that of the O-subjects was.

2.4.3.3 Leisure Activities with Entirely Open Courses

Leisure activities with entirely open and unpredictable courses are characterized by the fact that, as a rule, neither place(s), duration, nor possible contact persons are specifically known at the beginning of the "undertaking." Usually, there is a common meeting place as the starting point for further action. For the rest, there is no planning or preparation, not even in a short-term perspective. Moreover, the subject tries to avoid any kind of obligation.

Table 41. Leisure activities with entirely open and unpredictable courses (period of study)

	O-subjects (n=196)	G-subjects (n=200)
Corresponding leisure activities occurred for	85.7%	2.0%
In detail (multiple entries):		
Going to disreputable bars	84.7%	.0%
Going to meeting points in the "milieu" of train stations, amusement arcades, old towns etc.	61.2%	.5%
Aimless driving around with mopeds, motorcycles, or cars	58.2%	.0%
Going to meeting points or bars in the student or village "milieu"	.0%	1.5%

The *individual case studies* showed rather impressively that this specific kind of leisure behavior had already developed during childhood and early youth for many (especially O-)subjects. Leisure, for the subjects concerned, took place almost exclusively "in the streets" even during childhood. As children, they were "never at home," and their parents usually did not know where they were, whom they were with, what they were doing at the moment, or even when they would come home in the evening. The children or juveniles roamed about - always on the lookout for adventure and diversion - and frequently went to amusement arcades or even bars. They usually started to consume nicotine and alcohol intensively at an early stage and often committed first offenses, for example damage to property or petty theft. The radius of action of this kind of leisure behavior increased in the course of time. The juvenile was soon no longer satisfied with the area of his home town, but turned to the next larger town or even to a large city further away. Driving around with mopeds, later on motorcycles or cars, became more and more important.

In the course of time, these subjects spent more and more of their leisure time in the "milieu" (see also Sect. 2.5.3 below). In most cases, this also meant an at least latent but often real willingness to indulge in "excesses," in the form of excessive alcohol consumption or spending sprees (drinking up one's weekly pay, long taxi trips, etc.), or also quarrels or violent arguments.

Here and in the following, the "milieu" is to be understood as a specific kind of subculture which occurs in every city, but preferably and markedly in large and industrial cities: From the perspective of space, this subculture is limited to a block, a section of a town (e.g., parts of the old town of large cities) or only a few (disreputable) bars, pubs, amusement arcades, places of entertainment, etc. (mainly near the train station or the old town), where socially conspicuous or delinquent persons prefer to spend their time. Characteristic of this subculture is the basic willingness of the persons belonging to it to earn their living primarily or at least partially by committing offenses (in particular theft, robbery, receiving stolen goods, procuring, trading in weapons and drugs, forging documents) or prostitution. The persons concerned feel that they belong to this "milieu". This feeling does not relate to specific individuals but more to the place and the corresponding group of persons as a whole. Thus, even in a city they are entirely unacquainted with, persons familiar with these groups rapidly find the corresponding area where they can find like-minded people and think up, plan, and prepare offenses and dispose of the loot. Although they usually prefer the same places, these persons are not (occasional) visitors (frequently tourists) in nightclubs or other places of entertainment but rather the persons who frequent these places regularly. This environment and the contacts with the corresponding persons are in a certain sense the breeding ground for offenses, whether the offenses take shape in discussions, the individual joins in with others, has to "pull a job" to protect his reputation, or has to obtain money in some way to finance his life-style.

Available leisure time rarely sufficed for such undertakings. Consequently, at some time or other, the subjects extended leisure time not only at the expense of sleep, but also at the expense of the sphere of performance (see Sect. 2.4.2.2 above), until finally, the activities mentioned took up the entire social spheres as typical socially conspicuous behavior.

For the period of the study, four different fields of activities and places could be distinguished. These fields were partially interlocked in various ways (see Table 41).

This form of leisure activity as the predominant element of leisure organization occurred practically only for the O-subjects and then for the majority of them (86%). Only 28 O-subjects had never spent their leisure time in this way; about two-thirds (65%) of the remaining O-subjects demonstrated this behavior almost every day, almost one-third (31%) frequently, and only a few (4%) at the most occasionally.

A considerable number of G-subjects had also frequented such places out of curiosity, gone on a "spin" into the "milieu," or frequently driven around aimlessly with their mopeds, motorcycles, or cars for a certain period out of a certain passion for driving, particularly at the age of occupational training. As the focal point of leisure organization during the period of the study, however, such "milieu"-oriented activities occurred for only one G-subject. Another three G-subjects also frequently showed leisure activities with entirely open and unpredictable courses during the period of the study. However, they did not frequent the socially conspicuous, potentially criminal "milieu," but rather the student "milieu" (two subjects) or village bar "milieu" (one subject).

2.4.3.4 Structure and Course According to Age-groups

In the examination of the predominant manner of leisure organization at various ages, quite unequivocal trends appeared at an early age with respect to the subjects preferring a certain form of leisure activity (see Table 42).

Even at school age, the O-subjects preferred activities with entirely open and unpredictable courses. The older the O-subjects, the stronger this trend became at the expense of systematically pursued activities with definite courses. The G-subjects, in contrast, almost equally emphasized leisure activities with definite courses and courses inside certain limits, while activities with entirely open and unpredictable courses played an ever smaller role and were of practically no importance.

As this was an estimation of the *predominant* behavior during the corresponding interval, behavior patterns in leisure belonging to other forms cannot be excluded, in principle, for the

Table 42. Structures and courses of predominant leisure activities according to age-groups[a]

	School age (up to age 14)		Age of occupational training (age 15-18)		Period of study	
	O-subj (n=176)	G-subj (n=193)	O-subj (n=186)	G-subj (n=197)	O-subj (n=194)	G-subj (n=200)
With definite courses	25.0%	56.5%	17.2%	69.5%	4.6%	65.5%
With courses inside certain limits	24.4%	34.2%	22.6%	24.4%	11.9%	33.0%
With entirely open courses	50.6%	9.3%	60.2%	6.1%	83.5%	1.5%

Significance level: O-G: $p<.001$
[a] See GÖPPINGER 1980, p.301

individual subject. However, the *individual case studies* showed that the O-subjects whose predominant leisure activities had entirely open and unpredictable courses had practically no room left for other leisure activities and were not interested in a somewhat structured or surveyable organization of leisure. On the other hand, many O-subjects were interested in sports or hobbies at school age and during early youth. Yet the O-subjects increasingly neglected such activities, at the latest during adolescence, and finally gave them up entirely. For most O-subjects, however, behavior patterns with entirely open and unpredictable courses had already occurred to an extent beyond that common among the G-subjects during childhood. Finally, at adulthood, there were practically no structured activities, occasionally at best somewhat limited activities. As a rule, there was a rather obvious and almost comprehensive orientation toward the "milieu" of the old town with its places of entertainment, etc.

Though all three categories of behavior were also found rather frequently for the individual G-subject, structured, to some extent even particularly productive leisure activities played a much more important role for the G-subjects than for the majority of the O-subjects, even (at least temporarily, though not predominantly) for the G-subjects who were assigned to the second category in the statistical evaluation. Naturally, the specific activities changed in time according to the subjects' age and stage of development; yet it was striking how naturally the subjects took up new activities and tasks (and thus often responsibility) suited to their age.

2.4.4 Place of Leisure

Place of leisure was defined as the place where the subjects spent the main part of their leisure time. It was differentiated according to whether the subjects spent their leisure time predominantly *at home* or *away from home.*

For reasons of clarity, "at home" referred to the dwelling where a subject lived and slept as well as to the immediate environment belonging to the dwelling (e.g., garden, courtyard), if this environment offered any - in the individual case extremely varying - possibilities of developing leisure activities. All other places where leisure time was spent belonged to the category "away from home."

Quite a few subjects had places to live and sleep which could not be used for leisure activities at all or not without being disturbed because of crowded living conditions. This group is given additional attention (see Sect. 2.4.4.3 below).

The subjects (mainly O-subjects) who did not have a permanent place to live and sleep, and thus could not spend their leisure time at home according to the foregoing criteria, were disregarded for the corresponding age-group. During the period of the study, this occurred for no less than 51 O-subjects, who were "roaming about" with no fixed abode. Because of the only very limited comparability, one G-subject who was living in military barracks as a *Zeitsoldat* (a soldier who signs up for military service for a specific period of time) was not taken into consideration.

2.4.4.1 Place of Leisure According to Age-groups

There were obvious differences between the O- and the G-subjects for the different age-groups with respect to place of leisure as well (see Table 43).

The older the O-subjects, the more often they spent their leisure time away from home. The G-subjects, in contrast, predominantly spent their leisure time entirely or partially at home during all intervals of the study. A leisure organization *predominantly* away from home was only temporarily important at the age of occupational training, while it was exhibited by only a few G-subjects during the period of the study.

As to the limitation or extension of leisure time, several G-subjects showed increasing tendencies toward a leisure organization away from home at the age of

Table 43. Place of leisure according to age-groups

	School age (up to age 14)		Age of occupational training (age 15-18)		Period of study	
	O-subj (n=173)	G-subj (n=195)	O-subj (n=179)	G-subj (n=200)	O-subj (n=146)[a]	G-subj (n=199)
Predominantly at home	19.1%	27.2%	7.2%	14.5%	4.8%	36.7%
Equally at and away from home	43.9%	56.4%	42.5%	60.5%	19.9%	55.3%
Predominantly away from home	37.0%	16.4%	50.3%	25.0%	75.3%	8.0%

Significance level: O-G: $p<.001$
[a] Remaining group mainly without fixed abode

Table 44. Place of leisure according to whom subjects lived with (period of study)

	Subject lived predominantly[a]							
	With family of orientation		With family of procreation		With others		Alone	
	O-subj (n=74)	G-subj (n=62)	O-subj (n=28)	G-subj (n=104)	O-subj (n=15)	G-subj (n=12)	O-subj (n=29)	G-subj (n=21)
Place of leisure:								
Predominantly at home	1.4%	16.1%	17.9%	54.8%	6.7%	17.0%	.0%	19.0%
Equally at and away from home	20.3%	64.5%	35.7%	42.3%	20.0%	83.0%	3.4%	76.2%
Predominantly away from home	78.4%	19.4%	46.4%	2.9%	73.3%	.0%	96.6%	4.8%

Significance level: O-G: $p<.001$
[a] Subjects without fixed abode were disregarded

occupational training (without its being predominant); after this period, they pursued more leisure activities at home again. Leisure activities pursued predominantly at home during the period of the study increased for the G-subjects, in contrast to the O-subjects. This may well be due to the G-subjects' marrying in the meantime, which had far-reaching consequences in this context as well (see Sects. 2.4.4.2 and 2.5.6.2 below).

2.4.4.2 Place of Leisure According to Whom the Subjects Lived with

In order to examine to what extent the choice of place of leisure depended on the persons a subject shared his dwelling with, place of leisure was related to whom a subject lived with during the period of the study (see Table 44).

The O-subjects who were (still) single in their twenties showed a particularly strong tendency toward places of leisure *predominantly* away from home. This was not the case for practically all the single G-subjects. The G-subjects who lived with their families of orientation or with other persons (e.g., friends), as compared with all G-subjects, demonstrated a higher proportion of leisure activities away from home as a whole. The largest influence on place of leisure, however, was living with the family (of procreation), although the fundamental differences between the O- and the G-subjects became evident here again: In this subgroup as well, almost half of the O-subjects spent their leisure time predominantly away from the family and dwelling, while the corresponding G-subjects either stayed predominantly at home or were at home and away from home for equal amounts of time during their leisure time (usually together with their own families). This already suggests differences in the position of the family (of procreation) for the O- and the G-subjects, which is examined in more detail in the presentation of contact behavior (see Sect. 2.5.6 below).

The *individual case studies* showed that the specific atmosphere of the place of leisure played an important role for the subjects of both groups. The G-subjects often mentioned *Gemütlichkeit* or an individual and familiar area they liked and where they felt "at home." Insofar as the G-subjects spent their leisure time away from home, they usually went to places they (and their relatives) knew well, where they met a group of friends or acquaintances and were, in a certain sense, "integrated" (e.g., among a group of "regulars" or in a club house).

The O-subjects who spent their leisure time away from home mainly felt that sitting around at home was boring and "square." This "home" was occasionally disordered and often marked by quarrels and arguments (see Sect. 2.1.3 above). Yet nothing held the subjects at home even where there were ordered circumstances and the subjects had rooms to themselves; they felt an urge to go out. Their destination was usually rather indefinite when they left home and was often limited to leaving and waiting to see what possibilities might "open up" on the way.

2.4.4.3 Place of Leisure of Subjects with No Room at Their Disposal

The differences with respect to place of leisure between the O- and the G-subjects who had no room at their disposal at home at least temporarily during the period of the study showed that whether the subjects concerned spent their leisure time predominantly at home or away from home did not depend decisively on the room available for leisure activities (see Table 45).

The behavior of the subjects of the two subgroups with respect to the kind of place of leisure during the period of the study was almost the same as that of the corresponding total group. Insofar as a comparison was at all admissible considering the size of the subgroups, it was noteworthy that the subgroup of the G-subjects corresponded rather accurately to the distribution of the entire G-group, not only with respect to availability and courses, i.e., the criteria not necessarily connected with the kind of place of leisure, but also with respect to the place of leisure itself. In contrast, the O-subjects of the subgroup spent their time exclusively away from home, and with respect to availability and course of leisure activities, they tended even more plainly than the entire O-group to O-specific extreme forms.

2.4.5 Leisure Behavior and Social Class

Up to this point, leisure behavior was analyzed from abstracting points of view. Therefore, it can be assumed that circumstances such as education, belonging to occupational groups, and therefore also social class did not decisively influence

Table 45. Leisure behavior of subjects with no room at their disposal (period of study)

	O-subjects (n=196)	G-subjects (n=200)
No room at their disposal	19 (9.7%)	26 (13.0%)
Of these		
Availability of leisure time:		
Predominantly limitation	0	19
No limitation or extension	2	7
Predominantly extension	17	0
Structure and course of leisure time:		
Predominantly definite courses	0	18
Predominantly with courses inside certain limits	1	8
Predominantly with entirely open courses	18	0
Place of leisure:		
Predominantly at home	0	8
Equally at and away from home	0	15
Predominantly away from home	19	3

Table 46. Leisure behavior and (subject's) social class[a] (period of study)

	Upper lower class	
	O-subjects	G-subjects
Availability of leisure time:	(n=42)	(n=74)
Predominantly limitation	4.8%	64.4%
No limitation or extension	9.5%	34.2%
Predominantly extension	85.7%	1.4%
Structure and course of leisure time:	(n=45)	(n=74)
Predominantly definite courses	6.7%	62.2%
Predominantly with courses inside certain limits	8.9%	36.5%
Predominantly with entirely open courses	84.4%	1.3%
Place of leisure:	(n=40)	(n=73)
Predominantly at home	2.5%	35.6%
Equally at and away from home	20.0%	56.2%
Predominantly away from home	77.5%	8.2%

[a] For social class, see Sect. 2.3.4.1 above

the distribution in both groups, though the actual leisure activities of the subjects were certainly related to education and could thus be on a different "level." In *both* groups, there was a certain relationship between leisure behavior and subject's class, in that the middle class (O- and G-)subjects demonstrated the G-specific extreme forms of leisure behavior slightly more frequently than the lower lower class (O- and G-)subjects did. Yet the basic differences in leisure behavior between the O- and the G-subjects remained. This became particularly visible when the subjects of the *same* social class, e.g., upper lower class, were compared (see Table 46).

2.4.6 Leisure Behavior of Early and Late Delinquents

The late delinquents (O_2-subjects) differed in part considerably from the early delinquents (O_1-subjects) in their leisure behavior, as in the foregoing social spheres (see Table 47). While the behavior patterns characteristic of the O-group were already markedly present during childhood for the O_1-subjects, the O_2-subjects showed an obvious development from school age to the period of the study: At school age, their leisure behavior approximated that of the G-subjects; at the age of occupational training, they held a position between the O_1- and the G-group, at least with respect to availability and course of leisure (their place of leisure, in contrast, still corresponded fully to that of the G-group), while their behavior during the period of the study largely corresponded to that of the O_1-group in all respects.

The picture of the O_2-subjects' leisure behavior thus corresponds approximately to the somewhat more favorable general impression from the sphere of performance. Yet, while they also held a position between the O_1- and the G-subjects before the period of the study in the sphere of performance, this was no longer the case in the sphere of leisure. Together with the fact that the O_2-subjects had committed their first offenses an average of 4 years later, this might confirm - with certain reservations - the observations made repeatedly in the *individual case studies:* There is a close relationship between a certain form of leisure behavior and delinquency, and the conspicuousness in the individual social spheres possibly resulting in criminality appears in a certain chronological order (see Sect. 4.6 below).

2.4.7 The Leisure Syndrome

Although the criteria used relate to the same leisure behavior of the individual subject from the points of view of time, place, and content, they are largely complementary and do not necessarily imply each other. Thus, for example, an unstructured leisure behavior does not necessarily mean that a subject extends his leisure time at the expense of the sphere of performance. Even though the spatial aspect of place of leisure away from home and the extension of leisure time at the expense of the period of rest and sleep may frequently occur together with unstructured leisure activities, it is useful to examine to what extent the O-characteristic extreme forms of the variables "availability of leisure" and "structure and course of leisure activities" concurred for individual subjects.

The resulting *leisure syndrome,* consisting of the criteria "extension of leisure time predominantly at the expense of the sphere of performance" and "predominance of leisure activities with entirely open and unpredictable courses" (both criteria during the period of the study), turned out to distinguish clearly between the O- and the G-group (see Table 48; regarding its further importance, see Part IV, Sect. 2): During the period of the study, three-fourths of the O-subjects predominantly extended their leisure time at the expense of the sphere of performance and the period of rest and sleep and predominantly pursued leisure activities with entirely open and unpredictable courses. In contrast, this behavior was determined for only one G-subject (a student who idled away several terms). This leisure syn-

Table 47. (Predominant) Leisure behavior of O- and G-subjects and early and late delinquents

	O-subj	G-subj	Sig. O-G	O_1-subj	O_2-subj	Sig. O_1-O_2
Availability:						
School age	(n=177)	(n=196)		(n=107)	(n=70)	
Limitation	13.0%	27.0%		5.6%	24.3%	
Neither	40.7%	67.9%	++	30.8%	55.7%	++
Extension	46.3%	5.1%		63.6%	20.0%	
Training age	(n=189)	(n=193)		(n=113)	(n=76)	
Limitation	7.9%	35.2%		5.3%	11.8%	
Neither	33.3%	57.0%	++	20.4%	52.6%	++
Extension	58.7%	7.8%		74.3%	35.5%	
Period of study	(n=189)	(n=198)		(n=108)	(n=81)	
Limitation	4.8%	63.7%		2.8%	7.4%	
Neither	10.0%	33.3%	++	12.0%	7.4%	n.s.
Extension	85.2%	3.0%		85.2%	85.2%	
Structure and course:						
School age	(n=176)	(n=193)		(n=107)	(n=69)	
Definite courses	25.0%	56.5%		14.0%	42.0%	
Limited courses	24.4%	34.2%	++	17.8%	34.8%	++
Open courses	50.6%	9.3%		68.2%	23.2%	
Training age	(n=186)	(n=197)		(n=110)	(n=76)	
Definite courses	17.2%	69.5%		8.2%	30.3%	
Limited courses	22.6%	24.4%	++	14.6%	34.2%	++
Open courses	60.2%	6.1%		77.3%	35.5%	
Period of study	(n=194)	(n=200)		(n=110)	(n=84)	
Definite courses	4.6%	65.5%		2.7%	7.1%	
Limited courses	11.9%	33.0%	++	10.9%	13.1%	n.s.
Open courses	83.5%	1.5%		86.4%	79.8%	
Place of leisure:						
School age	(n=173)	(n=195)		(n=106)	(n=67)	
At home	19.1%	27.2%		9.4%	34.3%	
At/away from home	43.9%	56.4%	++	44.3%	43.3%	++
Away from home	37.0%	16.4%		46.2%	22.4%	
Training age	(n=179)	(n=200)		(n=107)	(n=72)	
At home	7.2%	14.5%		3.7%	12.5%	
At/away from home	42.5%	60.5%	++	29.9%	61.1%	++
Away from home	50.3%	25.0%		66.4%	26.4%	
Period of study	(n=146)	(n=199)		(n=83)	(n=63)	
At home	4.8%	36.7%		4.8%	4.8%	
At/away from home	19.9%	55.3%	++	16.9%	23.8%	n.s.
Away from home	75.3%	8.0%		78.3%	71.4%	

Significance level: *++*, $p<.001$; *n.s.*, not significant

drome therefore comprises - similar to the syndrome in the sphere of performance (see Sect. 2.3.4.6 above) - behavior patterns whose occurrence indicates a considerable danger of criminality.

This syndrome became even more significant when the concurrence of the opposite forms of the variables, which were characteristic *of the G-group*, was

Table 48. Leisure syndrome (period of study)

	O-subj (n=189)	G-subj (n=198)	O_1-subj (n=108)	O_2-subj (n=81)
(Predominantly) extension of leisure time at the expense of the sphere of performance *and* leisure activities with entirely open courses	75.1%	.5%	79.6%	69.1%

Significance level: O-G: $p<.001$; O_1-O_2: not significant

examined: While, during the period of the study, more than half of the G-subjects (53%) predominantly limited their leisure time and *at the same time* pursued structured activities with definite courses, such behavior occurred for only five O-subjects. (These five O-subjects were also not typical of the O-group with respect to their behavior in the other social spheres and with respect to their offenses. Their offenses included refusal to do alternative nonmilitary service, traffic delinquency in connection with aiding and abetting perjury, fraudulent insolvency of an artisan, and two cases of purely sexual delinquency, and therefore did not correspond to the delinquency predominating in the O-group - see Sect. 4.3.3 below).

2.4.8 Summary

The relevant results of the analysis of leisure behavior are as follows: In the course of the subjects' development in life, the fundamentally divergent orientation of the sphere of leisure of the two groups became increasingly obvious. The majority of the O-subjects tended more and more obviously, from school age, to age of occupational training, to the period of the study, toward leisure activities with entirely open and unpredictable courses, and they extended their leisure time at the expense of regular employment and of the period of rest and sleep. In the G-group, in contrast, there was an obvious increase in leisure activities which took place predominantly or at least largely at home and had definite courses or courses inside certain limits. Leisure time was regularly limited to a considerable extent by the subjects taking on the most varying commitments.

Here again, the differentiation of the O-group into early (O_1-subjects) and late delinquents (O_2-subjects) was quite impressive: The leisure activities of the O_2-subjects at school age and even at the age of occupational training (e.g., with respect to place of leisure) showed a tendency toward the G-subjects' behavior or - especially at the age of occupational training - occupied a midway position between the behavior patterns of the O_1- and the G-subjects. During the period of the study, a period during which most O_2-subjects had also committed offenses, the O_2-subjects' leisure behavior could no longer be distinguished from that of the O_1-subjects. Besides the basic differences between the O- and the G-group, this shows the close relationship between the O-specific leisure behavior and - at least certain kinds of - criminality (see also Sect. 4.6 below).

In the examination of whether the O-specific extreme forms of the evaluation criteria availability as well as structure and course of leisure activities concurred for the individual subjects, a leisure syndrome could be developed, which distinguished clearly between the two groups and which may well be a positive indicator of a danger of criminality.

Therefore, leisure behavior can be of considerable importance for (certain kinds of) criminality. Nevertheless, the criminological *literature* up to the early 1970s almost entirely neglected leisure in the lives of delinquents. The larger comparative studies do mention differences in organization of leisure, yet they are limited to only a few aspects of leisure behavior and mention leisure in passing, without aiming at a systematic analysis of the entire sphere of leisure.

Thus, apart from mentioning sporadically that the subjects frequently stayed away from work unexcused, the literature offers no points of view comparable to the criterion "availability of leisure time." On the other hand, numerous - more or less isolated - individual facts are mentioned, which coincide to a large extent with those mentioned in the present study as partial aspects of a more general discussion:

Place of leisure predominantly away from home, in the streets, in amusement arcades, in dance halls, etc. of the delinquent subjects at an early age is mentioned by the Centro Nazionale di Prevenzione e Difesa Sociale (1969, p.374), GLUECK and GLUECK (1974, pp.101 ff.), and WEST and FARRINGTON (1973, p.56; 1977, p.68). HEALY and BRONNER (1936, pp.44ff., 53ff.) generally noticed higher activity, increased flightiness, and less staying power of their delinquent subjects; this phenomenon may correspond to the O-subjects' rarely pursuing systematic leisure activities involving commitments. A similar dislike for such leisure activities was mentioned by GLUECK and GLUECK (1974, pp.101 ff.) and by SZEWCZYK (1974, p.26). Without giving an all-inclusive categorization, the Centro Nazionale di Prevenzione e Difesa Sociale (1969, p.368), GLUECK and GLUECK (1974, p.101), and WEST and FARRINGTON (1977, p.68) mention going to the movies, reading comics, gambling, going to discotheques, and parties as predominant leisure activities of their delinquent subjects; partially, the subjects' special interest in cinema and films is emphasized (HEALY and BRONNER 1936, p.72). An orientation toward the "milieu" is referred to by GLUECK and GLUECK (1974, p.102), in the sense that delinquents tended to go to deserted places or to stay in the streets or in amusement arcades where petty or even serious offenses were often committed.

2.5 The Sphere of Contacts

2.5.1 Preliminary Remarks

Delimiting the sphere of contacts is more difficult than delimiting, for example, the spheres of performance or leisure, considering the almost infinite number of contacts with other persons an individual establishes during his lifetime. This number - if the concept of contacts is extended accordingly - can total several dozens after one working day alone. Nevertheless, the contacts which are relevant to an individual and his development in life and at the same time typical of his integration in the social environment can be defined quite clearly in formal respect: On the one hand, normally, there are the contacts with the family of orientation, which are initially *given,* but can to a certain extent be fostered or neglected by the individual later on. On the other hand, there are the *self-chosen* contacts, which can be divided into contacts with friends and acquaintances, sexual contacts, and contacts with the family (of procreation) (see GÖPPINGER 1980, pp.301 ff.).

Considerable difficulties arise with respect to the interpersonal aspect of contacts, which can be marked by criteria such as feelings, spiritual or emotional ties, affection for other persons, etc. These aspects were covered in the investigations, explorations, and partially the other tests in the *individual case.* Categorizing such "soft" data is problematic, however, because of the danger of simulating an accuracy which is in no way justified (see Part I, Sect. 4).

The following presentation is therefore limited to a more *external-formal* examination of the subjects' contacts in their social spheres, whereas regular forms of contact and association with more or less definite courses, such as activities in clubs and organizations (see Sect. 2.4.3 above), and general contact criteria in the stricter sense (e.g., sociability, communication behavior) were not taken into consideration.

2.5.2 Contacts with the Family of Orientation

Contacts with the family of orientation are of a special nature in the sphere of contacts, insofar as a child is normally born into a family and remains bound to it in practically all respects, at least up to a certain age. Therefore, these contacts can be called "fated", or *given*, more legitimately than any other contacts later in life.

With respect to their attitudes toward persons of reference in the family, 36% of the O- and 48% of the G-subjects indicated a *special affection* for their (step)parents, siblings, and other close relatives during childhood and early youth. In contrast, 45% of the O- and 13% of the G-subjects regarded their contacts with their (step)parents as at least temporarily *marked by serious conflicts*. Serious conflicts with siblings and other close relatives were indicated by 10% of the O- and 3% of the G-subjects.

In this connection, the obvious differences between the two groups with respect to the subjects' age when they left home "for good" (see Sect. 2.2.2.6 above) should be mentioned, particularly since the separation, especially the O-subjects', often took place after conflicts with parents and then usually coincided with a complete rupture of any contacts with their parents' home.

In order to judge the further development of the relations between subject and family of orientation for the period of the juvenile's gradual separation from his family of orientation, it was examined to what extent a subject (still) spent his leisure time together with his family of orientation. A great many fewer O- than G-subjects spent their leisure time predominantly with their families (11% of the O- and 41% of the G-subjects) at (late) school age. At the age of vocational training, the proportion of subjects who spent their leisure time predominantly with their families of orientation decreased considerably in both groups, though, as before, more G- (18%) than O-subjects (2%) had such contacts. In later years, the importance of the family of orientation as the *predominant* sphere of contacts diminished further (see Sect. 2.5.4 below). Yet, of the subjects who lived at their parents' home during the period of the study (37% of the O- and 30.5% of the G-subjects), nearly half (45%) of the G-subjects spent at least *part* of their leisure time together with their families, as compared with only one-fifth (19%) of the O-subjects.

In the framework of the *individual case studies,* as well, relatively loose contacts to their families of orientation became apparent for most O-subjects, while deep, strong emotional ties were more the exception. In many cases, the O-subjects rejected a more than formal membership in the family: In the explorations and interviews, many subjects often expressed extremely negative opinions of individual family members and emphasized that they had separated themselves from their families at an early age. On the other hand, contacts were often reestablished during imprisonment, particularly since this made it possible to obtain privileges such as parole or temporary leave.

In contrast, a stronger cohesion in the family as well as a much more intensive integration of the subject in the family occurred for the majority of the G-subjects. This was shown not only in corresponding relations between the G-subjects and their families of orientation in the strict sense, but occasionally even in relations with other relatives and in-laws. Beyond a strong emotional component, a certain family-mindedness was expressed in everyday life, e.g., in standing up for other family members and in being willing to help each other, which was regarded as a matter of course.

2.5.3 Contacts with Friends and Acquaintances

As opposed to contacts with the family of orientation, contacts with friends and acquaintances are *self-chosen*. Occasionally during childhood or early youth, but usually later on with increasing independence of personality, self-chosen contacts can be of considerable and even decisive importance. Of course, relations with the family of orientation can be kept up, reestablished, or intensified in later years. In this way, in their organization, they usually assume the nature of self-chosen contacts. Since self-chosen contacts are particularly important for the individual personality as a whole and, at the same time, are much more specific and characteristic than the ones initially given, any differences between the groups of the study are all the more telling.

Such differences between the groups of the study occurred even in a purely quantitative respect: The O-subjects usually had a greater number of "acquaintances" of any kind than the G-subjects. This is mainly due to the very specific nature of these (loose or "milieu") contacts (see below) and their importance for the O-subjects. But only a qualitative examination, differentiating according to (family-external) stable contacts, loose contacts, and "milieu" contacts, proved to be adequate and sufficient to determine the specific social relations of the groups of the study.

In the following, *stable contacts* are relations of a personal nature where the partners know each other very well, and feel to a certain extent that they belong together and trust each other. Stable contacts therefore include boy- or girlfriend, friends of both sexes, close acquaintances, and family members who do not live in the same household. Usually, a part of leisure time is spent with these persons according to corresponding arrangements, either at home or away from home.

Such contacts were found for 70% of the G-subjects during the period of the study, most frequently with a group of close acquaintances (77%), followed by girlfriend (37%), one specific friend (29%), and family members who did not live in the same household (25%) (multiple answers). The O-subjects (45%) mentioned such contacts *much less frequently* for the period of the study. According to them, contacts with their girlfriends dominated (53%), followed by contacts with a group of close acquaintances (32%), with friends (27%), and with family members (11%).

In the *individual case studies,* however, an additional divergence became apparent, which throws a different light on these figures: It turned out, for example, that concepts such as "friend", particularly "girlfriend", differed in meaning and content, for the G-subjects in the sense of "stable" contacts, for the O-subjects more in the sense of "loose" contacts. Thus, a partner in a sexual relationship lasting a few days or even merely one night was already a "girlfriend" for the majority of the O-subjects, while the concept of girlfriend mostly involved a long-term, intensive, and not necessarily sexual relationship for the G-subjects. [These differing concepts are also expressed in the following, e.g., in the main kinds of contacts in various age-groups, (see Sect. 2.5.4 below) and in changes of sexual partners (see Sect. 2.5.5 below)].

Loose contacts with acquaintances are characterized by the fact that they go beyond, for example, a fleeting encounter in the street but mean much less than friendship. They are a more temporary, noncommittal relationship, where (short-term) undertakings, not (long-term) common personal-human interests are central and where new encounters - if they are thought about at all - are left to coincidence.

Naturally, the O- and the G-subjects all had such contacts. Yet, while they played a secondary role for the G-subjects, they were rather important for the O-subjects. On the whole, the impression arose that loose contacts had the same importance for the O-subjects as stable contacts had for the G-subjects.

"Milieu" contacts, which are closely related to certain leisure activities (see Sect. 2.4.3.3 above), are a special form of loose contacts. They are characterized less by the specific contact person than by the *places of contact,* which are "notorious" meeting points and where there is always "someone" to kill time or do "something" with. These meeting points are usually amusement arcades, movie theaters, or certain street corners at school age; later on, there is an orientation toward the "milieu" of the (large) city with socially conspicuous and delinquent persons. Such contacts usually last merely one evening and are succeeded by contacts of the same kind. Often, several such contacts exist at the same time in loose form. They are normally established quickly and are determined by a certain feeling of belonging to the "milieu" and its group of persons. With respect to this "milieu," the contacts generally have a stable element; the acquaintances as such - as individual personalities - are of practically no importance. The contacts are of an obviously utilitarian nature: Decisive for taking up contacts are mainly immediate (also material) interests, such as drinking together, contacting girls, finding a way to acquire money (quickly), or even only finding a place to stay for the night. The persons concerned are "important" only insofar as, with them or by way of them, additional possibilities in the subjects' own interest can be expected; the partners themselves are entirely interchangeable.

"Milieu" contacts can be regarded as specific to the O-subjects; four-fifths of them had such contacts more than once a week for a longer period of time. In the perhaps occasional visits to the "milieu" by the G-subjects, who mostly went there out of curiosity, there were almost no comparable contacts. The G-subjects often indicated that they had not even considered such possibilities. No G-subject expressed a feeling of belonging to the "milieu"; on the contrary, they felt repelled by its atmosphere after a short time. Even in the rare cases where G-subjects had had repeated contacts with the "milieu" temporarily, these contacts had played a minor role as compared with other forms of contact during that period.

2.5.4 Contacts According to Age-groups and to Whom the Subjects Lived with

The differing position of the various kinds of human relations for the O- and the G-subjects became even more striking in the examination of the *predominant* forms of self-chosen contacts at certain *age levels* (see Table 49; for the definition of the intervals, see Sects. 1.3 and 2.4.1 above).

For the O-subjects, (self-chosen) contacts with their families of orientation beyond the daily contacts contingent on living together - expressed, for example, in leisure activities undertaken together with the family - played a minor role from school age on. Even marriage had practically no effect on self-chosen contacts (in later years) with the family (of procreation). Very important throughout were loose and "milieu" contacts: Taken together, these contacts were the predominant form of contact during all three intervals examined here for two-thirds and three-fourths of the O-subjects, respectively. The shift from loose to "milieu" contacts in the course of time was noteworthy.

The differentiation of the O-group into O_1- and O_2-subjects showed that loose contacts had existed at school age in the same proportion for the O_2- as for the O_1-subjects. Later on, loose contacts did not lose importance in favor of "milieu" contacts to the same extent for the O_2- as for the O_1-subjects. Even during the period of the study, the O_2-subjects had practically as many loose as "milieu" contacts.

In contrast, loose or "milieu" contacts as predominant, determining contacts for a certain interval were of practically no importance for the G-subjects. Their contacts were almost entirely limited to their families of orientation (later on families of procreation) and to friends and close acquaintances.

The proportion of subjects who were more or less isolated during a certain period was small in both groups. During the period of the study there was no difference between the groups in this respect. About twice as many G-subjects as O-subjects had been more or less isolated at the age of occupational training, while the O-subjects predominated at school age.

The kind of *persons the subjects lived with* and the resulting possibilities of contacts with these persons plainly had no influence on the kind of contacts chosen elsewhere (see Table 50).

Thus, for the O-subjects who lived with their families of orientation or with other persons (not belonging to their families), such as acquaintances or friends, "milieu" contacts dominated by far and, together with loose contacts, were the predominant form of contact for about four-fifths of the subjects concerned. An even higher proportion of "milieu" contacts occurred for the O-subjects who lived alone. Yet these contacts were also predominant for more than half of the O-subjects who lived with their families of procreation.

For the G-subjects who lived with their families of orientation, with other persons (not belonging to their families), or alone, in contrast, there were predominantly stable contacts with friends and acquaintances or contacts with their families of orientation. The married G-subjects obviously concentrated their contacts almost exclusively on their own families. For only three G-subjects who lived alone did loose contacts play an important role. "Milieu" contacts did not occur as predominant form of contact; even for the G-subjects who lived alone, they did not occur to any extent worth mentioning.

Table 49. Predominant (self-chosen) contacts according to age groups

	School age (up to 14)				Training age (15–18)				Period of study			
	O-subj (n=188)	G-subj (n=200)	O_1-subj (n=110)	O_2-subj (n=78)	O-subj (n=191)	G-subj (n=197)	O_1-subj (n=113)	O_2subj (n=78)	O-subj (n=195)	G-subj (n=198)	O_1-subj (n=110)	O_2-subj (n=85)
Contacts with family of orientation and/or procreation[a]	11.2%	41.5%	5.5%	19.2%	2.1%	18.3%	1.8%	2.6%	4.1%	51.0%	3.6%	4.7%
Stable contacts with friends and acquaintances	14.4%	44.5%	13.6%	15.4%	17.3%	67.0%	13.3%	23.1%	8.7%	37.4%	5.5%	12.9%
Loose contacts with acquaintances	54.3%	6.0%	55.5%	52.6%	49.2%	5.1%	43.4%	57.7%	28.2%	4.0%	21.8%	36.5%
"Milieu" contacts	10.6%	.5%	15.5%	3.8%	26.2%	.0%	37.2%	10.3%	53.3%	.0%	63.6%	40.0%
More or less isolated	9.6%	7.5%	10.0%	9.0%	5.2%	9.6%	4.4%	6.4%	5.6%	7.6%	5.5%	5.9%

[a] For family of orientation, only self-chosen contacts

Table 50. Predominant contacts according to whom subjects lived with (period of study)

	Subject lived predominantly							
	With family of orientation		With family of procreation		With others		Alone	
	O-subj (*n*=74)	G-subj (*n*=61)	O-subj (*n*=29)	G-subj (*n*=104)	O-subj (*n*=20)	G-subj (*n*=12)	O-subj (*n*=71)	G-subj (*n*=21)
Predominant form of contact:								
Family contacts	2.7%	16.4%	20.7%	86.5%	.0%	8.3%	.0%	.0%
Stable contacts	12.2%	68.9%	17.2%	8.7%	25.0%	66.7%	1.4%	71.4%
Loose contacts	36.5%	3.3%	31.0%	1.9%	35.0%	8.3%	16.9%	14.3%
"Milieu" contacts	45.9%	.0%	24.1%	.0%	40.0%	.0%	77.5%	.0%
More or less isolated	2.7%	11.5%	6.9%	2.9%	.0%	16.7%	4.2%	14.3%

Significance level: O-G: $p<.001$

In the framework of the *individual case studies*, the impression repeatedly arose that the majority of the O-subjects had rarely had deeper emotional or spiritual-mental relationships but numerous superficial acquaintances. In contrast, the contacts of the G-subjects normally lasted longer; they often had someone with whom they had a deep and close relationship, whom they trusted, and from whom they did not separate easily. Casual acquaintances of the same type as those of the O-subjects rarely occurred for the G-subjects, not even for those who lived alone. It seems as if they did not even register these possibilities of contact as such; they were usually critical in selecting their friends and acquaintances, who only rarely - and then only temporarily - included a socially conspicuous person or a person who had repeatedly been convicted.

2.5.5 Sexual Contacts

As the sphere of sexuality is not free of taboos, the data on sexual contacts (besides the evaluation of records) was mainly collected in the psychiatric explorations. Only sporadically were *sexual variations and deviances* diagnosed, and their number was insignificant. For example, there were indications of homosexual contacts for only 21 O- and two G-subjects; only five O-subjects and no G-subject had ever worked as male prostitutes. Ten O-subjects and no G-subject had appeared as exhibitionists. No further sexual conspicuousness was mentioned; however, this was not the main focus of the interviews and explorations.

Up to the time of the study, the majority of the subjects had had *sexual intercourse for the first time.* On average, it took place considerably earlier for the O- than for the G-subjects (see Table 51).

While half of the O-subjects had had sexual intercourse for the first time by the age of 16, this was not the case for half of the G-subjects until somewhat after the age of 19. The median age of the groups of the study thus differed by 3.2 years. In contrast to other spheres, where the O_2-subjects initially demonstrated behavior similar to that of the G-subjects, they tended more toward the behavior of the O_1-subjects in this respect: The difference between the median age of the O_1- and the O_2-subjects was relatively small.

Table 51. Age at first sexual intercourse

	O-subj (n=176)	G-subj (n=195)	O_1-subj (n=102)	O_2-subj (n=74)
Up to the age of 15	52.3%	14.4%	59.8%	41.9%
Up to the age of 18	80.7%	49.2%	83.3%	77.0%
Up to the time of the study	93.2%	84.0%	94.1%	91.9%
Not yet	6.8%	16.0%	5.9%	8.1%
Median age of subjects (years)	15.9	19.1	15.6	16.5

Significance level: O-G: $p<.001$

Table 52. Age at first sexual intercourse in connection with social class and family background

	Median age (years)	
	O-subjects	G-subjects
Total group	15.9	19.1
Class of family of orientation		
Middle class	16.0	19.6
Upper lower class	15.8	18.3
Lower lower class	15.9	18.4
Family background		
Intact	16.8	19.4
Disrupted	15.6	17.1
Incomplete	15.5	19.0
Subject's class (only workers)	15.9	18.2
In comparison:		
Unskilled workers according to SCHMIDT and SIGUSCH (1971, p. 37 f.)		18.4

As it is occasionally stated in the literature that age at first sexual intercourse and sexual behavior as such depend to a large extent on which *social class* a subject belongs to or what kind of *family* he comes from, the median age of the groups of the study was examined to see whether the variables social class of family of orientation, family background, and subject's social class intervened (see Table 52).

It was shown that *social class of family of orientation* (see Sect. 2.1.2.1 above) was of practically no importance for the O-subjects with respect to age at first sexual intercourse, while the median age of the G-subjects from the lower class was about 1 year lower.

The effects of differing *family circumstances* led to a higher median age of both groups for subjects with an intact family background (see also Sect. 2.1.3 above). For disrupted family circumstances, the G-subjects in particular showed a clearly lower median age than the G-group as a whole. A structurally incomplete family of orientation had no influence in this respect.

As the differing *social stratification* in the O- and the G-groups (subject's social class according to class index; see Sect. 2.3.4.1 above) could have been responsible for the differences with respect to age at first sexual intercourse, the workers of both groups were compared. There was a - rather considerable - change for the G-subjects, but not for the O-subjects. Nonetheless, the median age of the two groups still differed by more than 2 years.

Finally, in order to take into consideration the differing composition of the "lower class" of the groups (the lower class O-subjects were mainly unskilled workers, the lower class G-subjects mainly skilled workers - see Sect. 2.3.4.1 above), the subjects of the study of sexual behavior of the "lower lower class" by SCHMIDT and SIGUSCH (1971) were taken as a further comparison group. The study had been conducted at approximately the same time as the Tübingen study and covered 150 unskilled workers between 20 and 21 years of age who, as the G-subjects, had been selected from the general population. In this comparison there was a clear difference between the median age of the O-subjects, even more so as the median age of the (unskilled) workers according to SCHMIDT and SIGUSCH (1971, pp. 37 ff.) was even somewhat higher than that of the (skilled) workers of the G-group.

In connection with first intensive sexual contacts, further differences became apparent between the O- and the G-subjects, for instance with respect to *partner in first sexual intercourse*. As these circumstances could not be clarified for all subjects, only tendencies can be presented in the following.

Differences as to the *age of the partner* in first sexual intercourse occurred insofar as the G-subjects more often had younger, the O-subjects more often older partners (see Table 53). However, it must be taken into consideration that first sexual intercourse occurred much later for the G- than for the O-subjects.

The median age of partners in first sexual intercourse was 18 for the G-subjects (the youngest partners had been 13 and 14, the oldest 32) and 19 for the O-subjects. The age distribution of the O-subjects was much more scattered: The youngest partners had been 7 and 11, the oldest 42.

The examination of the question whether a subject's first sexual intercourse was also his *partner's first sexual intercourse* showed relatively unequivocal tendencies as well: According to the subjects' information, this was so for only about one-third of the O- and two-thirds of the G-partners.

In the course of their further (sexual) lives, the O-subjects changed their sexual partners much more frequently than the G-subjects. Though one should certainly be somewhat skeptical about the indications of several subjects, especially when they mentioned a large number of sexual partners, rather obvious tendencies appeared, which should be reliable. According to their indications, three-fourths of the O-subjects had had *more than* three sexual partners, while almost three-fourths of the G-subjects indicated a *maximum* of three sexual partners up to the time of the study (see Table 54).

Here again, the number of sexual partners did not depend on the subject's social class or occupation. There was, however, a certain relationship between the age at first sexual intercourse and

Table 53. Age of partner of first sexual intercourse in comparison with age of subject

	O-subjects ($n=124$)	G-subjects ($n=110$)
Younger than subject	16.9%	43.6%
About the same age (maximum difference 1 year)	16.1%	20.0%
Older than subject	66.9%	36.4%
Median age of partners	ca. 19 years	ca. 18 years

Significance level: O-G: $p<.001$

Table 54. Number of sexual partners

	O-subjects ($n=140$)	G-subjects ($n=160$)
1- 3	24.3%	71.3%
4- 6	15.7%	12.5%
7-10	12.9%	8.8%
More than 10	47.1%	7.5%

Significance level: O-G: $p<.001$

frequency of changes of sexual partners. Thus, more than half of the 48 "early" O-subjects (first sexual intercourse before the age of 14) indicated more than 20 sexual partners and only one less than four sexual partners, while almost one-third of the 14 "early" G-subjects indicated more than 20 sexual partners and one-third less than four sexual partners. Of the "late" subjects (24 O- and 87 G-subjects who did not have first sexual intercourse until after the age of 19) three-fourths of the O-, yet more than 90% of the G-subjects had had less than four sexual partners; only one of these O-subjects indicated more than 20 sexual partners.

Closely related ($\overline{C}=.77$) to (large) number of sexual partners of the subjects were *contacts with prostitutes*. This does not mean, however, that the large number of sexual contacts with various sexual partners can be traced back to these contacts alone. More than half of the O-subjects with sexual experience had also had sexual contacts with prostitutes; in the G-group, in contrast, this was the case for only a minority of seven subjects.

The kind of sexual contacts thus corresponded to a large extent to the (nonsexual) forms of contact the subjects preferred: Insofar as could be determined in the *individual case studies,* the O-subjects preferred sexual contacts corresponding to the (nonsexual) loose or "milieu" contacts, while the sexual contacts of the G-group corresponded more to the (nonsexual) stable contacts.

2.5.6 Own Family (of Procreation)

At the time of the study, only one-fourth of the O-subjects, yet more than half of the G-subjects were married (three subjects in each group for the second time) or had been divorced in the meantime (concerning the family of procreation in general, see WITTMANN 1980).

For *age at marriage* (see Table 55), there were differences similar to those for age at first sexual intercourse, though the median age in the two subgroups did not differ as largely as the median age at first sexual intercourse.

The *median age of wives* diverged more than that of the subjects. The median age of the O-wives was 19, just as that of first sexual partners. The O-subjects, therefore, first turned to older and then to younger partners, while the G-subjects usually chose both partners in first sexual intercourse and wives who were younger or of the same age.

There was practically no divergence for the *age difference* between the spouses: 66% of the O- and 59% of the G-subjects had married younger partners. Large dif-

Table 55. Proportion of married subjects and age at marriage

	O-subj ($n=200$)	G-subj ($n=200$)	O_1-subj ($n=114$)	O_2-subj ($n=86$)
Married	23.0%	54.0%	19.3%	27.9%
Age at marriage (median)[a]				
Of subjects	20.9	22.4	20.6	21.6
Of wives	19.1	21.6	18.5	19.8

[a] In years

ferences in age (more than 5 years younger or older), however, occurred slightly more often for the O- than for the G-subjects.

Up to the time of the study, there were 56 *children* out of the 46 marriages of O-subjects and 129 children out of the 108 marriages of the G-subjects; thus, there was about the same average number of children per marriage in both groups (per O-marriage 1.22, per G-marriage 1.19 children). However, up to the time of the study, the O-subjects, including the single O-subjects, had a total of 50 illegitimate children; the G-subjects only two.

Certain differences occurred with respect to the number of children who had to be cared for in the family: Up to the time of the study, one or two children had to be cared for in 65% (30) of the O-families and in 72% (78) of the G-families, three or more in 22% (10) of the O-families and only 8% (9) of the G-families (the O-wives had brought 12, the G-wives two children into marriage). Thirteen percent (6) of the O-marriages and 20% (22) of the G-marriages were without children up to this time.

2.5.6.1 *Behavior Before Marriage*

Before marrying, the O- and the G-subjects who got married did not differ in behavior from the entire O- and G-group in the various social spheres.

For contacts and ties as well, there were essentially no other aspects than those concerning the entire group. More than two-thirds of the O-subjects who married had had sexual intercourse before the age of 16 and showed indications of early promiscuity. About one-fifth of them had an illegitimate child with another woman by the time they married, as opposed to two G-subjects. Early sexual relations including intercourse and frequent changes of sexual partners occurred for only eight of the married G-subjects. In contrast, 40% (43) of the married G-subjects had had first sexual intercourse with their later wives.

Insofar as could be determined on the basis of the information of the subjects or other persons, the *wives* of the subjects of both groups differed in premarital behavior patterns: More than one-fourth of the future O-wives had appeared, among others, as "quarrelsome," "unthrifty," or "sexually conspicuous" (frequent changes of partners), while such information existed for merely one G-wife.

The duration of acquaintance before marriage was frequently less than 6 months for the O-subjects; as a whole, 39% (18) of the O-couples, but only 12% (13) of the G-couples got married during the first 12 months of acquaintance. For 40% (44) of the G-marriages and 20% (9) of the O-marriages, there had been a close relationship for more than 3 years before the couples married. On the other hand, a large number of future wives in both groups (63% of O- and 42% of G-wives) had been pregnant before they were married. While pregnancy had been the decisive reason to marry for most of the O-subjects, most of the G-subjects concerned (93%) and their partners had already planned to marry, though at a later date.

The figures concerning duration of acquaintance before marriage were confirmed in the findings of the *individual case studies.* As rapidly as the majority of the O-subjects called an acquaintance a "girlfriend" (see Sect. 2.5.3 above), they also called such a relationship "engagement," in extreme cases after a few hours - in the momentary situation they meant this seriously. On the other hand, such "engagements" were just as quickly dissolved.

In accordance with the partially very short duration of acquaintance before marriage, the O-subjects did not *prepare for marriage* in the same way as the G-subjects did. Only six O-subjects (13%, of whom four were O_2-subjects) had saved money by the time they got married. Most O-subjects (36 subjects, 78%) had debts or current obligations, such as maintenance of an illegitimate child or installments to pay on a car. Typical preparations for marriage, such as security in employment, completing occupational training, saving for furniture, or finding an apartment, were usually of almost no importance for the O-subjects, while the marriage date of the G-subjects normally depended on such aspects. Thus, at the time of marriage, only one-fourth of the O-couples (12, of whom were O_2-couples), as opposed to 82% (89) of the G-couples, had their own dwellings.

2.5.6.2 Behavior During Marriage

The estimation of *marital relations,* which was made by both spouses, also differed considerably: Only 28% (13) of the O-couples (6 O_1, 7 O_2) but 91% (99) of the G-couples indicated that they had not had "any serious disagreements." "Seriously disrupted" marriages, characterized by frequent and partially violent arguments - mainly due to alcohol - which occasionally ended in a temporary or final separation (irrespective of the subjects' imprisonment - see Sect. 2.5.6.3 below) were reported by 72% (33) of the O- but only 9% (10) of the G-couples.

Although up to the time of the study marriage had not yet lasted more than 5 years for 70% of the O- and 59% of the G-subjects, the *courses of marriages* (for the O-subjects up to last imprisonment) could be roughly divided into two groups: "Intact marriages," where no significant, externally discernible disruption had occurred and which were termed well-balanced and harmonious by both subject and wife, occurred for 15% (7) of the O-subjects (of whom six were O_2-subjects) but 91% (98) of the G-subjects. In contrast, 85% (39) of the O- and only 9% (10) of the G-marriages were disrupted, meaning that vehement verbal, partially violent arguments occurred repeatedly and that the marriage was termed unhappy or more or less a failure by subject and wife.

This rather clear-cut trend in the groups also corresponds to the differences in the subjects' *social behavior during marriage.* About two-thirds of the O-subjects continued their earlier life-style with its specific conspicuousness, especially in the spheres of performance and leisure (for details, see Sects. 2.3 and 2.4 above). They continued to work irregularly and to spend their unstructured leisure time away from home. Because of their insufficient work performance, their families were frequently forced to give up their dwellings and go back to parents(-in-law) or to crude, simple dwellings. Half of the O-subjects did not live in dwellings appropriate to the size of their families during their entire married lives for much more than one year. Only a few O-subjects showed a sense of responsibility toward their wives (and children).

It is striking that - with one exception - in this respect as well as with respect to their premarital social behavior and preparations for marriage, six of the seven O-subjects (one O_1, six O_2) with intact marriages stood out very clearly in the O-group and were more similar to the G-group in their entire behavior. (Moreover, these subjects showed - with one exception - considerably less serious and frequent delinquency than the remaining O-subjects. Only one subject had committed several offenses against property and demonstrated considerably conspicuous behavior at work. The single O_1-subject with an intact marriage, whose first offense at 17 had been a traffic offense, was not seriously conspicuous in the various social spheres. Concerning delinquency as a whole, see Sect. 4 below).

The G-subjects' entire leisure time after marriage, especially when there were children, was concentrated on their families; they cared for their families and seemed to be fully aware of their responsibility. Even the G-subjects with disrupted marriages were rather similar to the G-subjects with intact marriages in this respect. It is striking that seven of these ten disrupted marriages were among the few G-couples who had married mainly because of a pregnancy. These subjects had taken up sexual contacts markedly earlier and had changed sexual partners more frequently before marriage.

The *individual case studies* in particular showed clearly that marriage was normally an important turning point in the lives of the G-subjects, while the lives of the majority of the O-subjects did not change in any essential respect. For example, as far as it could be ascertained, almost half (46%) of the married O-, as opposed to only 4% of the married G-subjects, had extramarital sexual relations.

However, particularly in disrupted marriages, the wives often demonstrated corresponding behavior patterns: 41% (19) of the O- and 3% (3) of the G-wives had become conspicuous through extramarital affairs or through "quarrelsome behavior," "throwing away money," or total neglect of the household.

There were differences between the O- and the G-group in connection with the *failure of marriage* as well: While violent arguments were normal in the disrupted marriages of the O-subjects, they occurred only occasionally in three of the ten disrupted G-marriages. In four disrupted G-marriages there were exclusively verbal arguments, and three couples separated by mutual consent without any previous serious arguments. The marriage of only one G-subject, who had married because of a pregnancy, had been marked by arguments from the outset; in contrast, this occurred for almost all the O-subjects concerned.

Up to the time of the study, 6% (6) of the G-, as opposed to 63% (29) of the O-marriages had ended in *divorce,* of these 20 before and 9 during the O-subjects' last imprisonment (see also Sect. 2.5.6.3 below). The proportion of divorced O_2-marriages was higher than that of divorced O_1-marriages (71% or 17 O_2- versus 55% or 12 O_1-divorces).

Eight of the divorced O-subjects had been divorced during the first 6 months of marriage, half of the O-subjects after about one year. The divorces were almost all the subjects' sole fault. In this context, criminality, which is easy to determine as a cause for divorce in civil suits, may well have been important. Official measures were taken against practically all divorced O-subjects for failure to pay maintenance; three subjects were sentenced for this reason.

The six G-couples were mainly divorced by mutual consent with both spouses equally at fault; no case of failure to pay maintenance became known either for the time before or after the divorce.

2.5.6.3 Marriage and Criminality

As the fact of survival or failure of a marriage in connection with criminality is repeatedly given some importance from several points of view, various aspects were examined for the subgroup of married O-subjects.

Most of the married O-subjects had already committed offenses before they married; only one-fifth of them did not begin committing offenses until after their marriage. For most of the O-subjects, the failure of their marriage (or their divorce) was simply another symptom of generally conspicuous behavior which repeatedly - and irrespective of marital status - led to their being sentenced and imprisoned. In no case was criminality a direct consequence of the failure of a marriage.

Only two O-subjects did not demonstrate increasing social conspicuousness and commit offenses until after they separated or were divorced from their wives. Yet there was a certain connection between failed marriage and criminality in several cases, insofar as three subjects were sentenced because they failed to pay maintenance to (former) relatives, and one other subject because he raped his ex-wife.

The *effects of imprisonment on marriage,* which are often said to be destructive, differed. Nine of the 29 O-divorces took place during the last imprisonment of the subject. These marriages had all been considerably disrupted before this time, and some of the couples had already been separated for quite some time.

The subjects' imprisonment either led to financial difficulties or reinforced the already poor economic situation of all O-marriages. However, several wives - particularly those whose marriages were no longer intact - frankly admitted that they could manage better with their social welfare benefits or the money they received from relatives than when their husbands had not been imprisoned.

The most serious problems resulting from imprisonment arose in the relations between the spouses and in their consequences. In this context, there were evident differences between intact and non-intact marriages (before imprisonment): The O-subjects with non-intact marriages were afraid that their wives - despite regular visits in prison - would take up sexual relations with other men. In requests for release from prison, these subjects mainly emphasized that their marriages were jeopardized by their imprisonment or that their children were suffering for lack of a father though they had never looked after their children before.

The O-subjects whose marriages were intact never questioned their marriages - despite the occasionally high (financial) burdens - and neither did their wives. They stood by their husbands, while the subjects did not doubt their wives' faith-

Table 56. Contact syndrome

	O-subj (n=149)	G-subj (n=198)	O_1-subj (n=90)	O_2-subj (n=59)
(Predominantly) loose or "milieu" contacts (period of study) *and* age at first sexual intercourse under 16 years or more than 6 sexual partners	59.7%	1.5%	66.6%	45.8%

Significance level: O-G: $p<.001$; O_1-O_2: $p<.02$

fulness and placed their greatest hopes for their own rehabilitation after release from prison in their wives and wives' assistance.

In short, therefore, there were no indications that there was a fundamental relationship between failure of marriage and criminality, or that (at least short-term) imprisonment had a basically destructive effect on marriage.

2.5.7 The Contact Syndrome

As in the spheres of performance and leisure, there were clearly divergent trends for the O- and the G-group with respect to the main criteria of evaluation in the sphere of contacts - for (nonsexual) contacts with friends and acquaintances as well as for contacts with the family (of orientation and procreation) on the one hand, and for (hetero)sexual contacts on the other hand. Here again, the extreme forms which were characteristic of the O-group could be taken together as a syndrome: The combination of mainly loose or "milieu" contacts during the period of the study, *as well as* first sexual intercourse before the age of 16 or more than six sexual partners up to the time of the study, distinguished the two groups especially clearly (see Table 56). This *contact syndrome* occurred for more than half of the O-subjects, but for only three G-subjects. In concurrence with the results obtained up to this point in the sphere of contacts, the O_2-subjects exhibited this syndrome less frequently than the O_1-subjects.

The contact syndrome, therefore - similar to the syndromes in the other social spheres - may well indicate behavior entailing a danger of criminality. [For its further importance (see Part IV, Sect. 2) exact figures are less important than the *early* age at first sexual intercourse - as compared with the general population - and the comparatively *frequent* changes of sexual partners.]

Like the characteristic behavior patterns of the O-group, the G-specific forms of various variables of nonsexual and sexual contact behavior can be summarized: Mainly family or other stable contacts during the period of the study as well as first sexual intercourse after the age of 20 (or no sexual intercourse up to the time of the study) and - also up to the time of the study - less than seven sexual partners. These criteria occurred for 50.5% of the G-subjects, as opposed to only 8.5% of the O_2-subjects and no O_1-subject.

2.5.8 Summary

There were quite obvious differences between the O- and the G-group's contact behavior as well. In concurrence with the O-subjects' frequently conflictual relations with their families of orientation (see Sect. 2.1.3.2 above), family-oriented or other close relations usually played a minor role for the O-subjects in later life as well. As a whole, there was a tendency toward frequently changing, superficial contacts, which were mainly utilitarian or "milieu" oriented. In the sexual sphere as well - besides having first sexual intercourse considerably earlier than the G-group - sexual relations were noncommittal; this noncommittal attitude continued almost consistently in their behavior after marriage. Marriage itself was rather unstable and not very strong.

In contrast, the G-subjects emphasized contacts with their families of orientation and particularly with their families of procreation, in addition to stable, strong relations with friends and acquaintances. In sexual behavior as well, they limited themselves to only a few partners before marriage; their marriages seemed to be more stable and strong than those of the O-subjects.

The differentiation of the O-group into early and late delinquents resulted - as in the other social spheres - in a certain midway position of the O_2-subjects in relation to general contacts: For the O_2-subjects, loose and "milieu" contacts played a much more important role than for the G-subjects. On the other hand, "milieu" contacts occurred somewhat less frequently for the O_2- than for the O_1-subjects. The O_2-subjects had stable contacts with friends and acquaintances more often than the O_1-subjects did. Sexual contacts in the broadest sense were more ambiguous: The O_2-subjects, on the one hand, started their first intensive sexual relations manifestly earlier than the G-subjects and were thus more similar to the O_1-subjects in this respect. On the other hand, their marriages could be termed intact much more frequently than those of the O_1-subjects, even if the divorce rate of the O_2-subjects as a whole was much higher than that of the O_1-subjects (and the G-subjects).

In the sphere of contacts as well, extreme forms of certain variables could be taken together as a syndrome, which consisted of loose or "milieu" contacts and, moreover, early first sexual intercourse or frequent changes of sexual partners.

The results on the contact behavior of the O-subjects correspond to a large extent to those of other comparative studies. GLUECK and GLUECK (1974, p. 102), HEALY and BRONNER (1936, pp. 52, 69 ff.), Statens offentliga utredningar (1971, p. 155; 1973 a, p. 216), WEST and FARRINGTON (1973, p. 156), and the Centro Nazionale di Prevenzione e Difesa Sociale (1969, p. 18) mention the "milieu" orientation of the contacts of their (delinquent) subjects and, in this context, the preference of socially conspicuous contact persons, while Statens offentliga utredningar (1973 a, p. 217) additionally emphasizes the flightiness and superficiality of these relations. For heterosexual behavior, early, frequently changing sexual contacts - also with prostitutes - are emphasized in particular for the delinquent subjects, as are early age at marriage, social conspicuousness of spouses, lacking stability and insufficient (also material) security of marriage with a lack of willingness on the part of the subjects to induce changes by their own initiative (GLUECK and GLUECK 1974, pp. 102, 161 ff.; OTTERSTRÖM 1946, p. 269; WEST and FARRINGTON 1977, pp. 54, 62). Also in concurrence with the results obtained in the present study, marriage alone is not regarded as a necessarily stabilizing factor in the lives of delinquents (HEALY and BRONNER 1926, p. 130).

3 Somatic, Psychiatric, and Psychological Aspects

3.1 Preliminary Remarks

3.1.1 On the Somatic Aspects

The medical assessment of the O- and the G-subjects was not aimed at an extensive diagnostic evaluation - i.e., one satisfying clinical criteria - as the Tübingen Institute lacked the necessary equipment. No relevant findings could be expected from a clinical-neurological examination alone without corresponding additional diagnostic procedures. Thus, only externally visible abnormal findings (such as physical impairments, deformities, anomalies of growth, and scars and tattoos) were noted. Electroencephalograms and echoencephalograms were recorded for most of the O- and the G-subjects. The latter examination, however, was soon discontinued, as the evaluation of the findings gave no new insights. On the other hand, chromosome patterns were examined after a certain time for 74 O- and 103 G-subjects.

3.1.2 On the Psychiatric and Psychological Aspects

On the basis of the impressions from the preliminary study and long-term personal experience with mental disorders of offenders, a frequent occurrence of *pronounced mental disorders* according to strict psychopathological criteria was not expected. Therefore, the psychiatric explorations were geared mainly to noting whether, in the area of transition between the normal and the abnormal (which is vague and cannot be defined clearly), there were predominant personality traits which were "diminutions" of certain mental disorders, whether there were any other kinds of conspicuousness, and whether there were any differences between the O- and the G-group in these respects. Furthermore, it was attempted, irrespective of psychopathological criteria, to obtain as complex a picture as possible of the life pattern of a subject. Anyone who has personally examined individuals not by accessing their personality with psychological tests alone knows how important these complex pictures are, but also how impossible it is to present them in detail (see Part III). In this respect, the following presentation must remain unsatisfactory for those mainly seeking countable facts.

In accordance with the aim of the Tübingen Comparative Study of Young Offenders, i.e., a substantially hypothesis free, descriptive presentation of the groups of the study by as unequivocal and verifiable facts as possible, *psychoanalytic methods* and theories were not considered. Further hypotheses deduced from other theories of personality were also disregarded. Only test procedures common at the time of the study were applied to verify any differences between the groups.

Therefore, the traditional procedure of *personality testing* was chosen. Projective procedures, not psychometric ones, were emphasized (Rorschach test, Wartegg design test, tree test). For the evaluation of intelligence, the WAIS was applied; it was and still is the most widely used test for this purpose. Two other tests (the Rosenzweig P-F test and the *Persönlichkeits- und Interessentest,* a test which measures personality traits and specific interests) were conducted with some of the subjects at a later stage.

The team members who had immediate contact with the subjects tried to collect the *impressions* they had of the subjects in the various study situations. They used terms which did not necessarily correspond to the scientific vocabulary of the related sciences of criminology. They covered, for example, the contact with the subject and his responsiveness and mood (see Sect. 3.4.1 below). Naturally, it was impossible to achieve the same degree of reliability and validity as with the data collected in the social spheres, considering that subjective impressions played a role in the judgments and no supplementary information from other sources was available (as for the investigations in the social spheres). Moreover, the training and practical experience of the team members concerned (psychiatrists, psychologists, and social workers) differed considerably, which may have influenced categories which are difficult to operationalize (e.g., "self-criticism"). Nevertheless, later on, the evaluation of the personality tests showed that the test results - insofar as they were related to criteria connected with these estimations - corresponded (at least in tendency) with the impressions of the team members.

3.2 Patient History and Physical Findings

Both the O- and the G-subjects ($n=200$ for both groups) rarely mentioned a family history of diseases known to have hereditary factors.

The O-subjects (9.5%) reported a history of various *somatic diseases,* such as diseases of the respiratory tract, heart, stomach, and bowels, more than twice as often as the G-subjects did (3.5%). There were no differences concerning the endocrine system.

Head traumata and concussions were mentioned more frequently by the O- (44.5%) than by the G-subjects (28.5%). However, one should be somewhat skeptical in believing the subjects' information on, for example, the occurrence of concussions: Repeated intensive questioning occasionally showed that the lack of memory (amnesia) after the would-be "trauma" had other reasons (often alcohol consumption).

Other diseases leading either to work inability for at least 3 months or to permanent impairment were mentioned by 10% of the O- and only 5.5% of the G-subjects.

As to *extremities* and *trunk,* impairments were noted more frequently for the G- (50%) than for the O-group (33%). Scars occurred more often in the O-group, usually as a consequence of accidents or brawls. When deformities, scars, and tattoos were taken together as externally visible abnormalities, the O-group clearly dominated (51.5% O; 19.5% G). *Tattoos* were found almost exclusively in the O-group (51 O; 1 G).

The predominance of somatic illnesses and consequences of head traumata mentioned in the personal histories of the O-subjects corresponded to some extent with the findings of GLUECK and GLUECK (1957) and, in more recent times, of LEWIS and SHANOK (1977). They found a higher occurrence of various diseases in offenders (such as chronic respiratory diseases, accidents, and operations). As a whole, however, the literature indicated no conclusive relationship between certain physical diseases and criminality. Furthermore, the findings of the Tübingen study do not permit the conclusion that the O-subjects had a *constitutionally* more delicate state of health than the G-subjects.

Assuming that the subjects' information on their personal histories was reliable, there were further circumstances in the overall view of both groups' life patterns which may account for the differences from another point of view, for example more inattentiveness toward oneself, also with respect to one's body. The O-subjects' numerous scars and frequent indications of concussions may be due to more frequent (traffic) accidents and brawls. Furthermore, the O-subjects' frequently insufficient physical hygiene and lack of health insurance may well be of some importance. During the years preceding the study, 68% of the O- but only 1% of the G-subjects had no health insurance or were irregularly insured. The lack of health insurance was due to various facts, especially to long periods of nonemployment, temporary labor, or imprisonment; nevertheless, it may also be the expression of a certain carelessness and lack of planning for the future, which was often ascertained for the O-subjects in other spheres as well, for example when a subject worked for a dubious company and did not pay any attention to whether he was registered with the social insurance plan. Not being insured may prevent the early detection and treatment of diseases and thus contribute to their deterioration or to their becoming chronic conditions.

Other findings and remarks by the subjects also spoke against a constitutional factor: The O-subjects mentioned high alcohol consumption much more frequently than the G-subjects (see also Sect. 3.4.2.3 below). A total of 68.5% of the O- and only 23.5% of the G-subjects termed themselves heavy smokers. Even when it was taken into consideration that the G-subjects might have glossed over such facts to present certain socially desirable criteria (although this might also apply for the O-subjects), a radical difference in the way of life of the O- and the G-subjects appeared on the basis of the remaining findings of the study (see Sect. 3.4.4 below and Part III). This may well be the explanation for the increased somatic impairments in the O-group.

Occasionally, the opinion (e.g., STUTTE 1974 and the literature mentioned there) is expressed that visible handicaps and abnormalities lead persons to join deviant groups by way of intermediate processes. These processes are still unclear, but can be called "problems of adaptation". The data showed clearly that scars and tattoos (which were usually acquired in prison) were almost always related to a conspicuous life pattern which had already existed for some time before. Tattoos in particular can demonstrate membership in certain groups, and - once existent - facilitate access or return to such groups.

The G-subjects did not consider physical impairments important to their *development,* while the O-subjects occasionally mentioned their importance for downward social mobility or for the impossibility of upward mobility (see Part III, Sect. 4.3.2.3).

3.3 Laboratory Tests

3.3.1 Cytogenetic Tests

In the mid-1960s, several publications discussed a possible relationship between chromosome aberrations and criminality. There were no studies of random samples of prisoners, however, or comparisons with corresponding control groups from the "average" population. The studies were limited to casuistic observations or selected serial examinations (e.g., according to the kind of offense or clinical-psychiatric findings). As there was no such selection in the Tübingen Comparative Study of Young Offenders, cytogenetic examinations were conducted by HABERLANDT (1970) for the subjects not yet examined (103 G- and 74 O-subjects); eight O- and three G-subjects demonstrated chromosome aberrations.

There was one pure XYY-pattern among the eight O-subjects, two mosaics with additional Y-chromosomes, two Klinefelter syndromes (XXY) and one mosaic with an additional X-chromosome. Two subjects exhibited structural changes in the set of chromosomes (abnormally large Y-chromosome). The three G-subjects with chromosome aberrations had two mosaics and one translocation; all three demonstrated above-average intelligence and were clinically normal; four O-subjects showed below-average intelligence. The offenses of the O-subjects with chromosome aberrations were property offenses, traffic offenses, bodily injuries, and sexual offenses.

A detailed examination of the individual chromosome aberrations resulted in differing physical and mental findings: While the structural chromosome aberrations exhibited by the G-subjects and several O-subjects were not - or only in a minor way - accompanied by any physical or mental impairment, the numeric aberrations (XYY and XXY) corresponded with a conspicuous physical habitus, disproportionate growth, and, in the mental area, inferior intelligence.

These few findings do not suffice for any general statement, for example on criminality (for details see HABERLANDT 1970; KLEIN-VOGLER and HABERLANDT 1974).

RUSELL and BENDER (1970) in particular studied criminality (and the resulting consequences) in connection with chromosome aberrations. JÖRGENSEN (1969) indicates that a "normal" set of chromosomes may contain abnormal genetic information which cannot yet be determined (for a survey of the literature see, for instance, BAKER et al. 1970; HABERLANDT 1970).

3.3.2 Electroencephalograms and Echoencephalograms

EEGs were recorded and evaluated by VETTER (1972) for 147 O- and 150 G-subjects. A total of 13 O- and 7 G-subjects exhibited pathological findings. One O- and one G-subject showed seizure patterns. The remaining subjects with pathological findings demonstrated variations which were higher than those of a normal EEG with respect to frequency and form of the various waves, though not always equidirectional. However, relevant differences which could be generalized were not found.

In the literature, it is occasionally claimed that the EEGs of offenders deviate from normal patterns more often than those of nonoffenders (WIENER et al. 1966, pp. 497 ff., for instance, describe a more frequent occurrence of slow waves in the EEGs of offenders). Nevertheless, the present results are not surprising considering how difficult the reliable evaluation of an EEG is. Normal EEG derivations alone offer a wide range of variations in wave amplitude and frequency as well as in stability of potential fluctuations. Furthermore, a clinically manifest organic disease of the central nervous system does not necessarily have to produce an abnormal EEG. On the basis of the EEGs in the Tübingen Comparative Study of Young Offenders, no statement can be made on the question of more frequent or even specific anomalies in the EEGs of offenders. (For a detailed bibliography, see VETTER 1972, SCHULZ and MAINUSCH 1969, and LOOMIS 1965).

The *echoencephalograms* also led to no meaningful results on differences between the O- and the G-group and were therefore discontinued at an early stage.

3.4 Psychiatric and Psychological Examinations

3.4.1 Impressions from the Examination Situation

In general *expressive behavior, manner of speaking,* and *rhetoric capability,* there were no differences worth mentioning between the O- and the G-subjects. *Speech defects,* especially stuttering, occurred for 5.5% of the O- and 1% of the G-subjects.

For the majority of both the O- and the G-subjects, the *contact with the interviewer* was good (85% O; 92% G). Inappropriate behavior such as lack of distance or extreme inhibition was demonstrated by 12% of the O- and 4% of the G-subjects.

Emotional responsiveness was also lower in the O-group, and the O-subjects were more frequently *affectively* labile. A *balanced, stable mood* occurred for 25.5% of the O- and 48.5% of the G-subjects, while *conditions of irritable mood* occurred more often for the O- than for the G-subjects (7.5% O; 1% G).

For 10% of the O- and 39% of the G-subjects, *memory functions* were good; for 21% of the O- and 6.5% of the G-subjects they were impaired. Correspondingly, *immediate retention* differed in the O- and the G-group: Good for 12.5% of the O- and 45% of the G-subjects, poor for 34% of the O- and 13.5% of the G-subjects.

In the estimation of *thought process,* a low faculty for adjusting and a tendency to cling to a subject, as well as occasional perseveration were found for 37% of the O- and 12% of the G-subjects.

There were obvious differences with respect to *judgment* and *self-criticism* as well: For 32% of the O- and 3% of the G-subjects judgment was poor; for 35.5% of the O- and 5% of the G-subjects self-criticism was poor.

3.4.2 Psychiatric Explorations

3.4.2.1 Psychoses

The presence of acute mental diseases was not to be expected, as offenders who are mentally ill are usually examined in the course of the criminal proceedings and are subsequently not sent to prison, while an acute psychotic state is usually recognized by the social surroundings and the person concerned treated (see also Sect. 3.4.2.3 below). Accordingly, during the period of the Tübingen study, a beginning *schizophrenic disorder* was suspected in only three cases (two O-, one G-subject); the disease actually developed in two of these cases. No *cyclothymic disorder* was diagnosed.

Moreover, one (G-)subject who had not been previously convicted demonstrated an obvious personality change and impaired intelligence after a serious *head trauma*; in the period that followed, serious social conspicuousness was noted, and the subject subsequently committed offenses.

3.4.2.2 Endoreactive Urges

Endoreactive urges are expressed in an uncontrollable need for activity accompanied by motoric agitation, impulsiveness, and the inability to maintain goal-directed behavior. These behavior patterns occur irregularly, sometimes for no apparent reason; they are often induced by external, often unimportant events and can occasionally be observed during childhood. The persons concerned stay away from work, want to leave: "I had to get away," or they walk away after an argument or a banal event that has irritated them. The duration of endoreactive urges differs. Usually, some kind of outburst takes place in the form of alcohol abuse, walking around uselessly, or driving away, often with a car stolen for this purpose and occasionally in connection with other offenses.

According to further observation of the subjects within the follow-up study, the endoreactive urges, and with them mostly criminality, seemed to subside toward the end of the subjects' twenties, making way for a certain indolence and inactivity.

The onset of these conditions, often unmotivated and difficult to understand, the increased motoric activity involved, and also the lack of, or at least the great difficulty in maintaining control suggest an underlying somatic process as well. As there has been no specific medical examination of this phenomenon to date, the relationship with mood lability of abnormal personalities (Schneider 1980; there is also a lack of systematic somatic studies) is as unclear as the relationship with minimal brain damage (among the multitude of publications on this subject, see Bresser 1965 and Lempp 1978, and the literature indicated there). Moreover, it cannot yet be decided whether the similar disorder described by several G-subjects and their parents, involving special difficulties in child rearing, corresponds to this phenomenon or whether there is any qualitative difference.

It is also impossible to determine exactly the percentage of O-subjects concerned, as the manifestation of such conditions was noted only in the course of the investigations and not all subjects were examined in this respect. About 10% of the O-subjects may have demonstrated endoreactive urges.

3.4.2.3 Other Mental Disorders

A certain degree of low intelligence was found in about 15% of the O- and 5% of the G-subjects, one O-subject being mildly mentally retarded. Thus, the O-subjects were more strongly represented in this respect (see also Sect. 3.4.3.2 below).

Other mental affections, such as *personality or neurotic disorders,* occurred only sporadically in both groups, the latter exclusively in the G-group. (The socially neglected O-subjects who are sometimes classified under the term "neurotic neglect" are not taken into consideration in this context.)

Although some of the offenses of the O-subjects can be described as reactions to (emotional) occurrences in the widest sense, for instance panic reactions *(Kurzschlußhandlungen),* it is worth mentioning that there was *no* such offense which, as a first offense after social inconspicuousness, led to a criminal *development* for *any* of the O-subjects.

In a few cases, however, social conspicuousness followed a particularly serious event (such as death of father or friend, or separation from fiancee) for both the O- and the G-subjects. For the O-subjects, however, social conspicuousness repeatedly meant staying away from work, roaming about, drinking, and landing in the "milieu," and finally criminality. The G-subjects concerned often demonstrated a prolonged depressive mood accompanied by a total withdrawal, while the sphere of performance was not seriously affected.

It became apparent that the O-subjects concerned had already been socially conspicuous before the event described as particularly serious.

In contrast, traits which might be called "*diminutions*" of typical and dominating traits of psychopathic personalities occurred more frequently. While all types of personality disorders were observed occasionally for the G-subjects, the following were often registered in the O-group: Personality traits that are found in their most marked form in personalities which are expansive (see PETRILOWITSCH 1966, pp. 65 ff.), labile of mood, explosive, lacking in willpower, susceptible, and attention seeking (see SCHNEIDER 1980), but also personalities which need recognition because of their self-experienced insufficiency. Furthermore, unscrupulous personalities (see GÖPPINGER 1960, pp. 82ff.) occurred in both groups. Yet this personality disorder was not relevant enough to be exclusively decisive for the lifestyle of the subjects.

In connection with offenses, *panic reactions* occurred frequently for O-subjects. Apart from bodily injury (violent offenses) and insults immediately following an event, there were problems in connection with earlier criminality (such as garnishment of wages, previous conviction becoming known, or police or probation officers turning up at the subject's place of work) or sometimes even relatively unimportant occurrences (e.g., trouble at work, quarrels with a girl or "buddy"). These problems or occurrences formed the beginning of a chain of events (leaving the job or apartment, going to one or more bars, considerable alcohol consumption) ending in offenses - possibly committed together with other "buddies" who had appeared in the meantime or who had been asked to help.

A total of 33 O-subjects and only one G-subject attempted to commit *suicide* one or more times. This information cannot be taken at face value, however, as the sincerity of a suicide attempt is difficult to estimate solely on the basis of the information of the person concerned. A comparison is even more difficult since most suicide attempts by O-subjects had taken place during previous terms in prison, and motivations other than the wish to die often played a role (e.g., the attempt to obtain special privileges or a transfer to a prison hospital, meaning better possibilities of escape). Insofar as the suicide attempts were not related to the specific situation in prison, they were mostly spontaneous reactions to events which were disappointing for a subject (e.g., unfavorable court sentence, infidelity of wife or her filing a petition for divorce, no mail). In no case was there any indication of a suicide attempt which was caused by illness (e.g., endogeneous depression) or which the subject had planned for a longer period of time, meaning that he had taken into account all circumstances of his life.

Drug consumption was indicated as temporary experimentation by several O- and G-subjects; drug addiction, however, did not occur for any of the subjects. There were no convictions for offenses connected with drug abuse either (see Sect. 4.3 below). This can be traced back to the fact that drug consumption was not yet widespread but was concentrated on certain population subgroups during the period of the study, i.e., the mid to late 1960s.

In contrast, *regular (considerable) alcohol consumption* occurred frequently (59% O; 9% G). A proportion (although a relatively small one) of the O-subjects could be termed alcohol dependent on the basis of their excessive and chronic consumption of alcohol. Some O-subjects had already been to a detoxification center. More important than alcohol consumption in the medical sense is the role alcohol played in connection with the social behavior and delinquency of many subjects (see Sect. 4.5.2 below and Part III, Sect. 3.3.3.3; see also KERNER 1972).

3.4.3 Psychological Test Findings

3.4.3.1 Preliminary Remarks

Besides the Hamburg-Wechsler intelligence test (WAIS), only projective tests were used to assess the personality of subjects, including the Rorschach test, the tree test, and the Wartegg design test (WDT). For a subgroup of the subjects, another projective test, the Rosenzweig Picture Frustration test (Rosenzweig P-F test), and a psychometric test, the *Persönlichkeits- und Interessentest* (PIT; a test which measures personality traits and specific interests) were applied.

One main feature of a projective test is that the subject is not aware of its aim or purpose. Therefore, purposeful distortion is not quite as easy as in personality questionnaires, whose intention can usually be perceived by the subject. Especially in connection with criminological and forensic/psychological problems, one must reckon with much more pronounced tendencies to distort. Therefore, projective methods seem to be the best way to gain access to the personality of an offender (despite the objections which - at that time fewer than today - are raised).

3.4.3.2 Conduct and Results of the Psychological Tests

The *Hamburg-Wechsler intelligence test for adults* (WAIS), which was used to measure *intelligence*, consists of a number of verbal and performance subtests, e.g., information and similarities on the one hand and picture completion and block design on the other. From the statistical point of view, the WAIS results in an intelligence quotient (IQ) between 91 and 109 for 50% of the population (WECHSLER 1964, p. 52), the remaining IQs being in equal proportions (25%) above and below.

The O-subjects' median total IQ value was obviously lower than the G-subjects' (O=92.8; G=103.9). The differences between the O- and the G-subjects were more marked for the verbal scale (O=92.0; G=104.4), less marked for the performance scale (O=94.7; G=103.0).

In both groups, 50%-60% of the subjects belonged to the median intelligence range, while the G-group (34% G; 8% O) was overrepresented in the upper range

(IQ above 109) and the O-group (41% O; 11.5% G) in the lower range (IQ under 91). With respect to IQ, there were no differences between the O_1- and the O_2-group.

One O-subject was mildly mentally retarded (IQ under 63) and 13.5% of the O-subjects belonged in the category of very low intelligence (IQ up to 80). Only 3.5% of the G-subjects had an IQ between 70 and 80.

A further differentiated analysis, i.e., calculating various indices on the basis of individual WAIS subtests, concentrated particularly on power of concentration, judgment of social situations, and signs of mental deterioration. It became apparent that there were no significant differences between the groups with respect to power of concentration. Judgment of social situations, however, was visibly poorer for the O- than for the G-subjects; similarly, there were more frequent signs of deterioration of mental capacity for the O-subjects (17%) than for the G-subjects (5%). (According to the interpretation of the test, this means that there is an impairment of intelligence performance which usually does not occur until a later stage of life.)

Among the tests used for *personality diagnostics,* the *Rorschach test* was used to assess the "entire personality," not isolated aspects.

The subjects interpret unstructured visual material in the form of colored and black-and-white ink blots. How a subject processes this visual material reflects the structure and dynamics of his personality.

There were differences between the groups for only a very few categories. With respect to the basic attitude of the personality toward ego and environment (experience type), more O- than G-subjects (46.5% O; 29% G) were extremely extratensive (according to the evaluation of the Rorschach test suggested by BOHM 1967): This experience type is characterized, among others, by a more stereotyped intelligence, more reproductivity, a more outward- than inward-turned life, a more extensive than intensive rapport; furthermore, persons characterized by these criteria have a large number of acquaintances but only superficial ties. In a differentiation between the O_1- and the O_2-group, this type occurred even more frequently for the O_2-subjects (41% O_1; 53.5% O_2). The marked numerical differences for the extreme form of extratension between the O- and the G-group decreased, however, when subjects with less marked extratensive tendencies were also considered (69.5% O; 59.5% G).

Affective adaptability was poor for 75.5% of the O- and 44.5% of the G-subjects, while it was normal for 11% of the O- and 23% of the G-subjects. There was no difference between the O_1- and the O_2-group.

Regarding ability to establish social contacts, the groups of the study did not differ. However, it is striking that in the O_1-group, as opposed to the O_2-group, there was a tendency toward more frequent difficulties in establishing social contacts.

Both tests in which the subject has to draw, the *Wartegg design test* (WDT) and the *tree test,* aim - as the Rorschach test - at gaining access to the entire personality.

In the *Wartegg design test,* the subject has to complete eight unfinished drawings. The evaluation takes place according to qualitative categories. In the *tree test,* the subject draws a tree; in the evaluation, traits of the drawing as symbols in space, graphology, and formal individual traits of the tree design are taken into consideration.

Neither test offered any results which could be interpreted. Only differences for individual traits were noted. Their significance remained unclear even after an extensive evaluation (in the WDT there were differences for seven of the 26 traits; in the tree test for 23 of the 89 traits).

In contrast to these nonconclusive results, the *Persönlichkeits- und Interessentest* (PIT), the only psychometric test, demonstrated several differences between the two groups, although it was applied to only a small number of subjects.

The personality scales of the PIT (the interests scales were not assessed), on the basis of the test sheets of 42 O- and 47 G-subjects, showed that the self-description of the G-subjects, as opposed to that of the O-subjects, was rather inconspicuous. The G-subjects found themselves to a larger degree not depressive, not schizoid and not paranoid. With respect to vegetative stability and social attitude, the G-group scored visibly higher than the O-group.

The *Rosenzweig P-F test* was also conducted only for subgroups of 71 O- and 104 G-subjects.

This test aims particularly at assessing individual reactions to frustrating conditions. It consists of cartoon drawings of various situations which depict an individual with other persons in a frustrating situation. The remark of one person is given, and the verbal answer of the other person has to be filled in. The essential criteria of evaluation are direction of aggression and reaction pattern.

This test did not reveal any obvious differences. However, the G-group, as opposed to the O-group, tended to have higher rates of outward aggression, while the O-group more often demonstrated a circumvention of aggression. With respect to reaction patterns, the O-subjects mentioned the solution of the frustrating situation more often, the G-subjects the obstacle.

3.4.3.3 Critical Evaluation of the Findings

The *personality tests* used in the Tübingen Comparative Study of Young Offenders were only rarely capable of differentiating between the O- and the G-subjects. The same holds for the O_1- and the O_2-subjects. Any test-diagnostic differences found in the structure of the personality were contradictory and could not be uniformly interpreted.

As opposed to the personality assessment, the examination of *intelligence* offered unequivocal differences. The O-subjects, as compared with the G-subjects, had a lower average intelligence rate, a result which remained after further differentiations according to possible differences in capabilities. Nevertheless, it is erroneous to conclude that intelligence is of special importance with respect to criminality, considering the complexity of human experience and behavior. Besides differing intellectual-cognitive requirements, personality-specific aspects play an important role, as do the manifold individual experiences with the specific "environments" of a person.

Intelligence became apparent in many different ways. For instance, the subjects with an IQ of 91-109, who were about equally represented in both groups, differed considerably with regard to their success at school: Practically all G-subjects had completed (at least) the *Hauptschule,* while approximately half of the O-subjects had not (see Sect. 2.3.2.1 above). Intelligence is of greater importance, however, if it ranges far below the average norm at the borderline toward mental retardation; this was the case for only six O-subjects.

A comparison with the results of *other studies* showed the following: The present results concerning *intelligence* correspond to those of other studies, according to which offenders have a low median IQ (among others CONGER and MILLER 1966, p. 74; FERRACUTI et al. 1975, p. 46; WEST and FARRINGTON 1973, pp. 84ff.; WOLFGANG et al. 1972, pp. 61 ff.; differing results: MCCORD and MCCORD 1959, pp. 65 ff.). Furthermore, the poorer results of prisoners in the *verbal* part and the relatively better results in the *performance* part correspond to the results of other studies on offenders which tested intelligence with the WAIS (among others FERRACUTI et al. 1975, p. 46).

A comparison of the findings on *personality structure* in other multifactorial studies is practically impossible: On the one hand, some studies concentrated on traits of temperament, others on motivational factors; on the other hand, too heterogeneous methods were applied (partially strictly psychometric, partially projective methods). This causes additional problems regarding the validity of results (see Sect. 3.4.3.1 above).

3.4.4 Attitudes Related to a Specific Life-style

While neither the psychopathological aspects (see Sect. 3.4.2 above), nor the psychological tests (see Sect. 3.4.3 above) made it possible to determine definite mental particularities which clearly distinguished the two groups, it was possible to discern, particularly in the psychiatric explorations, behavior patterns connected with a certain life-style of the O-subjects. The patterns did not occur for the G-subjects, at least not in this manner and not as frequently. However, these patterns were not immediately assessable as psycho(patho)logical criteria, for example by determining traits of personality, but could only be described in more detail after a careful observation of a subject's social behavior as a whole:

This typical conspicuousness manifests itself in the end as an "*unchecked living in the immediate present*", characterized by a short time perspective, a deficient sense of reality, and the absence of planning in life. This is mainly marked by a subject's seeking immediate satisfaction of his present wishes and spontaneous needs - without regard to negative consequences of a physical, material, or ideal nature for himself and others. This is related, on the one hand, to an attitude which, together with a low tolerance for stress, leads the subject to avoid what is required of him if any problems arise, without considering subsequent, possibly much more serious difficulties. On the other hand, an attitude which can be described by an inadequately high level of aspirations, a paradoxical expectation of adaptation, and a demand to be free from any ties also becomes apparent.

This conspicuousness can be recognized on the basis of repeated behavior patterns in the longitudinal section of life. It is typical of the O-subjects insofar as it did not occur for G-subjects in the same marked form. It occurred for the *majority* of the O-subjects, not for all of them (for more details on the attitudes accompanying or determining the social behavior of the subjects concerned, see Part III, Sect. 3.3.3).

3.5 Summary

In an overall view of the somatic, psychological, and psychiatric findings, no results appear which would allow a convincing differentiation between the O- and the G-group.

In the somatic area there are several differences, but they must be doubted to some extent, as they rest solely on the information of the subjects as regards, for example, previous illnesses or accidents. There is no reliable medical confirmation of these indications. Apart from this, the findings are not at all uniform; they are partially even contradictory and, moreover, too insignificant in number to allow any acceptable scientific conclusions. Thus, the somatic findings cannot be interpreted in the sense that the O-subjects are more conspicuous, constitutionally and somatically, than the G-subjects. Laboratory tests do not lead any further in this respect, either.

In principle, the same holds for the findings obtained by the traditional methods of psychiatric and psychological examination. If existent, differences were very slight or unspecific in their importance for criminality. Thus, for example, the importance of intelligence is weakened by the fact that the O- and the G-subjects of medium intelligence exhibited differing developments in the entire sphere of performance.

The endoreactive urges are a special aspect. However, the criteria for these conditions became visible only in the course of the examinations. Therefore, further, more differentiated studies are necessary. For the time being, it is not certain whether the same phenomenon occurs for the G-subjects in some form as well; it is a finding which deserves further research, particularly from a medical point of view.

Unequivocal and also criminologically important differences between the O- and the G-group did emerge, however, from the conspicuousness found in social behavior which is not exclusively related to the physical or mental disposition of the subjects. They are the expression of specific attitudes connected with the life-style of the subjects and correspond in the final analysis to the findings in the various social spheres (see Sect. 2 above and Part III).

4 The Sphere of Delinquency

4.1 Preliminary Remarks

The presentation of delinquency in the longitudinal section of life is aimed at characterizing the O-group as compared with other offenders and showing relationships with the O-subjects' social behavior (in particular, see Sect. 4.4 below).

First, the O- and the G-subjects' pre-delinquent and delinquent behavior patterns before the age of criminal responsibility are compared (see Sect. 4.2.1 below). These patterns have already been mentioned sporadically with regard to the social spheres. Then, the O- and the G-subjects' actual delinquency at responsible age is presented, i.e., including the delinquency which remained undetected or was not punished (see Sect. 4.2.2 below).

Only the registered delinquency of the O-subjects is analyzed in detail (see Sect. 4.3 below and the more detailed presentation of KESKE 1983). It should be noted once again that the O-subjects represented a large section of (recidivist) offenders, not offenders as a whole. The present selection covers, so to speak, the broad "medium range" of criminality: Neither petty crimes (by disregarding offenders sentenced to less than 6 months) nor a certain section of major crimes (by disregarding offenders sentenced for capital crimes) were taken into consideration (see Part I, Sect. 2.3). In view of these selection criteria, a comparison with the G-subjects is both useless and impossible - unlike in the preceding sections. Although the G-subjects were not a group of nonoffenders but a cross section of the general population, the relatively small number of offenders (47) in the G-group made a differentiated analysis very problematic. The delinquency and related social conspicuousness of the G-group are therefore presented separately (see Sect. 4.7 below).

The findings on the delinquency of the O-subjects were extracted chiefly from the extensive records. The findings mainly relate to kind, extent, and course of delinquency. The criminological appearance of the offense (see Sect. 4.5 below) and the modalities of the "last" offense in connection with the subjects' specific circumstances in life is given special attention (see Sect. 4.6 below).

4.2 (Pre-)Delinquent Behavior and Actual Criminality

4.2.1 Social Conspicuousness and "Offenses" During Childhood

As the age of criminal responsibility basically starts at 14, criteria of criminal law are not applied to corresponding acts by children in official proceedings - as they are in registered delinquency. Thus, it is usually difficult to distinguish considerable social conspicuousness from "offenses."

Table 57. Social conspicuousness and "offenses" during childhood

	O-subjects		G-subjects	
A: *Conspicuousness at home up to the age of 13*	(*n*=196)[a]		(*n*=200)	
1) Inconspicuous	43.4%		91.0%	
2)[b] Insincerity, disobedience, quarrelsomeness, running away	29.1%		6.5%	
3)[b] Theft, deceit	27.5%		2.5%	
B: *Conspicuousness outside home up to the age of 13*	(*n*=200)		(*n*=200)	
1) Adjusted, inconspicuous	30.0%		47.0%	
2)[b] Minor theft, insolence, smoking, alcohol consumption	8.5%		28.0%	
3)[b] Roaming about, persistent truancy, damage to property, sexual conspicuousness	20.0%		16.5%	
4)[b] Theft, deceit, extreme pugnacity	41.5%		8.5%	
C: *"Offenses" at and/or away from home up to the age of 13*	O-subj (*n*=196)	G-subj (*n*=200)	O_1-subj (*n*=113)	O_2-subj (*n*=83)
Theft, deceit, extreme pugnacity; (A3 and/or B4)	49.5%	10.5%	65.5%	27.7%

Significance level: $p<.001$

[a] Four children who grew up in homes were disregarded

[b] Only subjects who are not covered under 3) and 4) are considered under 2), correspondingly for 3) with respect to 4)

Therefore, the partially serious social conspicuousness of the O- and the G-subjects during childhood, which corresponded to the concept of "delinquency" in Anglo-American usage, was not differentiated according to aspects of criminal law but according to degree of seriousness. In Table 57 conspicuousness at home and away from home in the various spheres was taken together (see Sect. 2 above).

Conspicuousness at home occurred chiefly for the subjects who were not supervised by their parents or whose parents were socially conspicuous (see also Sect. 2.1 above). Theft and fraud usually meant taking often considerable amounts of money, for example from the household cash box, or deceiving the persons rearing the subject - partially by sophisticated methods.

More than half of the G-subjects and 70% of the O-subjects demonstrated *conspicuousness away from home*. The actual differences became apparent when the conspicuousness was differentiated: The G-subjects became conspicuous by pilfering (e.g., stealing fruit) or by impertinence, smoking, or drinking alcohol. Only rarely did they demonstrate serious kinds of conspicuousness, in particular theft, fraud, or extreme pugnacity. In contrast, such conspicuousness occurred very frequently for the O-subjects, for instance in theft of valuable objects or theft under difficult circumstances, forging signatures, and bodily injury in connection with brawls.

Furthermore, these "offenses" were often related to other kinds of serious social conspicuousness, particularly roaming about, which again was connected with persistent truancy, deceiving parents or teachers, and "offenses" (see also the "socioscholastic syndrome," Sect. 2.3.2.3 above).

As a whole, the examination of "offenses" at home and away from home showed that there was an obvious relationship with later delinquency (see also

Sect. 4.4 below). Two-thirds of the O_1-subjects, who were first convicted between the ages of 13 and 17, had already become conspicuous during childhood. The O_2-group (27.7%), in contrast, was much closer to the G- (10.5%) than to the O_1-group. Evidently, the G-subjects' conspicuousness was chiefly sporadic and did not lead to recidivist criminality (see also Sect. 4.7 below).

This fact shows that an "offense" during childhood as such is of no importance unless it occurs together with further social conspicuousness (on the relationship between "childhood delinquency" and criminality, see in particular the study of TRAULSEN 1976).

Considerable conspicuousness during childhood in general and "offenses" in particular led to *measures by official authorities* only for a certain percentage of the O-subjects (21.5%). Schools usually reacted initially with school-internal measures even for "offenses" (see Sect. 2.3.2.4 above). The youth welfare office, with or without the approval of the subjects' parents, prompted a committal to a home or reform school for 16 O-subjects but no G-subject [see also Sect. 2.2.2.3 above; regarding committals to reform schools from the age of 14 on as a penalty under the Juvenile Court Act *(Jugendgerichtsgesetz)* or Youth Welfare Act *(Jugendwohlfahrtsgesetz),* see Sect. 4.3.1 below].

4.2.2 Registered and Nonregistered Delinquency at the Age of Criminal Responsibility

As expected, most of the O-subjects - besides the numerous offenses they had been sentenced for - and the G-subjects - several of whom were also previously convicted - had committed offenses which remained undetected (on the methodological aspects, see Part I, Sect. 2.1.2). The question arose whether the officially registered delinquency of the subjects, documented in their criminal records, corresponded in tendency to the whole of their offenses or whether their registered delinquency presented an entirely distorted section of their entire offenses. It was of special interest to determine whether the considerable differences between the O- and the G-subjects would disappear at least partially with respect to actual delinquency. For this purpose, the analysis of the subjects' registered delinquency was supplemented by an examination of the offenses they had actually committed. Yet such an examination is always of limited validity for lack of objective data as well as for other reasons (see below).

SCHÖCH (1976) examined the actual delinquency, i.e., registered and nonregistered delinquency together, of the G-subjects of the Tübingen Comparative Study of Young Offenders and of a group of prisoners corresponding to the criteria of the O-group. The extent of delinquency in the two groups was compared.

This study was not begun until the final stage of the investigations of the Tübingen Comparative Study of Young Offenders, and only 154 G-subjects could be taken into consideration. Only 39 of the O-subjects could be examined, too few for a differentiated statistical analysis. Therefore, 103 inmates of the penal institutions at Ludwigsburg and Rottenburg who were between 20 and 30 years old and had been sentenced to a term of at least 6 months (and, as a rule, at the most one year) were selected instead, in early 1974. The most important results were compared with those of the O-group, and they did not differ in tendency.

Almost all of the G-subjects (99%) indicated that they had committed at least one of the offenses inquired into at least once. Yet there were considerable differences in view of structure, seriousness, and frequency of offenses. The extent of the subjects' delinquency was measured with an index related to seriousness and frequency of offenses (see SCHÖCH 1976, remark 27). This showed that the average extent of delinquency of the prisoners (index score 28) was seven times as high as that of the G-subjects (index score 4) during the 12 months preceding the study. For the total period, the difference diminished somewhat; this may be related to lack of memory (see below). Furthermore, particularly serious offenses were mentioned almost exclusively by the prisoners (see Table 58).

These differences between prisoners and general population *cannot be traced back to a class-specific delinquency:* In the G-group alone, delinquency was approximately evenly distributed among all social classes (according to "Scheuch-Index," see SCHÖCH 1976, p. 220). Independence of social class became even more obvious in a comparison of the extent of delinquency of the *lower class subjects* of both groups (see Table 59).

Here again, it is obvious that prisoners usually belong to the lower class but that the extent of their delinquency is not at all typical of the lower class (the same holds for social conspicuousness, see Sects. 2.1.3.4, 2.3.4.2, and 2.4.5 above).

As a whole, it became apparent that the actual delinquency of the prisoners differed widely from that of the general population in *qualitative* and *quantitative* respects (also in the lower class). According to HINDELANG et al., these differences may well even be considerably greater as, even if the subjects are willing, their ability to provide correct information on their actual delinquency decreases the more registered offenses they have committed (see HINDELANG et al. 1981, pp. 214 ff.).

Table 58. Serious offenses according to information of subjects[a]

Subjects indicated: "Yes, committed at least once"	Prisoners	G-subjects
Aggravated theft	77%	9%
Motor vehicle theft	63%	12%
Fraud	35%	9%
Robbery	20%	4%
Rape	8%	1%

[a] See SCHÖCH 1976, p. 223 (section of Table 7)

Table 59. Delinquency index of lower class subjects according to information of subjects[a]

Index Score	0-4	5-9	10 or more
G-subjects ($n=51$)	33%	61%	6%
Prisoners ($n=64$)	8%	14%	78%

[a] During the last 12 months; see SCHÖCH 1976, p. 220

Also with respect to the familiar methodological problems related to determining nonregistered delinquency, a limitation to an analysis of registered delinquency seemed appropriate, given the above results. Moreover, the correctness of the information on nonregistered delinquency could not be verified reliably on the basis of further sources of information, in contrast with the other spheres, especially that of registered delinquency. This lack of information from other sources also made it impossible to obtain as comprehensive and differentiated a picture as the one of registered delinquency, which was documented by an average of 50 pages per criminal proceeding.

4.3 The Entire Registered Delinquency of the O-Subjects and Its Sanctioning

4.3.1 Sanctions and Imprisonment

It was expected that the selection criteria for the O-group would mean that many subjects had already had a "criminal career." The sentencing policy in the Federal Republic of Germany at the time of the Tübingen study was such that a prison sentence was usually only executed if other kinds of punishment or measures had not been "successful" or if execution of a prison sentence was necessary considering the seriousness of the offense (as a general preventive measure). Thus, it was not surprising that most of the O-subjects had been convicted several times and had previously received "light sanctions": Including the sentence leading to the imprisonment in the penal institution of Rottenburg, 89% of the O-subjects had already been sentenced at least three times by juvenile or criminal courts (including decisions according to §§27 and 47 in connection with §45 of the Juvenile Court Act); 70% of the subjects had even been sentenced four or more times.

The first sanction had chiefly been relatively lenient and only rarely (11.5%) led to a longer imprisonment: a prison sentence for juveniles for nine subjects and imprisonment without probation for 14. The majority of the subjects (63.5%) had already started their criminal careers as juveniles or adolescents and had been sentenced according to the Youth Welfare Act. Sentences according to the Criminal Code consisted mainly of imprisonment (70%). Longer prison sentences were rarely imposed: The longest sentence for 47% of the subjects had been one year, while only 21% were sentenced to prison for more than two years. Fines (imposed in 30% of the offenses) were also relatively low: 64% of the subjects had never received a fine greater than DM 200.

Apart from weekend arrest, more than three-fourths (78.5%) of the O-subjects had already been *in prison before* the term of imprisonment leading to their selection for the Tübingen study (including pretrial detention), 57% of all O-subjects for at least one month. The average length of imprisonment per term was 6 months, the average total length of imprisonment 16 months.

A total of 44.5% of the subjects had been sent to prison for the first time before the age of 19 (see Table 60), and 23 subjects had spent more than one-fourth of the time from the age of 14 (age of responsibility) to the time of the study in prison, two subjects even more than half.

Table 60. Age at first detention or imprisonment[a]

	O-subjects (n=200)	cum%[b]
14 years	2.0%	2.0%
15 years	4.5%	6.5%
16 years	11.0%	17.5%
17 years	9.0%	26.5%
18 years	8.5%	35.0%
19 years	9.5%	44.5%
20 years and over	34.0%	78.5%
No detention or imprisonment before the present one	21.5%	
Total	100.0%	

[a] See KESKE 1983, p. 56
[b] Cumulated, i.e., the subjects of the preceding age-group are included

If the time spent in reform schools or other closed institutions is included, the number of O-subjects who were never imprisoned decreases to 40 (20%). Yet it must be considered that, even as juveniles, i.e., having reached the age of criminal responsibility, seven subjects were committed to reform schools under the Youth Welfare Act - this in addition to the 58 orders for correctional education under the Juvenile Court Act (see also Sect. 2.2.2.3 above). Including the time spent in reform schools, more than 26 subjects had spent more than one-fourth and 11 subjects more than half of their lives in imprisonment from the age of 14 on, two subjects even more than 85%.

4.3.2 Frequency and Seriousness of Offenses

On average, the O-subjects had been sentenced for a total of 14 (cumulative) offenses (including the sentence leading to their "last" imprisonment). More than half of the subjects had committed more than ten offenses, one-fourth even more than 17, according to their criminal records. The opportunity to commit offenses depends not only on the age of the subjects, but also on how much time they spent in prison. Therefore, the *relative frequency of offenses* of the subjects was calculated per year they were not in prison; this led to an average of four offenses per year. It was shown that a rather considerable number of subjects (30.7%) had committed five or more offenses and more than 60% at least three offenses per year out of prison (see Table 61).

The *damages* caused by property and fraudulent offenses amounted to an average of DM 350; they were less than DM 100 in half of the offenses (calculated according to the value of money in 1970). In only a very few offenses (10%) did the damages exceed DM 1000 (see also Sect. 4.3.5 below). The damages for the victim were not very high in the majority of the other offenses, either (see KESKE 1983, pp. 103 ff.).

Table 61. Annual average of offenses from first registered offense on[a]

	O-subjects ($n=186$)[b]
1 offense	19.9%
2 offenses	21.5%
3 offenses	22.0%
4 offenses	5.9%
5-6 offenses	10.8%
7-12 offenses	13.4%
More than 12 offenses	6.5%

[a] See KESKE 1983, p. 118
[b] As 14 subjects had spent less than 1 year out of prison, they were disregarded

Nonetheless, the total damages were rather high because of the large number of offenses. Thus, it was not so much the *seriousness* of the individual offenses as the *large number* of offenses which finally led to the subjects' being committed to prison.

4.3.3 Typical Offenses

About half (48%) of all of the O-subjects' offenses were *offenses against property*. Most of the O-subjects (89%) had (at least also) been punished for offenses against property (see Table 62). A total of 47% of the subjects committed primarily offenses against property (i.e., more than 50% of the offenses they committed were offenses against property), and these offenses made up more than one-third of the total delinquency of another 11%. Offenses against property consisted mainly of *theft* (for a separate examination of this group, see LIN 1972); 85% of all subjects with offenses against property (also) committed simple theft, 69% (also) aggravated theft (see Table 62).

The subjects chiefly stole objects and money for their own immediate use or consumption (for details, see Sect. 4.5 below). Frequently, the subjects stole objects in or attached to motor vehicles or the motor vehicles themselves. Aggravated theft usually meant (nocturnal) entering or breaking into sales rooms, bars, weekend houses, office or production facilities (often those of former employers), or cars.

The second-largest group of offenses was *traffic delinquency* (20% of all offenses). Two-thirds (67%) of all O-subjects had been convicted for one or several such offenses. A total of 81% of the subjects had been punished for driving without a driver's license, about one-third (33.6%) of them for bodily injury by negligence or for negligent homicide in traffic accidents. Drunken driving, hit-and-run driving, and other kinds of dangerous driving occurred relatively seldom (see Table 62).

It was striking that offenses *in connection with a motor vehicle* (34% of all offenses distributed among 71.5% of the O-subjects) constituted a large section of total delinquency; 62.5% of the O-subjects had been sentenced *solely* for unau-

Table 62. Distribution of individual offenses and offense groups among O-subjects[a]

Offense[b] (according to *Strafgesetzbuch*)	Subjects concerned (n=200)	Subjects for whom this category covers more than 50% of their total offenses	Subjects for whom this category covers 100% of their total offenses	Average number of offenses per subject concerned
1. *Property offenses (in the wider sense), §§ 242ff.*	178	94	8	8.8
Of which Robbery, extortion[c]	30			1.2
Aggravated theft	122			5.5
Simple theft	152			4.4
Unauthorized use of vehicle	48			1.7
Embezzlement	44			1.6
Receiving stolen property	15			1.3
2. *Fraud and dishonest dealings, §§ 263ff.*	95	12	-	4.0
3. *Sexual offenses, §§ 173ff.*	36	7	-	3.8
Of which Rape, indecent assault	10			2.0
Indecency with minor	13			3.0
Homosexuality	7			4.0
Exhibitionism	10			5.1
Procuring	1			1.0
4. *Purely violent offenses, §§ 123f., 185ff., 211ff., 303f.* (except in connection with traffic)	104	5	2	2.9
4.1. Offenses against persons	72			2.3
Of which Injury	54			1.7
- Homicide	4			1.0
- Grievous and dangerous bodily injury	26			1.3
- Minor bodily injury	30			1.8
Coercion, deprivation of liberty	16			1.5
Insult	27			1.9
4.2. Other violent offenses	56	-	-	2.3
Of which Damage to property	37			2.0
Unlawful entry	35			1.5
5. *Traffic offenses*	134	9	-	4.5
Of which Negligent bodily injury or homicide	45			1.2
Failure to stop after or to report an accident	25			1.2
Drunken driving	31			1.5
Other dangerous driving	15			1.1

Table 62 (continued)

Offense[b] (according to *Strafgesetzbuch*)	Subjects concerned ($n=200$)	Subjects for whom this category covers more than 50% of their total offenses	Subjects for whom this category covers 100% of their total offenses	Average number of offenses per subject concerned
Driving without a driver's license	109			3.2
Driving with a noninsured or improperly registered vehicle	31			3.8
6. *Other offenses*	89	-	2	not calculated
Of which Forging documents §§ 267 ff.	38			2.0
Failure to fulfill a maintenance obligation § 170b	13			2.0
Resistance to state authority	7			3.1
Perjury §§ 153 ff.	5			1.4
Offenses against military criminal code	15			1.7
Refusal to do alternative nonmilitary service	2			1.0
Offenses in codes other than the criminal code (not in connection with traffic)	25			1.5

[a] Multiple entries possible; see KESKE 1983, p. 120
[b] Nominally coinciding offenses are counted separately
[c] Extortion and robbery are taken together, as in the police statistics *(Polizeiliche Kriminalstatistik)*

thorized usage or theft (for temporary use) of a motor vehicle or driving without a driver's license or with a vehicle not properly licensed; more than half of them had also stolen motor vehicles.

These were often offenses called "joy-rider" delinquency in the American literature (concerning this concept, see GIBBONS 1977, pp. 308 ff.). In this context, the interest of the offender was mainly driving as such and not the material value of the object (of theft). This "motor vehicle delinquency" - although generally regarded as a typical juvenile offense - was committed as frequently by adolescents and adults as by juveniles: The proportion of subjects for whom "motor vehicle delinquency" was registered was approximately the same in all age-groups (between 56% and 58%). However - as opposed to typical joy-rider delinquency - such offenses did not occur alone, but were accompanied by a varying number of "classic offenses."

Almost half (47.5%) of the O-subjects had committed *fraudulent offenses,* which made up 12% of all offenses. Only 12 subjects primarily committed fraudulent acts; for another three subjects, fraudulent offenses made up more than one-third of their offenses.

As a rule, these fraudulent offenses were not sophisticated. They were similar to theft delinquency in the absence of planning and the way they had been carried out (see also Sect. 4.5 below): In more than three-fourths of the offenses contracts had not been complied with, bills or services not paid, or borrowed objects not returned; in 15% of the offenses, objects stolen by the subjects (including stolen checks) had been turned to account. The remainder consisted to a large extent of mainly occupation-oriented, small-scale cheating.

Violent offenses against persons were relatively rare (5.3% of all offenses). Nevertheless, 36% of the O-subjects had been sentenced for offenses against persons, chiefly for simple bodily injury.

The occasion of these offenses was often an argument in public. In half of the offenses the injuries had been so slight that no medical treatment had been necessary. In only one case (aiding and abetting infanticide) was a person killed with intent. The absence of willful homicide offenses was to be expected, however, on the basis of the selection criteria, as offenders who had committed capital crimes had not been taken into consideration (see also WULF 1979).

Sexual offenses made up a relatively small proportion of the total delinquency of the O-subjects (4.2%); 18% of the subjects had (also) been convicted for sexual offenses. Only seven subjects, however, had primarily committed sexual offenses, four offenses on average. Especially homosexual and exhibitionist acts occurred repeatedly (see Table 62).

4.3.4 The Spectrum of Delinquency of the Individual Subjects

Almost two-thirds (65%) of the subjects had been sentenced for the same category of offenses in more than half of their convictions. The subjects who had primarily committed *offenses against property* (47%) and fraudulent offenses (6%) dominated (see Table 62). Particularly these subjects had also committed an above-average number of offenses (61% more than ten offenses); subjects who had primarily committed other offenses had committed less offenses (88% no more than ten).

Though a number of subjects had primarily committed offenses of one category, a considerable *breadth of variation* in the offenses was rather characteristic of the O-subjects. The more offenses a subject had committed, the more marked was this variation ($\overline{C}=.77$; see KESKE 1983, p. 127). Even when traffic offenses were disregarded, only 31 subjects exclusively committed offenses belonging to *one* common object of legal protection: 18 subjects were exclusively sentenced for offenses against property, three for fraudulent offenses, three for sexual offenses, four for bodily injury, two for refusal to serve in the armed forces or to do alternative nonmilitary service, and one for failing to fulfill his maintenance obligation (from the legal point of view, the elements of an offense often realized in coincidence were disregarded, e.g., deprivation of liberty in rape, or forgery of documents in fraud; see KESKE 1983, pp. 151 ff.).

Even if several subjects had primarily or exclusively committed offenses belonging to one category, they generally did not limit themselves to one specific kind of offense of the category. An exception were *sexual offenders*. Although they were frequently sentenced for a violent offense (insult or bodily injury) committed in coincidence, they usually committed only one specific kind of sexual offense.

Only the offenders who had been convicted for sexual abuse of or indecency with children had additionally (in coincidence or in plurality of acts) committed other sexual offenses (for details, see KESKE 1983, pp. 135 ff.)

4.3.5 The Development of Relative Frequency and Seriousness of Offenses

The majority of the subjects (57%) were convicted for the first time as juveniles, i.e., before the age of 18 (O_1-subjects, see also Sect. 1.3 above). The remaining subjects (O_2-subjects) had no criminal record until they were adolescents ($n=49$) or adults ($n=37$). It should be noted that a subject's first registered offense was not necessarily the first one he committed (see Sect. 4.2.1 above).

From their first registered offense on, the majority of the subjects (53.5%) demonstrated an *increasing relative frequency of offenses* (i.e., related to the time they were not in prison). Yet an obvious intensification of offenses did not occur until adulthood for all subjects (see Table 63).

This does not mean, however, that there was a continuous development in the sense of a steady increase of offenses. More than half of the subjects (53.5%) did not commit any (registered) offenses for prolonged periods of time; almost half of these subjects (47%) had intervals without offenses of more than 3 years. A total of 27 of the subjects with "interruptions" were O_1-subjects who had not committed any registered offenses for an interval of at least 4 years. Their delinquency as juveniles was thus an early delinquent phase not immediately related to the offenses they committed later on. But during the following period as well, their relative frequency of offenses was visibly lower than that of the other O-subjects (see Table 63).

During the periods when the subjects did not commit any offenses, 48.5% of the subjects also exhibited changes in their social behavior, especially in the spheres

Table 63. Development of relative frequency and seriousness of offenses

		Average relative frequency of offenses[a] at the ages of			Average seriousness of offenses[b] at the ages of		
		14–17	18–20	21–PS[c]	14–17	18–20	21–PS[c]
Subjects with first registered offenses as							
Juvenile ($n=114$)	$=O_1$	1.4	1.3	2.6	2.2	2.5	3.3
Adolescent ($n=49$)	$=O_2$	-	1.2	2.1	-	2.3	3.2
Adult ($n=37$)	$=O_2$	-	-	2.0	-	-	3.3
O_1 without interruption ($n=87$)		1.8	1.9	3.1	2.2	2.4	3.2
O_1 with interruption[d] ($n=27$)		.7	.1	1.3	1.8	3.1	3.5

[a] Offenses per year the subject was not in prison
[b] For property and fraudulent offenses (1 point equals a value of up to DM 10, 2 points up to DM 100, 3 points up to DM 350, 4 points up to DM 1000; see SCHINDHELM 1972, p. 98)
[c] Period of study
[d] Interval without offenses of at least 4 years

of family, contacts and performance. Most of the subjects exhibited a stabilization of the sphere of performance, and a considerable number of them ties with a special person of reference.

The development of the *seriousness of offenses* also showed an increasing tendency for all categories of offenders. The amount of damages in the property and fraudulent offenses sentenced last had more than doubled as compared with the first offenses. A differentiation into the individual categories of offenders showed that, on the one hand, the later the subjects committed their first registered offense, the more serious the property and fraudulent offenses were at the beginning of a subject's "criminal career," expressed in points according to the index of SELLIN and WOLFGANG (1964; adapted to the situation of the Federal Republic of Germany, see SCHINDHELM 1972; see also KESKE 1983). On the other hand, the individual groups demonstrated a comparable seriousness of offenses at the same age (see Table 63).

4.3.6 The Development of Offense Types

The structure of the O-subjects' delinquency changed in the course of their criminal careers, as a comparison of the offenses in the subjects' first and last convictions showed (see Table 64).

In particular, property and sexual offenses played a much more substantial role in the total delinquency in the last than in the first convictions of the subjects. This also holds when traffic offenses, which took up a much larger proportion of the first than of the last offenses, are disregarded.

Among the last convictions, the offenses against property were mainly aggravated theft, whereas simple theft dominated in the first convictions. Furthermore, for the last offenses, robbery, extortion, and fraudulent offenses gained importance. Here, the O_1- and the O_2-subjects differed in the way the structure of their

Table 64. Kind of offenses at first and last conviction[a]

	Most serious offense			
	At first conviction		At last conviction	
	(n=200)	(n=157)[b]	(n=200)	(n=198)[b]
Fraudulent offenses	7.0%	(8.9%)	9.0%	(9.1%)
Property offenses	47.5%	(60.5%)	69.5%	(70.2%)
Of these: Robbery and extortion	2.5%	(3.2%)	7.5%	(7.6%)
Aggravated theft	9.0%	(11.5%)	49.0%	(49.5%)
Simple theft	25.0%	(31.9%)	11.0%	(11.1%)
Sexual offenses	4.5%	(5.7%)	10.0%	(10.1%)
Other offenses against persons	5.5%	(7.0%)	4.5%	(4.6%)
Traffic offenses	21.5%	(-)	1.0%	(-)

[a] See KESKE 1983, p. 185
[b] Traffic offenses were disregarded for these figures

delinquency developed: The O_1-subjects had almost exclusively committed offenses against property as juveniles, mainly simple theft. From age-group to age-group, the proportion of aggravated theft increased, fraudulent offenses increasing as well. Correspondingly, the breadth of variation, i.e., the heterogeneity of offenses, rose. The O_2-subjects, however, showed less preference for offenses against property, while fraudulent delinquency played an important role at the beginning of their criminal careers, as opposed to the O_1-subjects.

4.4 The Total Delinquency and Social Conspicuousness of the O-Subjects

The O-group itself was not a homogeneous one. Divided according to criteria of delinquency, the subjects demonstrated differences in social conspicuousness as well. Differentiating between the O_1- and the O_2-subjects alone proved to be extremely useful in all social spheres. A further differentiation of the O-subjects according to onset and development of criminal career and to the character of their offenses also showed differences in the extent of social conspicuousness (see Table 65). This became particularly obvious for "offenses" during childhood (see Sect. 4.2.1 above), for the conspicuousness taken together in the syndrome of lacking occupational adaptation in the sphere of performance (see Sect. 2.3.4.6 above) as well as for the behavior patterns characterizing the leisure and the contact syndromes (see Sects. 2.4.7 and 2.5.7 above).

Accordingly, it became apparent that it was important at what age a criminal career had started: The earlier a subject had committed his first (registered) offense, the more probably had he committed "offenses" during childhood and the more often did he exhibit the performance syndrome, which relates to difficulties in the entire sphere of performance. This relationship was not as obvious for the contact and leisure syndromes. As the contact syndrome related partially and the leisure syndrome exclusively to the period of the study, the differences in conspicuous behavior between early and late delinquents tended to diminish (see Sects. 2.3.4.9, 2.4.6, and 2.5.7 above). For the (relative) frequency of offenses, which was closely related to the onset of criminal career, there was a comparable tendency: The more frequently and rapidly offenses were committed, the more strongly the subjects exhibited these kinds of social conspicuousness.

When the O-subjects were differentiated according to the structure of their delinquency, obvious differences appeared only if the large group of subjects who committed (at least also) *property and fraudulent* offenses was considered as a whole and compared with the remaining group. The subjects without property or fraudulent offenses mainly did not demonstrate as serious kinds of social conspicuousness. Their offenses, however, were rather heterogeneous. Because of the small numbers of subjects, it is impossible to make any unequivocal statement. Yet the subjects who committed only one kind of offense - apart from traffic offenses - seem to be worth mentioning: The four subjects sentenced exclusively for sexual offenses (two subjects for rape, two for exhibitionism) and the two subjects convicted for refusal to serve in the armed forces or to do alternative nonmilitary service demonstrated none of these serious kinds of social conspicuousness, and

Table 65. Delinquency patterns and social conspicuousness of O-subjects

	"Offenses"[a] up to 14 years		Performance syndrome[b]		Leisure syndrome[c]		Contact syndrome[d]	
All subjects	(n=196)[a]	49.5% (97)	(n=199)[b]	42.7% (85)	(n=189)[c]	75.1% (142)	(n=149)[d]	59.7% (89)
Age at onset of delinquency								
14–15 years	(n= 67)	74.6% (50)	(n= 67)	53.7% (36)	(n= 63)	79.4% (50)	(n= 55)	65.5% (36)
16–17 years	(n= 46)	52.2% (24)	(n= 46)	53.2% (25)	(n= 45)	80.0% (36)	(n= 35)	68.6% (24)
18–20 years	(n= 47)	31.9% (15)	(n= 49)	37.5% (18)	(n= 46)	63.0% (29)	(n= 36)	47.2% (17)
21–29 years	(n= 36)	22.2% (8)	(n= 37)	16.2% (6)	(n= 35)	77.1% (27)	(n= 23)	52.2% (12)
Frequency of offenses								
a) Number of offenses								
Up to 10 offenses	(n= 98)	38.8% (38)	(n= 98)	30.6% (30)	(n= 94)	68.1% (64)	(n= 74)	54.1% (40)
More than 10 offenses	(n= 98)	60.2% (59)	(n=101)	54.5% (55)	(n= 95)	82.1% (78)	(n= 75)	65.3% (49)
b) Relative frequency of offenses[e]								
Low (up to 1.6)	(n= 60)	35.0% (21)	(n= 60)	28.3% (17)	(n= 56)	58.9% (33)	(n= 47)	53.2% (25)
Medium (1.7–3.4)	(n= 61)	54.1% (33)	(n= 63)	50.0% (31)	(n= 61)	73.8% (45)	(n= 45)	62.2% (28)
High (3.5 and more)	(n= 61)	62.3% (38)	(n= 63)	54.0% (34)	(n= 58)	89.7% (52)	(n= 46)	67.4% (31)
Property and fraudulent offenses								
Yes	(n=178)	52.3% (93)	(n=185)	45.6% (82)	(n=173)	79.2% (137)	(n=135)	63.7% (86)
No	(n= 19)	21.1% (4)	(n= 19)	15.8% (3)	(n= 16)	31.3% (5)	(n= 14)	21.4% (3)
"Motor vehicle" offenses								
Yes	(n=122)	54.1% (66)	(n=124)	50.0% (62)	(n=121)	80.2% (97)	(n= 90)	67.8% (61)
No	(n= 74)	41.9% (31)	(n= 75)	30.7% (23)	(n= 68)	66.2% (45)	(n= 59)	47.5% (28)

[a] See Sect. 4.2.1 above
[b] See Sect. 2.3.4.6 above
[c] See Sect. 2.4.7 above
[d] See Sect. 2.5.7 above
[e] 14 subjects who had spent less than 1 year out of prison were disregarded; see Sect. 4.3.2 above.

none of the offenders sentenced exclusively for violent offenses (four for minor bodily injury) were conspicuous in the sphere of performance, although two were conspicuous in the sphere of leisure. Of the group of subjects with property and fraudulent offenses, the three offenders who committed only fraudulent offenses differed from the others in that they committed offenses related to their occupations; of these three, only one demonstrated conspicuous behavior in the sphere of leisure.

The group of subjects with *motor-vehicle delinquency,* which was extracted irrespective of categories in criminal law (see Sect. 4.3.3 above), showed an obviously higher extent of social conspicuousness as compared with the other subjects.

These results point relatively roughly to relationships between social conspicuousness and criminal career or certain criteria of offenses. However, this says nothing about the specific interplay between social conspicuousness and the development toward the individual event of the offense (see Sect. 4.6 below).

Unlike social conspicuousness, there were no differences which could be uniformly interpreted for other more external or formal criteria, such as the subject's social class. Regarding intelligence as well, there were practically no differences; for example, the subjects who had also committed fraudulent offenses were only minimally more intelligent than the remaining O-subjects; even the IQ of the three purely occupation-related "defrauders" (98.7) was lower than the average IQ of the G-subjects (see Sect. 3.4.3.2 above).

4.5 The Criminological Appearance of the O-Subjects' Offenses

4.5.1 Criminological Content and Dimension of the Appearance of the Offense

The nature and character of the offenses the O-subjects committed did not become visible beyond legal or formal criteria until the appearance of the offense was examined from a criminological angle. The presentation of the actual event of the offense (see Sect. 4.5.3 below) is divided into the outward appearance of the offense, the object of the offense, the commission of the offense, the modus operandi, the role of the victim, and, where determinable, the dynamics of the offense. Furthermore, the integration of the event during the time (immediately) preceding (see Sect. 4.5.2 below) and following (see Sect. 4.5.4 below) the offense is considered (see GÖPPINGER 1980, pp. 687 ff.). The analysis of the period following the offense concentrates particularly on the reaction of the offender, such as flight or measures to suppress evidence, and on the subject's attitude to the offense after its commission. The analysis of the period preceding the offense concentrates in particular on the immediate relationship between a subject's general behavior, contact persons, alcohol consumption, or mood and the offense.

The following presentation is limited mainly to the "last" offenses of the subjects - in a certain sense representative of all other offenses (see, also for the following, MASCHKE 1986). In order to show the development of the subjects with respect to the commission of offenses as well, previous offenses are referred back to for the most important criteria.

The "last" offenses were basically taken from each subject's last sentence. Offenses which were concurrent in criminal law were considered one offense, the kind of offense being defined according to the main emphasis of the event of the offense. For whole series of offenses, the first offense of the series was considered, for different kinds of offenses which took place within a short period of time, the offense whose documentation was most detailed was taken (especially in view of the periods preceding and following the offense). This choice did not take into consideration the offense which was most characteristic of the individual subject or the (normatively) most serious offense.

The 200 "last" offenses were - with the exception of three traffic offenses - committed with intent. There were 128 offenses against property, 24 fraudulent offenses, 18 sexual offenses, 13 violent offenses, 6 offenses in connection with refusal to serve in the armed forces or to do alternative nonmilitary service, 4 traffic offenses, 3 failures to fulfill maintenance obligations, 3 perjury offenses, and one forgery of documents. The average age of the offenders when they committed the offenses was 23.4 years.

For a number of these offenses, some aspects of the criminological appearance of the offense were not taken into consideration due to the nature of the aspect, for example, the time immediately preceding the offense for continuing offenses such as failure to fulfill maintenance obligations, or the outward appearance of the offense for forgery of documents, perjury offenses, or offenses in connection with refusal to serve in the armed forces or to do alternative nonmilitary service.

4.5.2 The Period Immediately Preceding the Offense

The central question for the period immediately preceding the offense was whether there was a direct relationship between a subject's general behavior, not necessarily directed at the realization of an offense, and the offense itself. Such a relationship became most obvious in **offenses which were committed jointly**: These offenses were practically an inevitable result of the preceding form of leisure organization and contacts: In 73 of the 76 joint offenses, the participants were the contact persons of the subject in connection with going to bars (in about half of the cases in the "milieu") before the offense was undertaken. It was especially significant that in all of the 14 cases in which the subject met previous acquaintances from reform schools or prisons, these acquaintances also participated in the later offense. Moreover, the (12) offenses where roles were differentiated among the groups of offenders belonged to the above cases. For the rest, most (54 of 76) of the joint offenses were committed by casual groups or "cliques" which had formed temporarily while frequenting bars; nine of the offenses were committed by spontaneous groups which had developed in the actual situation of the offense. For one offense, the group could not be categorized.

The examination of the O-subjects' *previous offenses* showed that the form of participation varied for most of the offenses; only 4.5% of the subjects had acted exclusively in groups, 20.5% of the subjects exclusively alone. Other persons had participated in half of the offenses committed by juveniles and adolescents, as compared with one-third of the offenses committed by adults. As a whole, particularly the subjects who had primarily committed property offenses acted jointly (53%), whereas 80% of the subjects who had (primarily) committed fraudulent or sexual offenses had mainly committed their offenses alone.

As in the "last" offenses, the participants in previous offenses had also mainly been loose leisure acquaintances; 10% had been fellow inmates of reform schools or prisons whom the subjects had gone to see after being released or whom they had met in the "milieu," 15% fellow employees, and 10% relatives. In about half of the offenses, the participants had met each other more or less by chance, and the acquaintance had been limited to a one-time cooperation for the purpose of committing an offense. Nonetheless, a prolonged cooperation with one specific person was observed insofar as some subjects had committed several offenses (which had not necessarily succeeded each other immediately) with the same accomplices in the course of their criminal careers. For 70% of all joint offenses, the size of the group had been limited to two offenders, who had mainly not defined any roles or planned any details of the offense before committing it. In about 20% of the offenses, three or more offenders had gotten together to commit chiefly aggravated theft, robbery, bodily injury, and damage to property. Actual gang delinquency in the sense of a relatively stable group of more than two persons who demonstrate a feeling of solidarity and get together for the purpose of committing offenses (see GÖPPINGER 1980, pp. 559 ff.) occurred very rarely: Only 10% of the O-subjects had belonged to such a gang at some point in time. These subjects all had violent offenses among their previous convictions, though they had also primarily committed offenses against property.

A direct relationship between general behavior and committing an offense also became apparent as regards **alcohol consumption** preceding the offense: As far as could be determined, alcohol consumption of some kind had preceded 70% of the "last" offenses. In more than half of the offenses it was considerable, i.e., the subjects had had more than five bottles of beer, or the per mil blood-alcohol concentration (insofar as it was stated in the records) had been 1.5 or more. In about three-fourths of the joint offenses, the participants had also consumed alcohol. This rate of alcohol consumption usually corresponded to the subjects' (or participants') normal rate, without special occasion or intention (see also Sect. 3.4.2.3 above). In only two cases could it be assumed that the effect of alcohol was induced expressly in view of the offense to be committed. Another five subjects wanted to "solve" an acute problem or mood in this way.

Alcohol had also played a significant role in *previous offenses*. Its importance for the commission of offenses could be determined only by indications in records stating that the offenders had gone to bars, etc., and could thus not be determined accurately enough. When only the sentences expressly mentioning the influence of alcohol were considered, about two-thirds (65%) of the subjects had been sentenced at least once, half of them even several times for offenses they had committed under the influence of alcohol; according to his records, one subject had committed all his offenses after considerable alcohol consumption. Not only the subjects who were alcoholics (see Sect. 3.4.2.3 above) had committed their offenses under the influence of alcohol, but also almost half (44%) of the subjects who drank only occasionally. Above-average frequency of alcohol consumption was noted by the courts or the police for bodily injury and sexual offenses, while the sentences and records of interrogation rarely considered the influence of alcohol in the commission of fraudulent offenses, even if there were specific indications.

Finally, the subjects' **mood** before the offense played a considerable role: 15 subjects indicated that they had been angry, mad, or considerably annoyed, with or without occasion, during the hours or even days preceding their "last" offenses.

A total of seven subjects had shown signs of general irritability before the offense; some said that they had been "fed up with everything." Eight subjects indicated that they had been dejected or depressed because of a definite event; one subject said, in contrast, that he had been in extremely high spirits. In five offenses, motoric agitation, impulsiveness, and inability to maintain goal-directed behavior were determined, which the subjects could not explain and which suggested endoreactive urges (see Sect. 3.4.2.2 above).

Several of these complex circumstances occurred in varying intensity and may even have reinforced each other reciprocally immediately before the offense. The danger of committing an offense was thus near at hand. Yet this says nothing about the **actual way the offense came about:** In about 40% of the offenses, a subject recognized and seized a good opportunity - for example an object for theft or a sexual "object"; 17% of the offenses were entirely spontaneous, which does not mean that the subjects had not been basically willing to commit an offense. Four percent of the subjects indicated that they had had an indefinite "feeling that something was going to happen that day" - for example when they had left home. A total of 15% had planned committing a (mainly property or fraudulent) offense ("pulling a job" to get money); another 24% had definite ideas about the offense before they committed it.

Accordingly, only about three-fifths of the "last" **offenses were planned.** For more than half of the offenses, planning the specific deed meant "having a look" at something to see whether there was anything worth stealing, "getting even" with someone, or "trying it" with a woman. Barely 30% of the "last" offenses were thoroughly planned, and alternative methods had been considered in only 4%. Only for these last eight offenses did the planning and preparations include the possibility of being caught in the very act, procuring an alibi, and measures to suppress evidence, or flight. For property and fraudulent offenses in particular, it would seem likely that the subjects would have some idea as to how stolen goods or advantages should be used. Yet it became apparent from the indications and behavior of the subjects and the kinds of stolen goods that the subjects had not thought about the stolen goods and their use at all in 15 of these offenses.

In *previous offenses,* perpetration according to a plan was also more the exception than the rule for 15% of all offenses committed by the O-subjects; another 29% of the offenses had been roughly planned. Mainly, however, offenses were committed "by chance" (11.5%), or "good opportunities" were seized (39.5%). In most cases, however, there had been a latent willingness to commit an offense, although this willingness was not directed at a definite offense. Another 5% of the offenses were committed "in the heat of passion" in the widest sense. The planning of offenses was dependent on age: The proportion of (at least roughly) planned offenses rose from 32% to 44% at adulthood for the O_1-subjects, while the O_2-subjects had planned about half of their offenses from the outset.

4.5.3 The Event of the Offense

The evaluation of the **outward appearance of the offense** showed that the *days on which offenses were committed* were rather evenly distributed among the days of the week; there was no concentration of offenses during the weekend, for example. This was not surprising, considering that, in the end, the majority of the subjects had no ordered sphere of performance with a corresponding structuring of time. About 60% of the O-subjects had not worked on the day they committed the offense, either because they had stayed away from work unexcused or on the pretext of being ill, or because they had no longer been working regularly at all at that time; for one-third of the subjects there had been a shift of their entire daily routine, their day usually beginning in the afternoon and ending early in the morning.

With respect to the *time of day* offenses were committed, there was a concentration of offenses during the night, in particular between 10 p.m. and 3 a.m., while only a few offenses were committed between 3 a.m. and 6 a.m. This shows once again how frequently there is a relationship between committing offenses, not only offenses against property, and going to bars (with the corresponding contacts).

The distribution in percent of the *places offenses were committed* among urban and rural areas agreed to a large extent with the corresponding distribution of official place of residence or actual place of abode (see Sect. 2.2.3 above) as well as last place of leisure. Almost two-thirds of the subjects committed their "last" offenses at the place they were living or at least staying for a few days and also spending their leisure time immediately before the offense. For another 17%, the subject's last place of leisure coincided with the place he committed the offense. For only 9% of the subjects were all three places in different municipalities. Furthermore, the *place of offense in the stricter sense* (i.e., street, neighborhood, etc.) was often very close to the previous place of leisure: It was identical in 28% of the offenses, and the place of the offense could be easily reached on foot in another 43%. In only 28% of the offenses was the last place of leisure so far away from the place the offense was committed that a motor vehicle was necessary to get from one to the other.

A total of 12% of the offenses were committed in the subject's own neighborhood, 29% in business or shopping areas or in the downtown bar districts, about 25% in neighborhoods other than the subject's, about 15% in industrial zones or shopping centers at the edge of town, and another 15% in colonies of summerhouses or weekend houses or in the countryside. The remaining offenses were immediately associated with traffic.

Thus, to a large extent, the offenses - according to aspects relating to place - occurred in the subjects' *immediate social environment*. This became especially obvious for burglary: Numerous objects had already been known to the offender in some form; for example, the objects of theft were at a former place of work, or the offender came back to the bar he had just left to steal something. Especially remarkable was the importance of cars: In about one-fifth of the offenses against property, cars played a role as the immediate object to be stolen or to break into (see Sect. 4.3.3 above).

Although the "last" offenses took place mainly in the immediate social environment, only 20% of the offenders had been well acquainted with their **victims** before the offense; the rest had known the victims slightly (14%) or not at all (28%), or the victims were anonymous (38%) (concerning the relationship between offender and victim, see GÖPPINGER 1980, pp. 594ff.). Even in the sexual offenses, which are often regarded as offenses of the immediate environment, about two-thirds of the victims were not known to the offenders. The victim as an individual was not only unimportant and entirely interchangeable in property and fraudulent offenses, but also in most of the sexual and violent offenses: The offense could just as well have been directed against another person. In only 16% of the "last" offenses did the offender seek a particular victim (mainly offenses against persons, in two cases burglary as "revenge").

In the *previous offenses,* the proportion of entirely interchangeable victims increased to 92%, the victims of sexual offenses being almost as interchangeable (92%) as the victims of property and fraudulent offenses (about 96%), usually even if the offenders did know the victims beforehand. Most of the offenses, however, were directed against unknown victims (55%); a certain exception were the sexual offenses, in the sense that the victim was more frequently (60%) known to the offender before he committed the offense.

An *offense-specific behavior of the victim* with respect to facilitating or actively contributing toward the offense was determined in only 3% of the cases. A marked *offender-victim affinity,* in the sense that offender and victim were "partners" in the offense and that it was a matter of greater physical or mental faculties or of chance who became the victim and who the offender (see GÖPPINGER 1980, pp. 596ff.) could be assumed for three (violent) offenses.

For the **commission of the offenses** there were no special aspects, beyond the circumstances which were necessary to make the offenses amount to the corresponding legal definition. The *modus operandi* showed no particularities for two-thirds of the subjects either. A total of 14% of the offenses were marked by a rather differentiated procedure, another 14% by especially brash methods. The procedure was particularly naive or even simple in about 7% of the offenses. Insofar as the offenses were *planned* in detail at all (besides a noncommittal reflection), the *commission of the offense* corresponded with the plan in 85% of the offenses; in only one case did it go further, and in the remaining cases it did not correspond to the plan.

A total of 17.5% of the offenses developed a certain degree of *own dynamics.* This made the offender lose control of the course of the offense, at least partially. In 11 of these cases, the dynamics of the offense were due to actions of the offender, in another 11 to actions of the victim (especially self-defense) or to the offender being caught in the very act. In two cases (one sexual and one violent offense), the course of the offense escalated because of the offender and the victim together.

4.5.4 The Period Following the Offense

How unimportant, in part almost "normal" an offense was for many of the subjects was shown not least in the way the subjects behaved after the offense: Mainly, there were no special **reactions** differing from the subjects' usual behavior. Only 7% of the offenders exhibited behavior which could be called "losing one's head". Of the 23 offenders (11.5%) who were caught *in the very act,* 11 tried to avoid being apprehended by the police by fleeing or hiding, one offender put up resistance, and the remaining subjects did not resist being arrested at all. About three-fourths of the subjects were not arrested until after the *police had investigated* the offense. A total of 14 subjects voluntarily gave themselves up to the police after some time - one, who had to expect being arrested soon, immediately after committing the offense. *Measures to suppress evidence or preparations for escape* were undertaken by relatively few offenders: 12% took to flight after the offense, over and above leaving the place where the offense was committed; 13.5% took some kind of measures to suppress evidence.

In the property and fraudulent offenses, the **stolen goods** - if there were any (not so in about 20% of the offenses) - were turned to account immediately and used for the *satisfaction of immediate needs:* Motor vehicles were used to drive around in, stolen alcohol and food consumed, or money used to purchase alcohol, cigarettes, etc. In only five cases were the stolen goods hoarded for no obvious reason or given away with no apparent advantage. Insofar as the stolen goods were obtained in offenses committed jointly, they were divided equally in 80% of the offenses; in 7% the share of the subject was smaller, in 13% larger than the shares of the participants.

Of the 72 subjects (36%) who were immediately confronted with the person of the victim in the course of the (property, sexual, violent) offense, only six took care of the victim either immediately after the offense or later on. Other attempts at *redress* were an exception (7% of the offenses).

In the framework of the investigations, it was attempted to get to know the **subjects' attitudes** toward their "last" offenses after they committed them. Statements made to the police and the court were disregarded, as the subjects may well have made these statements to protect themselves, considering their situation. In view of the many previous (and in some cases subsequent; see Sect. 4.6 below) offenses they had committed, the subjects often no longer precisely remembered the specific offense or remembered it only after some reflection or after being provided with further information. In about 24% of the cases, the offense seemed to have left no impression. For the rest, the subjects mainly limited themselves to justifying the offense, glossing over the information of the court, or denying having committed the offense (39%); 17% of the subjects felt self-pity, especially with respect to the sentence they had to serve. Apart from some cases which cannot be clearly classified, only nine subjects indicated repentance or (later) pity for the victim, though there had been an immediate, partially severe confrontation between offender and victim for a number of "last" offenses. On the other hand, seven subjects whose "last" offenses had been offenses against property were relatively consternated by the fact that they had committed offenses at all, or these "last" offenses in particular.

4.6 The Development of Offenses out of Certain Situations in the O-Subjects' Lives

A further aim of the study was to gain access to the actual interplay between a certain behavior and the event of the offense (see MASCHKE 1986) beyond the statistical correlations between socially conspicuous or O-characteristic behavior patterns and criminality (see Sect. 4.4 above). For this purpose - again representative of all other offenses - it was examined how long before the "last" offenses acute conspicuousness had occurred in the social spheres by referring back to the days and weeks preceding the "last" offense of each O-subject. The conspicuous behavior patterns in the *spheres of leisure and contacts* at the time of the offense could be traced back furthest, whereas the situation in the *sphere of performance* at the time of the offense (about half of the O-subjects exhibited conspicuousness such as nonemployment or staying away from work unexcused or on the pretext of being ill) had existed in this acute form for only a few days or at most a few weeks before the subjects committed their "last" offenses. This does not mean, however, that there had been no conspicuousness in sphere of performance before, for example conspicuousness indicating the presence of the syndrome of lacking occupational adaptation (see Sect. 2.3.4.6 above). The situation in the *sphere of abode* was less unequivocal, although there had been an acute deterioration during the weeks and months preceding the offense for about one-third of the subjects (for ten subjects only during the days preceding the offense), who had given up their abode and roamed about or found temporary places to sleep.

Nevertheless, the O-subjects were also heterogeneous insofar as not *all* "last" offenses developed from such critical situations and not *all* social spheres were affected in this way during the period preceding the offense for most of the subjects.

Even for the O-subjects who had developed criminal careers in the sense of repeated convictions and serving of sentences (see Sects. 4.3.1 and 4.3.5 above), the O-characteristic behavior patterns noted in the individual social spheres did not always occur in the same extreme form. Repeatedly, there were periods during which the subjects had at least made attempts to change their behavior. In contrast, there were also times during which the individual subjects had expressed O-specific behavior patterns very obviously, which, as a rule, led to delinquency (again) at some time.

Despite a certain arbitrariness of the specific kind of offense and the multiformity of the actual courses of occurrences and situations in life, it was possible - beyond the rough division into property, fraudulent, sexual, violent, etc. offenses (according to the kind of object of legal protection violated) - to determine comparable situations in life leading to offenses. In accordance with the degree of logical consistency with which a certain life pattern or even only a particular social situation led to an offense, a broad spectrum resulted: The cases where the offenses seemed almost inevitable constituted one extreme, since the corresponding life pattern could be kept up only by the commission of an offense. The cases where the current social situation of the subject in no way indicated a "danger" of criminality formed the other extreme. The following "typical" forms occurred:

For a group of 30 O-subjects (15%) whose "last" offenses had been against property, the offenses were *practically inevitable* on the basis of the subjects' behavior, mainly in the spheres of performance and abode, and therefore also in the sphere of leisure, as a consequence of a total shift in their daily routines. Their *life-style* had gotten the subjects into a *critical situation:* They no longer had the means to support themselves. Thus, they had the choice of changing their life-style fundamentally by taking any job they were offered (which was basically possible at that time due to full employment) or by obtaining the means they needed by committing an offense. As the first alternative was out of the question, owing to the vicious circle they were caught up in, they committed an offense.

In detail, there were the subjects who had no fixed abode and who were "on the road" without working, either because they had just been released (two subjects) or had just escaped (five subjects) from prison or reform schools or had decided to give up job and dwelling to "see things," "go to sea," "take a trip," etc. (eight subjects), or because they had had no fixed abode or income for quite some time but had found food and drink and temporary places to sleep in some way and had now lost these opportunities (15 subjects). These subjects thus lived "from hand to mouth." In this situation, some subjects could remain without committing an offense for some days, others for merely a few hours (especially after being released or escaping from prison): The subjects soon committed offenses to satisfy their elementary needs, especially offenses in the form of - usually at least roughly planned - simple theft, burglary, or unlawful entry to obtain money, food, a place to stay at night (mainly in weekend houses), or a means of transportation (bicycle, moped, car). Apart from two subjects who were arrested immediately after the offense, the "last" offenses of 28 subjects (according to the selection, as first offenses of series - see Sect. 4.5.1 above) were the "first" ones of series of similar offenses, which were their means of supporting themselves until they were arrested.

Offenses also developed from a similar critical situation caused by changes in all social spheres for several other subjects: for four, a fraudulent offense (cheating hotels and restaurants and defrauding a car-rental service) and for three draftees, desertion. These offenses were also the first ones in series of fraud and theft to satisfy elementary needs.

Also closely related with their previous life-style, which, however, had already lasted for some time, were the "last" offenses (against property) of a group of 27 O-subjects (13.5%). Yet for this group, it was not so much a (self-induced) social exigency or the satisfaction of elementary needs as it were *unrealistic (material) aspirations* and a lack of willingness either to realize aspirations by working accordingly or to reduce expectations which were important (for the criteria "inadequately high level of aspirations", see Sect. 3.4.4 above and Part III, Sect. 3.3.3.3). But also for this group, breaking out of one's life pattern in favor of a total change and new orientation was irrelevant.

Because of their difficult financial situation (in about two-thirds of the cases due to insufficient work performance) or their aspirations (about four-fifths of the subjects had spent money "unnecessarily," particularly for leisure, during the period preceding the "last" offenses), the subjects decided to improve their financial situation by committing offenses: Apart from two cases of robbery or extortionary robbery, these were usually planned burglaries (especially of factory buildings or scrap-yards, where large amounts of scrap metal were stolen), half of which were committed jointly in a relatively differentiated way (organization of instruments, means of transportation, etc.), and the commission and planning had largely been identical. The stolen goods were usually sold immediately - mainly to fences the subjects already knew. The first such offenses led to further offenses of the same kind in two-thirds of the cases.

A comparable situation was noted for another 17 subjects whose "last" offenses were fraudulent ones. In order to improve their financial situation, they had committed check and credit fraud or had defrauded their employers or clients.

A third group also demonstrated serious social conspicuousness in the various social spheres. Decisive for the offense, however, was less the general situation in life than the specific situation immediately before the offenses: They were almost necessarily connected with going to a bar in the evening, (considerable) alcohol consumption, and, in most cases, contacts with buddies and "carousers." After such a "half-started evening" and thus a basically *unsatisfactory leisure situation*, something "had to happen" - often out of a combination of boredom and an urge for activity. This would not necessarily have meant an offense (for others); however, in the framework of the subjects' basic view of life and their value orientation, this did lead to illicit (and punishable) acts. The behavior of the individual subjects of this group was very heterogeneous; there were mainly offenses against property, but also a large number of sexual and violent offenses.

For one subgroup (13 O-subjects), good opportunities were spontaneously seized after extensive carousing and considerable alcohol consumption. In nine cases, shop windows were robbed on the way home at night, usually without prior reflection or planning; in four cases, fellow carousers or passersby were robbed, also relatively spontaneously.

Of the 13 violent offenses, eight were committed in a similar situation: Brawls ensued with fellow carousers, or passersby were abused or attacked (usually on the way home).

For a second subgroup (22 O-subjects), the idea of "pulling a job" developed in discussions with buddies and fellow carousers, or relatively concrete ideas of offenses were discussed and the decision taken to commit the offense. The offenses (mainly stealing from vending machines and burglaries of offices, warehouses, factories, or cars) were planned and considered. Half of these offenses were marked by a differentiated, sometimes even sophisticated procedure. Their purpose was always to obtain money. In 80% of these cases, similar offenses were committed in the course of the following days or weeks.

In another case, a similar situation led to the - very differentiated - planning and realization of the kidnapping and rape of a prostitute among a group of carousers.

The third subgroup - relatively homogeneous with respect to the way the offenses were committed - covered 22 O-subjects who, after going to a bar and consuming alcohol, yet without any discernible influence by fellow carousers or buddies and without any other participants, seized or looked for a good opportunity or relatively purposefully committed a planned burglary either in the bar or on the way home. Here again, the "last" offenses were the first ones in series of similar offenses in about half of the cases.

The situation of three sexual offenses where a female passerby was raped while the subject was on his way home from a bar is comparable to the preceding one.

For a last group, the commission of the "last" offenses was even more limited to the actual situation and much less related to the general situation in life than for the aforementioned groups. The offenses could thus not be traced back to the subjects' other circumstances in life. These offenders (15) seized specific, "tempting" *opportunities in their immediate social environment.*

Insofar as offenses against property were concerned (11 cases), the subjects had free access to the place of the victim and knew their way around. They were regarded as belonging there and were trusted or at least not distrusted. The offenses were mainly spontaneous and thoughtless simple theft (in another four cases fraudulent acts) at the expense of relatives, fiancees, girlfriends, fellow employees, employers, schoolmates, or landlords. The stolen goods were usually insignificant, and the subject was almost inevitably suspected.

A "tempting" situation in the immediate social environment also led to three sexual offenses (sexual contacts with stepsister, mother, or nephew) and one violent offense ("rearing" the child of a girlfriend by maltreatment).

For the remaining 32 O-subjects (16%), the "last" offenses could not be categorized according to these aspects. The offenses, ranging from traffic delinquency to sexual offenses, perjury and failure to fulfill a maintenance obligation, and attempted homicide, as well as the situations in life and personal circumstances connected with the offenses form a wide spectrum. At one extreme there were the eight subjects whose offenses were connected with a deviant sexual drive (three exhibitionists, four pedophiles, and one fetishist). At the other extreme there were the two Jehovah's witnesses who refused to do alternative nonmilitary service: They committed their offense out of an entirely inconspicuous social situation, although not by chance, but because of a rational decision on the basis of ethical principles.

The center of this broad spectrum of situations in life and courses of occurrences were the four "typical" forms described in detail above. Most (84%) of the "last" offenses could be assigned to one of these categories. In these offenses it was an external - self-induced - exigency, an incomplete and thus unsatisfactory (social) situation on the evening of the offense, a "tempting" opportunity in the immediate social environment, or unrealistic aspirations which led to the offenses. These offenses had in common a close relationship with the *specific life-style of the subjects*; partially, they were even typical of them (for a complex, overall view of the offender in the context of his social relationships, see Part III). Thus, as in the other spheres, an "unchecked living in the immediate present" became apparent with many offenses: the desire to satisfy immediately spontaneous desires and needs arising from the momentary situation regardless of any harmful effects (see Sect. 3.4.4 above). People with a socially customary life-style and a corresponding value orientation, in contrast, would probably not have perceived the "good" opportunity as such, just as they would not end an unsatisfactory leisure situation in this way or realize their aspirations by committing offenses or even have a life pattern leading to a crime-prone exigency (see also Part III, Sect. 4.3).

4.7 The Registered Delinquency of the G-Subjects

4.7.1 Offenses and Sanctions

Up to the time of the study, 47 G-subjects had been previously convicted. The extent of previous convictions of the G-subjects (23.5%) was somewhat lower than that of the corresponding population, which, according to Keske (1979), is an average of 25% to 30% for the Federal Republic of Germany (for possible reasons for this, see Part I, Sect. 2.3). Of the G-subjects with previous convictions, 32 had been sentenced exclusively for traffic offenses, 15 for "classic" offenses (five of these additionally for traffic offenses).

The *"classic" offenses* were mainly offenses against property (six cases of simple theft, one case of aggravated theft, and one aggravated embezzlement). Furthermore, there were two cases of dangerous bodily injury, one attempted aggravated indecency with minors, two cases of unlawful entry, and two insults.

Six of the G-subjects previously convicted for "classic" offenses had already had a criminal record: One subject had committed a "classic" offense, five subjects traffic offenses (of these three repeatedly, i.e., up to four times). The traffic offenses were never immediately related to the commission of a "classic" offense.

With respect to the *criminological appearance* of these "classic" offenses, almost half were committed *jointly*, some with only one partner, some also with a clique. The G-subjects, however, always played a less important role in the group or were hangers-on. It seems noteworthy as well that the subjects' average age when they committed the offenses was 18 for those who committed offenses jointly and 22 for those who committed the offense alone.

The G-subjects' offenses were mainly not even roughly *planned*. The subjects seized "good opportunities" (particularly where offenses against property were concerned), acted spontaneously (for the violent offenses, e.g., in the form of brawls in bars, insulting police officers during an inspection, refusal to leave a bar) or participated in offenses organized by third persons (stealing cigarettes from vending machines and breaking into summerhouses or weekend houses under the influence of a clique). The *commission of the offenses* was more awkward than sophisticated. Not least for this reason, the subjects - if they had not been caught in the very act - were soon arrested by the police. The value of the *stolen goods* in the offenses against property ranged from DM 3 to DM 400, with one exception (DM 1200; embezzlement of musical instruments bought under reservation of ownership). Most of the stolen goods were used immediately. Except for two cases of theft at a subject's place of work, the victims were not known to the subjects.

Seven G-subjects were sentenced according to the Juvenile Criminal Code (two reprimands, two fines, two weekend arrests, and one order to perform work), eight subjects according to the Criminal Code: six to a fine (average DM 270) and two to a prison sentence on probation.

The delinquency of the G-subjects who had been sentenced *exclusively* for offenses in connection with *traffic* consisted of the following: 18 cases of negligent bodily injury, six cases of drunken driving, five cases of failing to stop after an accident or to report an accident, two cases of driving without a driver's license, and six other traffic offenses. Four subjects had been previously convicted for the same kind of offense once, two subjects twice. The average age of the subjects when they committed the offenses was 21.6 years for these "traffic delinquents," as opposed to 20 years for the subjects with "classic" offenses.

4.7.2 The Social Conspicuousness of the Previously Convicted G-Subjects

As (recidivist) criminality was usually accompanied by serious social conspicuousness in the O-group, it could be assumed that this would also be so for the G-group - though to a lesser degree. At first sight, the G-subjects seemed to form a relatively homogeneous group with respect to the extremes of the O-group: Only four of the 47 previously convicted and three of the 153 not previously convicted G-subjects exhibited one of the syndromes of social conspicuousness (see Sects. 2.1.4, 2.3.4.6, 2.4.7, and 2.5.7 above). Though the lives of the G-subjects with previous convictions was thus not marked by social conspicuousness, the period during which the offense was committed was characterized by a certain conspicuousness in the social spheres. The following differences became apparent:

The "*traffic delinquents,*" i.e., the subjects who had been convicted exclusively for offenses in connection with traffic, did not differ from the remaining G-group; offenses were committed out of an otherwise inconspicuous social life pattern (regarding the criminology of traffic offenses, see also GÖPPINGER 1960).

Some of the G-subjects with "*classic*" *previous convictions* - in particular those who had committed offenses against property - demonstrated behavior patterns comparable to those of the O-group, at least temporarily. These disruptions were chiefly less intensive and extensive than those of the majority of the recidivist O-subjects (sentenced for property and fraudulent offenses): Three of the eight G-subjects punished for offenses against property were conspicuous in the spheres of performance, leisure, and contacts during the period when they committed the offense.

The subjects had mainly hung out with previously convicted "buddies" or hoodlum gangs during their leisure time and had consumed an increased amount of alcohol; one subject had then frequently stayed away from work, one had often come to work late and one had given up his job without any prospect of a new one. The offenses were committed under the influence of the "buddies" or hoodlum gang.

The conspicuousness of three subjects sentenced for offenses against property and two sentenced for violent offenses was limited to the spheres of leisure and contacts (especially in the form of excessive alcohol consumption and frequent "milieu" contacts). These G-subjects with "classic" previous convictions had had contacts with previously convicted or other conspicuous persons during the period when they committed the offenses. They had come into contact with the "milieu" by chance together with others (e.g., fellow employees). It seems noteworthy that the four G-subjects who were members of a hoodlum gang definitely left these groups after they committed the offense or after they were convicted. In other respects as well, the delinquent G-subjects showed a rather obvious stabilization in their social behavior after the commission of the offenses or after the court proceedings.

4.8 Summary

By reason of the selection criteria for the O-group, it was to be expected that the O-subjects - apart from the offenses leading to their selection for the study - would show a higher extent of delinquency than the G-subjects. On the one hand, this was confirmed by the fact that almost two-thirds of the O-subjects had started their "criminal careers" as juveniles or adolescents and had been repeatedly convicted for numerous offenses. On the other hand, on the basis of an additional study, it could be assumed that, irrespective of registered delinquency, the *actual extent of delinquency* (i.e., registered and nonregistered offenses together) was much higher for the O- than for the G-subjects or the general population with respect to seriousness and frequency of offenses. Furthermore, it was shown that the O-subjects, particularly the O_1-subjects, had been more seriously conspicuous during childhood than the G-subjects in the sense of "offenses" or social conspicuousness.

Offenses against property in the form of simple or aggravated theft, followed by traffic, fraudulent, violent, and sexual offenses were typical of the *registered delinquency* of the O-subjects. Offenses involving motor vehicles held a special position in total delinquency. The subjects concerned not only committed "joy-rider" offenses, but "classic" ones as well. Despite an obvious emphasis on certain offenses, the O-subjects' spectrum of delinquency was marked by a certain breadth of variation; only exceptionally did a subject limit himself to offenses against one specific object of legal protection.

The numerous offenses (the average O-subject committed four offenses per year he was not in prison) were not very serious when considered individually; taken as a whole, however, they amounted to considerable total damages. The offenses mainly occurred rather arbitrarily, out of a situation, and were not planned in any detail; often, the subjects simply seized good opportunities. Of much greater importance for offenses were the contacts with certain people during the period immediately preceding the offense and alcohol consumption in particular. The offenses themselves usually occurred - from the point of view of place - in the immediate social environment of the subjects, usually rather incidentally and in a very unsophisticated way. The victims were mainly entirely interchangeable, and the stolen goods obtained in the property and fraudulent offenses mostly served to satisfy immediate needs.

In the course of their criminal careers, the structure of the delinquency of the O-subjects changed mainly in favor of offenses against property. Sexual offenses also increased in importance in total delinquency as compared with the first sentences of the subjects. The majority of the O-subjects showed an increasing relative frequency and seriousness of offenses, particularly at adulthood. These developments did not take place steadily and continuously; there were repeated intervals without registered delinquency, and almost all of the O-subjects demonstrated intervals without any offenses during which there were changes in other social spheres as well.

The *relationship between delinquency and social conspicuousness* was also shown in other respects: The differentiation of the O-group into early and late delinquents yielded visible differences in all social spheres. A more detailed differentiation was made according to age at first offense. It became apparent that conspicuousness in the sphere of performance, as expressed in the performance syndrome, as well as "offenses" during childhood, were all the more marked the earlier a subject had committed his first offense. Not as obvious was the relationship between the leisure and contact syndromes and age at first offense. Subjects without property or fraudulent offenses were less conspicuous as a whole; subjects with "motor vehicle delinquency," in contrast, were very markedly conspicuous.

The relationship between social conspicuousness and delinquency often became even more obvious in the analysis of the situations in life out of which offenses were committed: Apart from a few exceptions, the period of the offense was mainly characterized - as compared with the period before - by more marked social conspicuousness in one or more social spheres. Essentially, four "typical" courses of occurrences could be distinguished, to which 84% of the "last" offenses could be assigned: One course was a social exigency the subjects themselves had induced by a certain life-style, an exigency which could be resolved only by the commission of an offense, since the subjects had become used to the specific life-style and adhered to their value orientation. Then there was the "half-started" and not entirely satisfactory course of an evening, during which - after alcohol consumption, often among "buddies" - "something" had to happen. Furthermore, there were unrealistic aspirations or "tempting" opportunities in the immediate social environment. The decisive point was that these situations would presumably have been solved differently, i. e., not through the commission of offenses, by persons with another life-style and value orientation.

The offenses of the O-subjects mainly reflect behavior patterns similar to those in the other social spheres (see Sect. 3.4.4 above): In many of their offenses, an "unchecked living in the immediate present" became apparent as well: a short time perspective and a low tolerance for stress. Furthermore, for the subgroup of the subjects who had committed property offenses or fraud, the offenses were directly related to their "inadequately high" level of aspirations. On the whole, the impression arose that the offenses were not an alien, but a "normal" element in the lives of most (but not all) O-subjects, belonging to their specific way of life as did their remaining (socially conspicuous) behavior patterns.

In contrast, the offenses of previously convicted G-subjects (23.5%) did not fit into their lives as a whole in a similar way. Although the 15 G-subjects previously convicted for "classic" offenses had partially shown considerable conspicuousness during the period when they had committed the offenses, the conspicuousness and the offenses themselves were isolated episodes in their lives. The offenses, or their punishment, were a turning point, insofar as the subjects' behavior largely consolidated during the period that followed. The behavior of the G-subjects whose offenses were connected exclusively with traffic did not differ at all from that of the entire G-group: They demonstrated no serious social conspicuousness before, during, or after the period of the offenses.

Alone by reason of the specific selection criteria for the groups of the study - related to the measure of punishment and thus also to delinquency for the O-group - a direct comparison between the results on the sphere of delinquency of the O-subjects and the corresponding results of other multifactorial studies was impossible. Here, in particular, was the problem that statutory definitions of offenses and sanctions in the various legal systems cannot be compared; this was apparent in the Anglo-American concept of "delinquency". In the *literature,* information usually does not go beyond a statement of the (delinquency-specific) selection criteria and some individual aspects concerning the criminological appearance of the offense. Also, aspects comparable to the present ones concerning situations in life and courses of occurrences are only rarely considered. WEST (1982, pp. 24 ff.), for example, discusses this area extensively and mentions as reasons for committing the offense (a) enjoyment, (b) group solidarity, and (c) the desire for material gain. Attitudes possibly connected with a specific way of life and underlying offenses are considered in *Statens offentliga utredningar* (1971, pp. 154 ff.), where it is indicated that most offenses showed traces of immaturity and inability to control impulses and desires.

5 Survey of the Individual Findings

A complex view aimed at the *integration* of the individual results of the present chapter soon reaches its limits on the statistical level. Combining only a few characteristics from all individual spheres to see whether they occur for each individual subject would automatically entail very small subgroups, and finally only individual cases. This dilemma also applies in principle for studies with a significantly larger number of subjects. The solution provided by multivariate methods such as factor analysis, which calculate statistically related characteristics as "factors" - whether they *actually* occur together for each individual subject or not, was not applied in the present study as a matter of principle (see Part III, Sect. 1) and for methodological reasons (see Part I, Sect. 4). Instead, links connecting the individual spheres are established, as has already been done in part (see Sect. 2 above), and the *concurrence of particularly important criteria* from the various spheres is examined (see Fig. 1).

The **medical, psychiatric, and psychological eaminations**, which were not and did not claim to be exhaustive, provided only a few findings which distinguished clearly between the groups. In the *somatic area* (see Sects. 3.2 and 3.3 above), damage to the extremities and the trunk occurred clearly more often in the comparison (G-)group, while, on the basis of the information of the subjects (which could not be verified), internal illnesses and head injuries, as well as externally visible somatic conspicuousness more frequently occurred in the offender (O-)group. However, the number of subjects concerned was partially very small. Moreover, the interpretation of these findings should also take into account the entirely different life-styles of the two groups - that of the O-subjects involved many more risks - which may have had physical effects (e.g., head injuries). The somatic examinations did not point to any relationship between the investigated conspicuousness and criminality. The EEG examinations and cytogenetic tests did not lead to any meaningful results in this respect, and the *psychopathological examinations* (see Sect. 3.4 above) did not provide for any scientifically meaningful differentiation between the O- and the G-subjects either. Alcohol (and drug) consumption as a problem of *addiction* was of practically no importance, though the O- and the G-subjects' form and extent of drinking differed considerably. This was closely related with their remaining social behavior and partially with the commission of offenses (see Sect. 4.6 above). The endoreactive urges, which occurred frequently for the O-subjects, but whose genesis is yet unclear, were of special importance.

With the *psychological tests,* it was possible to distinguish between O- and G-personalities in individual respects. The differences were not uniform, partially even contradictory, and thus did not lead any further. The examination of intelligence, in contrast, showed unambiguous differences: Compared with the G-subjects, the O-subjects had a visibly lower average intelligence, mainly due to an overrepresentation of subjects with an IQ under 90. In the medium range (91-110), both groups were almost evenly represented. The fact that the subjects of medium intelligence from the O- and the G-group performed very differently in school showed how unimportant intelligence alone is.

That the psychological tests and psychopathological examinations did not provide many important results only means that no essential differences in personality could be found *in the situation of the examination itself*, with the given methods. However, on the basis of the behavior patterns of the O-subjects which occurred time and again in certain social situations, *specific attitudes* became apparent which went together with their conspicuous social behavior or constituted its foundation. In its extreme form, this conspicuousness was expressed in an *unchecked living in the immediate present,* without any structuring or planning and marked by an immediate satisfaction of needs and corresponding actions and attitudes (see Sect. 3.4.4 above). Not all O-subjects could be characterized in this way. Yet, the older the subjects, the more marked these occurrences became and the more social spheres were concerned, so that this conspicuousness applied to the majority of the O-subjects.

Accordingly, the findings throughout the *social spheres* presented a relatively uniform picture. The O-subjects were seriously conspicuous in all the spheres as compared with the general (G-)population, increasingly so the older they were. The earlier and more marked the conspicuousness, the earlier did delinquency occur.

In the **sphere of the family of orientation** (see Sect. 2.1 above), the O-subjects were mainly subject to more strains in external and internal circumstances. On average, their families had a lower socioeconomic status and demonstrated various problems of adaptation more frequently and markedly: For almost half of the O-subjects, the persons rearing them were socially conspicuous or delinquent, and just under 30% of the O-subjects had lived in inadequate housing conditions for more than 6 years. Also with respect to internal circumstances, where functional aspects were much more important than structural-formal ones, the O-subjects more frequently exhibited unfavorable conditions: most of them were reared inconsistently; almost half of them had parents whose relationship was disrupted; half of them were inadequately supervised. Several subjects also actively avoided any attempts to supervise them.

Although these difficult external and internal family conditions occurred more frequently for the lower-class O-subjects, they could *not* be interpreted *as (lower-) class specific:* In the G-group, the same strains were distributed irrespective of social class (see Sect. 2.1.3.4 above). As a whole, the variable social class was shown to be *criminologically unspecific* in all social spheres. But conditions of socialization as such were also generally too unspecific in their importance for (later) criminality. On the one hand, a considerable number of O-subjects grew up in well-ordered family circumstances, and the late delinquents in particular (O_2-subjects, see Sect. 1.3 above), who were convicted for the first time after the age of 18, mainly did not exhibit such unfavorable conditions. On the other hand, many G-subjects were also subject to such strains.

Nonetheless, the concurrence of certain factors which turned out to be both factually important and distinguishing in the statistical sense was of considerable importance. This was shown in the *syndrome of family strains* (see Sect. 2.1.4

above), which consists of difficult external (socio)economic conditions, social conspicuousness or criminality of a person rearing the subject, and lack of supervision of the subject. As only one-fifth of the O-subjects demonstrated the syndrome, it is impossible to speak of a concurrence typical of the O-group. Yet the small number of such G-subjects, (2, or 1%) allows the conclusion that the absence of recidivist criminality must be regarded as an exception if the syndrome occurs.

In the **sphere of abode** (see Sect. 2.2 above) it was shown that the O-subjects had more frequently grown up in homes or with persons other than their parents, but that the majority of both groups had grown up in their families of orientation. Yet the families of orientation of the O-subjects lost their relevance much earlier: Somewhat more than half of the early (O_1-subjects, see Sect. 1.3 above) and somewhat less than half of the late delinquents (O_2-subjects) had left their parents' homes for good before the age of 17. The O-subjects did not change their places of abode significantly more frequently than the G-subjects at school age. The period that followed, in contrast, especially the period after the subjects left home, was marked by a higher mobility of the O-subjects, which even led to a temporary lack of abode for a considerable number of them. The O-subjects' own sphere of living was usually of short duration and often insufficiently furnished. The O-subjects' heightened mobility went in the direction of large cities, especially for those subjects whose actual places of abode did not correspond to their official places of residence or who had no fixed abode at all. The remaining O-subjects also preferred places of leisure in large cities.

The O-subjects' increasing instability in the sphere of abode corresponded to a large extent with that in other social spheres. It was opposed to the G-subjects' high stability of abode with a varied social integration.

The **sphere of performance** was marked by conspicuousness even at *school* (see Sect. 2.3.2 above). The majority of the O-subjects, but only barely one-fifth of the G-subjects, demonstrated conspicuous behavior at school, which included considerable truancy and offenses committed at school; the difference was even greater for more serious forms of conspicuousness. The conspicuous behavior of the O-subjects was also related to their lack of success at school (more than half of the O-subjects, as opposed to one-tenth of the G-subjects, did not manage to complete the *Hauptschule).* The earlier the first conspicuousness, the more frequently did failures occur. At the same time, there was a relationship with circumstances at home: The subjects who were conspicuous at school were mainly not supervised by the persons rearing them or avoided supervision. Of particular importance was the *socioscholastic syndrome* (see Sect. 2.3.2.3 above), consisting of serious school-internal and -external conspicuousness. The syndrome occurred for no G-subject and for (only) 15% of the O-subjects.

In *occupational life* (see Sects. 2.3.3 and 2.3.4 above), the O-subjects demonstrated even more substantial shortcomings than at school as compared with the general population. These were partially a continuation of difficulties at school, partially a consequence of downward occupational mobility. Although a large number of O-subjects started occupational training, many of them stopped, usually during the first year. Further downward mobility ensued, and at the time of the study, three-fourths of the O-subjects held the position of unskilled workers.

This downward occupational mobility or lack of occupational success, which occurred irrespective of social class, was the expression of a lack of stability that pervaded the entire sphere of performance. It was regularly accompanied by frequent job changes, irregular employment or periods of nonemployment, and negative behavior during occupational training or at work, often preceded by negative conspicuous behavior at school. The foregoing kinds of occupational conspicuousness form the criteria of the *syndrome of lacking occupational adaptation* (performance syndrome, see Sect. 2.3.4.6 above). The syndrome can be regarded as specific to the O-group, as besides one G-subject, it concerned only O-subjects. As in the sphere of the family of orientation, where the late delinquents mainly came from families living in ordered circumstances, they initially differed in a positive sense from the early delinquents in the sphere of performance as well. After behaving mainly inconspicuously at school and completing school successfully, they were also more successful in occupational training, less conspicuous in the sense of negative occupational behavior patterns, and still occupied a higher occupational position. During the period preceding the study, however, their behavior approached the negative picture of the early delinquents in this sphere. (Serious) criminality was not necessarily accompanied by a lack of occupational adaptation in the *entire* sphere of performance: Only 58% of the early and as few as 31% of the late delinquents exhibited *all* negative extreme forms of this syndrome (the extent of occupational conspicuousness was much more pronounced immediately before the "last" offense, see Sect. 4.6 above). Yet, if these symptoms occur, they may well be a very strong indicator of (recidivist) criminality, as they were practically nonexistent in the general (G-)population.

The development in the **sphere of leisure** (see Sect. 2.4 above) corresponded largely to that in the sphere of performance: The leisure behavior of the O-subjects increasingly lost continuity and structure. The G-subjects mainly exhibited leisure behavior characterized by a frequent limitation of leisure by the assumption of various obligations and by leisure activities at home or equally at home and away from home, with definite courses inside certain limits. The O-subjects tended more and more, from school age to age of occupational training and to the period of the study, to extend their leisure time at the expense of regular employment and to engage in leisure activities away from home with entirely open and unpredictable courses. Initially, the late delinquents differed in a positive sense from the early delinquents, but their leisure behavior approached that of the early delinquents during the period preceding the study. At that time, three-fourths of the O-subjects exhibited the leisure syndrome (see Sect. 2.4.7 above), which consists of the negative extreme forms of the two criteria (a) availability of leisure time and (b) structure and courses of leisure activities. This syndrome may be regarded as specific to and typical of the O-subjects, as it was practically nonexistent in the general (G-)population.

The **contacts** of the O-subjects also lacked stability and continuity (see Sect. 2.5 above). The initial contacts with the family gave way to self-chosen contacts earlier and to a greater extent than in the G-group. As a rule, contacts changed more frequently, were more likely to be utilitarian and superficial and were increasingly oriented toward the "milieu." With respect to sexual partners as well, the contacts of the O-subjects were rather noncommittal; first sexual intercourse was earlier and the number of sexual partners greater than that of the G-subjects. Finally, up to the time of the study, fewer O- than G-subjects were married, and the O-subjects' marriages were disrupted or failed more often. Again, the late delinquents differed positively from the early delinquents in that they generally separated from their parents' homes later and had fewer changing relationships and fewer "milieu" contacts. Of special importance was the combination of the most important criteria of contact behavior, whose negative extremes form the *contact syndrome* (see Sect. 2.5.7 above). This syndrome may be regarded as specific to the O-group; it occurred for 67% of the O_1- and 46% of the O_2-subjects, but for only 1.5% of the G-subjects.

According to the foregoing findings, the *O-subjects were an extreme group* forming a strong contrast to the general (G-)population. Yet the G-group was in no way homogeneous, as might appear on the basis of the comparison with the O-group; on the contrary, it reflects - as "general population" - a broad spectrum of (also conspicuous) social behavior: A small, but not negligible percentage of the G-subjects exhibited even the most serious conspicuous behavior characteristic of the O-group. This was not so for the **specific syndromes** in the individual social spheres. They were formed in such a way that the most distinguishing and factually important findings of the various spheres concurred. These syndromes either did not occur or occurred for a maximum of 1.5% of the G-subjects (most of whom were also convicted for an offense), yet did occur for a substantial percentage of the O-subjects. These syndromes should not be seen in isolation. Just as the social spheres, which were separated solely for analytical purposes, form a unity (see Sect. 1.1 above), the criteria relating to a sphere included in the syndromes are interrelated.

Figure 1 attempts to present graphically how, in the development of their lives, an increasing number of O-subjects demonstrated the syndromes in the corresponding stages and spheres, until 75% of the O-subjects (80% of the O_1- and 69% of the O_2-subjects) demonstrated the leisure syndrome - which, as opposed to the performance and contact syndromes, covers only the period immediately preceding the study. The differing development of the O_1- and O_2-subjects is particularly noteworthy.

In the examination of how the individual syndromes "overlap," i.e., to what extent the subjects demonstrated several syndromes, it became apparent that there was only a small "hard core" of subjects (11% of the O_1-subjects and no O_2-subject) who were conspicuous throughout - from the syndrome of family strains to the socioscholastic syndrome to the syndromes of the spheres of performance, contacts, and leisure.

The individual syndromes are related to each other in different ways. A particularly strong correlation was found between the performance and leisure syndromes and between the contact and leisure syndromes: 93% of the subjects with a performance syndrome and 92% of those with a contact syndrome also exhibited a leisure syndrome. Conversely, a certain percentage (17.5%) of the subjects with a leisure syndrome did not demonstrate a contact or a performance syndrome. There was a relationship in the longitudinal section of life as well: 60% of the subjects with a socioscholastic syndrome also exhibited a performance syndrome later on.

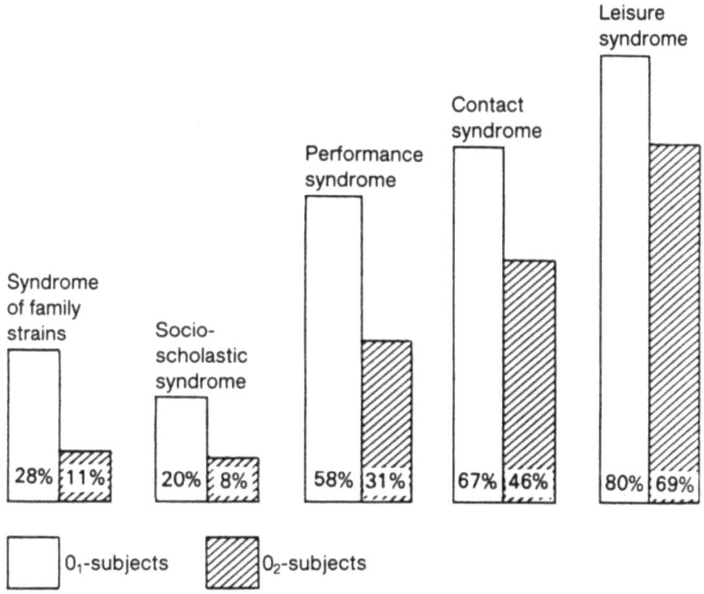

Fig. 1. Overview of syndromes from the individual spheres of live

In the **sphere of delinquency** (see Sect. 4 above), a direct comparison between the O- and the G-group was made only for "offenses" during childhood, which occurred for 66% of the O_1-, 28% of the O_2-, and 11% of the G-subjects (see Sect. 4.2.1 above). For registered delinquency (nonregistered delinquency, which also showed serious differences between O- and G-subjects, was disregarded, see Sect. 4.2.2 above), the *O-subjects were studied separately.* It was shown that the O-group was not homogeneous with respect to social conspicuousness. Even in the social spheres, the division of the O-group into early (first registered offense before the age of 18) and late delinquents (first registered offense at the age of 18 or later) yielded obvious differences. These results were confirmed in a more detailed differentiation according to age at the onset of delinquency: The earlier the subjects had committed their first registered offense, the earlier and more marked was their social conspicuousness. The structure and development of delinquency differed according to onset of "criminal career," particularly with respect to the relative frequency of offenses. In contrast, the differentiation of the O-group according to kind of offenses did not lead much further. Apart from a few "monotropic" offenders, particularly offenders who committed fraudulent and sexual offenses, who also differed (positively) with respect to social behavior, there were chiefly *"polytropic" recidivist offenders,* with property delinquency predominating, followed by fraud and traffic delinquency. The numerous offenses (an average of four per year) were usually not serious taken individually, but did amount to considerable total damages. They usually occurred without any planning out of a certain situation, for example after going to a bar and consuming a considerable amount of alcohol, and were directed against arbitrary objects. Correspondingly, if offenses were committed by groups at all, they were generally only arbitrary ones, and the victims were entirely interchangeable. In view of this dominating lack of planning and arbitrariness of offenses, the sphere of delinquency fits into the picture of the remaining social spheres. The specific interplay between social conspicuousness and criminality became even more obvious in the analysis of the situations in life out of which the "last" offense had been committed (see Sect. 4.6 above). Some (typical) forms could be elaborated. While the offense developed out of the entire life pattern with a certain inner logical consistency in one case, the specific situation before the offense, whether an "opportunity" in the immediate social environment, or the company of "buddies" and alcohol consumption in bars, or (less frequently) the rational decision to obtain money, was decisive for the commission of the offense in other cases.

As recidivist criminality was usually accompanied by serious social conspicuousness in the O-group, it was to be expected that this would also be the case for the *G-group* - though to a lesser extent. At first view, the G-subjects seemed to be a relatively homogeneous group with respect to the extreme forms of the O-group. In a differentiated analysis, however, a certain variation became apparent - though on another level. There were no differences between the G-subjects without previous convictions and the G-subjects previously convicted for traffic offenses. The G-subjects who *had previously been convicted for "classic delinquency"* differed more pronouncedly: In detail, it was shown that offenses committed by juveniles were mainly accompanied by (temporary) conspicuousness in the spheres of leisure and contacts (apart from one case of a performance syndrome), and that offenses committed by adults usually occurred out of an otherwise relatively inconspicuous social behavior.

On this level of the analysis, the following *results* may be stated: (Considerable) social conspicuousness is a good *indicator* of degree and extent of criminal development. Generally, and thus necessarily summarily, it can be said that:

The *early delinquents,* who more often came from disordered family circumstances, usually became conspicuous at early school age and increasingly deviated from normal social behavior - measured in terms of the general (G-)population - the older they were, until, in the end, they demonstrated a social conspicuous lifestyle pervading all social spheres (see also "The continuous development toward criminality beginning during early youth", Part III, Sect. 4.4.2).

For the *late delinquents,* who mainly grew up in ordered family circumstances, a socially conspicuous development did not begin until later on, and, for a large proportion, did not increase until adolescence or adulthood (see also "The development toward criminality beginning during adolescence or the early years of adulthood", Part III, Sect. 4.4.3).

The previously convicted *G-subjects* (as well as several "atypical" O-subjects) usually remained socially inconspicuous or became only temporarily or partially conspicuous, particularly in the sphere of leisure, rarely in the sphere of performance. This corresponded to the nature of their criminality (see also "Criminality as a sudden event", "Criminality in the course of personality maturation", and "Criminality despite no other conspicuousness"; Part III, Sects. 4.4.4, 4.4.5, and 4.4.6).

III Complex, Overall View

1 Methodological Considerations

1.1 Limits of Statistical Analysis

The limits to which statistical analysis is in principle subjected became apparent to all those who were concerned with the individual case investigations forming the source material of the present study. As any statistical analysis entails a certain loss of reality, such an analysis could be only *one* means among others of obtaining knowledge. Similar reservations were mentioned by HEALY and BRONNER (1926, p.209; 1936, p.33), who also based their study on individual case investigations.

The immanent limits of statistical methods became apparent even before the search for complex relationships began, i.e., in the relationships between certain variables and criminality: It can only be determined whether there is a relationship between two variables which is not simply a random one; all other possibilities of interpretation remain open. Even for relationships which are considered statistically significant, there is a certain, often considerable number of cases which demonstrate the same "characteristics" without the subjects having become recidivist offenders - apart from the theoretically possible exceptions (see, for instance, BUIKHUISEN 1979, p.37). Thus, the statistically correct statement that a relationship between a certain characteristic and criminality is not a random one does not signify very much. It can even be trivial or misleading if the "characteristic" has an entirely different or even opposite effect - depending on the further individual situation.

Part of the deficiencies deriving from the analysis of relationships between no more than two variables are supposedly avoided by the more complex statistical methods, which consider a number of variables. The large multifactorial studies in particular (see, for example, WEST and FARRINGTON 1977, p.146; GLUECK and GLUECK 1974; CONGER and MILLER 1966; FERRACUTI et al. 1975, pp.129ff.) tried to show relationships between the facts they had collected in this way. Yet precisely for this purpose, statistical methods are insufficient. In simply additive or numerically weighted indices (or prediction tables) and in classical multivariate methods such as factor analysis, assumptions are made about the object which artificially adapt it to the statistical instrument. When, for example, various variables are combined to form an index, which is then used as a measure of the "danger" of or "predisposition" to delinquency (in the sense of a prediction table), it is assumed in the simplest - and also most frequent - case that the individual variables are related in an additive way (the more characteristics occur, the greater the danger of criminality). Furthermore, it is tacitly assumed that the mere occurrence of each individual characteristic alone is important. Finally, it is also assumed that the *direction* in which all variables take effect as regards their relationship with delinquency is the *same*. Other statistical methods are based on similar assumptions. Moreover, the *static* perspective of the additive model is not overcome. Where the dynamics of the time element are to be determined, for example in the path model, the priority in time of the individual variables must first be defined, which means that a necessary and decisive precondition consists of insecure theoretical assumptions, which are themselves not verified.

Much more modest, but substantially less problematic are the statistical methods which do not measure relationships between variables but - expressed in a simplified way - count persons (subjects) who exhibit certain combinations of characteristics. This enables verification of whether variables which, individually seen, are each related to delinquency coincide for the subjects concerned or whether they are randomly distributed. This, however, says nothing about how the variables affect each other. These reservations also hold for the syndromes described in Part II (in particular, see Part II, Sect. 5).

On the whole, therefore, there are very strict limits to statistical analysis as soon as one goes beyond questions of frequencies and into questions of weighting, importance, and *actual interplay* among various variables. There is no way to weight the individual variables other than according to the strength of the statistical relationships or to a general measure defined in advance. This is also true for all imaginable technical models, such as differentiating statements on the interplay among the individual variables by way of moderator variables. Thus, it remains unresolved whether a single variable may make a whole group of other variables irrelevant in the *individual case* or whether a series of variables which are irrelevant when regarded individually may be of decisive importance when they occur together in a certain way. Such indications arose repeatedly in the individual case studies; they are included in the complex, overall view of the present chapter.

1.2 Limits of Individual Case Studies

Within the framework of individual case studies, it is possible to retain the proximity to reality which is necessarily lost in the preparation of information from statistical points of view.

These are not only the advantages of more detailed information and proximity to life, which are normally expected of individual cases studies in empirical social research. Applying them as a methodological aid in empirical social research guarantees that the actual investigations do not miss reality in the "explorative" preliminary phases. Later on, they fill the gaps of interpretation in the statistical analysis by "illustrative" description and show how the actual relationships can be imagined (see the "illustrative cases" of GLUECK and GLUECK 1974, pp. 250 ff.; POWERS and WITMER 1951, pp. 189 ff.; FERGUSON 1952, pp. 67 ff., 83 ff., 96 ff.; ROSENQUIST and MEGARGEE 1969, pp. 470 ff.; MCCORD and MCCORD 1959, pp. 41 ff., 118 ff.; HEALY and BRONNER 1936, pp. 92 ff.).

As useful as this function of individual case studies to complement a statistical analysis seems, their specific kind of knowledge is rarely used for the actual scientific results. As opposed to probability statements of statistical analyses, individual case studies enable comprehension of the *inner logical consistency* of an occurrence. Comprehension in this sense does not mean simply the consideration of "subjective meaning," possibly even limited to the time preceding the offense, but an objective examination of the offense in its connection with the offender in the context of his social relationships. In other words, this means that the offense should be seen as "meaningfully related with the internal and external situation of the offender" (EXNER 1939, pp. 16ff.; trans.). In this way, it is possible to make specific statements on the importance of individual circumstances for the entire occurrence within the framework of an individual case study - given the knowledge of the necessary facts and the necessary experience in the matter.

Despite the great relevance of individual case studies on the basis of this means of obtaining knowledge, it should not be forgotten that no general statements can be made on the basis of *single* individual case studies. This becomes apparent in the multifactorial comparative studies, whose "illustrative cases" are entirely separated from the main body of the statistical evaluation (typical in this respect are, for instance, ROSENQUIST and MEGARGEE 1969, pp. 470ff., and FERRACUTI et al. 1975, pp. 138ff.).

As long as no general statements can be made on the basis of individual case studies, the problem of the isolated coexistence of different means of obtaining knowledge, which are reciprocally related with respect to advantages and disadvantages, remains unresolved: On the one hand, in the statistical analysis, objectivity and possibilities of generalization are paid for by trivialism or a lack of reality, on the other hand, specific and essential individual case studies are inevitably not generally valid.

1.3 Conception of Ideal Types

In the present study, extensive and differentiated investigations were conducted for all of the 400 subjects. Therefore, neither theoretical presuppositions nor individual illustrative case "histories" had to be referred to for the interpretation of frequencies: It was possible to take recourse to the knowledge gained from all individual case studies. With the exception of the - simple - statistical analysis itself, all steps in forming indicators, classification, etc. and in fact the entire "processing" of the individual findings were also marked by this knowledge. In this respect, the dilemma between proximity to reality and possibilities of generalization was smaller from the outset than is commonly assumed in the methodology of social sciences. Even so, the statistical analysis could not overcome the basic limits of this kind of evaluation.

Therefore, the *knowledge of relationships* which were comprehendible in their inner logical consistency in the individual case study had to be elaborated in such a way that the criteria of reality *and* validity were equally respected. This was attempted by "condensing" the wealth of information from the individual case studies into special kinds of rules. First steps toward this "condensing" were specific comparisons between O- and G-subjects, by which it was attempted to find the criteria essential to criminality. These comparisons were conducted on different levels in breadth and depth: from a tiny section of a life pattern to a complex comparison of the cross and the longitudinal section of life. In this way, findings which would have been lost in general statistical statements (such as the fact that a fair number of G-subjects also showed social conspicuousness - and delinquency

- while many late delinquents initially did not) became the fertile starting point for new comparisons, for example, between the O- and the G-subjects with externally similar situations and differing developments. Recognizing these possibilities of comparison as such would not have been possible without the knowledge of the individual case studies and of their connection with the whole.

First, the O- and the G-subjects were described in a contrasting way on a systematic basis. The descriptions were subdivided according to the various spheres (see Sect. 2 below). In the *cross section,* this comparison was "condensed" even further by extracting the (criminorelevant) constellations (see Sect. 3.3 below). In the longitudinal section, overview forms were prepared for each subject, containing the various events in life schematically in chronological order. An important intermediate step in the search for courses of development as a whole (see Sect. 4.4 below) was the formation of "twin" pairs. This enabled comparison of the differing reactions of the O- and the G-subjects to similar situations (see Sect. 4.3 below). In this context, it became increasingly apparent how necessary it was to consider patterns of relevance and value orientation as important *internal facts,* despite a considerable insecurity in determining them (see Sect. 5 below).

The presentation of these results only insufficiently expresses the actual procedure of obtaining knowledge. The extremely tedious process of getting to know the individual cases, attempts to systematize, critical discussions among team members, and renewed verification by referring back to the individual case studies cannot be described in detail in such a way that the actual creative element becomes apparent.

If one attempts to classify methodologically the rules obtained from experience in this way, the *conception of ideal types* as discussed by Max WEBER in his *Gesammelte Aufsätze zur Wissenschaftslehre* (1973, first 1922; see also BOCK 1983), and particularly as taken over by Karl JASPERS, seems best suited. The basic dilemma which arose from the limits of both statistical analysis (see Sect. 1.1 above) and individual case study (see Sect. 1.2 above) was also WEBER's starting point in his methodological reflections on the conception of ideal types. In his view, the dilemma could be resolved if there was an "interpretation of a coherent course of conduct" which is "adequate on the level of meaning" on the one hand and "a causally adequate interpretation of the same phenomenon" on the other. "The interpretation of a sequence of events will be called causally adequate insofar as, according to established generalizations from experience, there is a probability that it will always occur in the same way." (WEBER 1968, p. 11). The correspondence of these two aspects was precisely the intention of "condensing" rules from experience. These rules were still to have the decisive advantage of individual case studies, namely to be a means of obtaining knowledge about courses of occurrences which are *comprehendible* in their inner logical consistency. At the same time, they were to be valid as *rules* established *on the basis of* and verified *in* all individual case studies.

Terming these rules "ideal types" or "ideal-typical" does *not* mean that they are *merely convincing constructions* of relationships. On the basis of the *actual* courses of occurrences in the individual case studies, it could be constantly verified whether the relationships whose inner logical consistency was immediately apparent actually occurred.

It must be considered, however, that *ideal types are necessarily abstractions,* albeit of a *special kind:* The concept shows the characteristic essence of a phenomenon by disregarding anything which is *also* (regularly) given in everyday life. In other words: *In the ideal type, the essential characteristics of the occurrence are intensified and become the pure, ideal form, which occurs at best as an extreme case.* Thus, it becomes an "absolute" measure for determining how pronounced an occurrence is. This necessarily means that *each* examination of *actually* occurring circumstances can only lead to an indication of the extent to which the observed phenomena approximate the (conceived) ideal type. Ideal types thus have a *dual aspect*; this is what JASPERS means when he says that "their truth rests on the inner connectedness of the meaningful whole; their reality, except in the rare borderline case, rests on the fragmentary emergence of the type which is limited in reality by other factors, not to be understood in terms of the type, which cannot therefore exert sole influence" (JASPERS 1963, p.434).

Thus, whenever this necessary verification of actual circumstances became necessary in the present study, the pure, extreme form could not be meant either. This was especially the case where, in the framework of such a verification, the "presence" of one or the other criteria was concerned (for details, see Sect. 3.3.2 below).

The exact opposite occurs when the ideal type itself is used as a *methodological* aid to find the specific form of the corresponding criteria in an *individual case,* as is done in Applied Criminology (see GÖPPINGER 1985). In Applied Criminology, it is always the pure, ideal form which is meant; the comparison of the individual case with the extreme serves to determine the degree of approximation or deviation. This also means that the individual case is not related to the "ideal type" by deduction or subsumption, but that there is a greater or smaller difference which can be recognized only in an individual examination.

Closely related to this dual aspect of ideal-typical concepts are, first of all, any *statements on relationships between certain forms of social behavior and criminality.* They are always related to the examination of the actual circumstances and not to the (merely psychological) evidence of the inner logical consistency of the relationship.

Statements of this kind are *in no way related to a deterministic concept of causes.* A phenomenon such as recidivist criminality (for example, that of the O-subjects) is part of a potentially unlimited complex of conditions and consequences. Whenever *the* cause of *the* offense is examined, for instance, in monocausal theories of criminality, "last" points are sought, for example, in social or biological structures, to explain criminality. The issue of such "last" causes is consciously left unresolved here. Instead, we proceeded backward from the fact of criminality, asking: Are there criteria or constellations (of social behavior) in this potentially unlimited complex of conditions which are causally essential or important or which are more or less irrelevant? An answer to such questions appears possible whenever certain forms of phenomena occur (almost) exclusively in courses leading to (recidivist) criminality. If it is additionally possible to determine not only that such a causal relationship exists but that, at the same time, there is a comprehendible, meaningful relationship between the causally important criteria of social behavior and criminality, these are the cases where there is a true correspondence between adequacy "on the level of meaning" and "established generalizations" (see above). These cases are presented here in particular in the criminorelevant constellations (see Sect. 3.3 below).

But even the determination of such a relationship says nothing about which underlying causes led to the presence of such constellations or courses of development for one subject but not for another. The - theoretically unlimited - causal regress *must end* when the specifically *criminological* importance of individual facts can no longer be determined; this is the case the more one moves away from criminality in time and goes back to given social or even psychological or somatic circumstances. *In the present study, no statements are made on "causes" in this sense.*

2 Comparison of Ideal-typical Behavior of O- and G-Subjects

2.1 Preliminary Remarks

The attempt to contrast the ideal-typical behavior patterns of the O- and the G-subjects may lead to considerable misunderstandings: Particularly in this context, there is a great danger that the differences will be considered normative, i.e., that the behavior of the G-subjects from the general population will be regarded as "ideal" in the sense of "positive" and the behavior of the offenders (O-subjects) "ideal" in the sense of "negative". Such misinterpretations are all the more probable as the specific behavior patterns concerned are *actually judged* "positive" and "negative", socially and culturally. *Therefore, it must be strongly emphasized that the findings underlying the following comparison were not determined from a normative point of view, but derived from experience. They are to be seen in this way alone.*

The following comparisons are called "ideal-typical" in the sense that they show the two extreme poles of criminorelevant behavior, between which there is a broad range of behavior patterns; the behavior patterns of the majority of the subjects are near one of the two extreme forms. "Intermediate" forms are consciously disregarded; in other words, it was not taken into consideration that not all subjects demonstrated a smaller or larger proportion of the presented "extreme" behavior patterns - not even approximately. This was true not only for the behavior patterns which turned out to be relevant (i.e., which distinguished best the two groups) in Part II, but also and all the more so for facts which were not considered in the statistical analysis, since the majority of the subjects were not concerned at all. These facts, if they occurred, were important for a judgment of the corresponding sphere: They fit into the overall picture.

This does *not* mean that *all* behavior patterns occurred for the individual subject, not even in a moderated form. With respect to the O-group, this becomes particularly obvious for the late delinquents (O_2-subjects), who mainly remained inconspicuous during their youth: O-ideal-typical behavior patterns are characterized by the earliest possible and most marked social conspicuousness. In the G-group as well, there was no subject who exhibited all the elements of G-ideal-typical behavior. Furthermore, there were several G-subjects who showed O-specific, and also several O-subjects who showed G-specific behavior patterns. This has already become apparent in the presentation of frequencies in Part II. The following comparison consciously abstracts from these actual circumstances.

The actual value of the following ideal-typical behavior patterns is to be seen as regards their (methodological) application in the analysis of individual cases (for details, see GÖPPINGER 1985). Determining specific behavior in view of its position between the two extreme poles leads to a differentiated (though not quantified - as is usual in psychology) profile of individual social behavior.

2.2 A Synopsis of Ideal-typical Behavior Patterns

2.2.1 The Behavior of the Subjects in Connection with (Parental) Child Rearing During Childhood

O-ideal-typical	*G-ideal-typical*
Active avoidance of parental supervision or exploitation of a lack of supervision in all respects	Acceptance of parental supervision or search for contact with an (ordered) family (e.g., of a friend) if no ordered family sphere
Deception and overreaching of persons rearing the subject, or intensification of inconsistent child rearing by clever tactics and by playing off persons rearing the subject against each other (who cannot "cope with" the subject)	Basic openness toward persons rearing the subject and no exploitation of inconsistent child rearing
Persistent refusal to assume tasks and obligations (suited to the subject's age) and avoidance of corresponding responsibility	Voluntary and willing assumption of tasks and obligations (suited to the subject's age) or search for tasks for which the subject feels responsible

2.2.2 The Sphere of Abode

O-ideal-typical	*G-ideal-typical*
Frequent changes of abode (together with the family) even during childhood or going back and forth between parents, relatives, foster parents, and homes	Growing up in parents' home and no long-term absences from home during childhood
Early committal to a home because of intolerable behavior and/or indications of neglect	
Running away from homes repeatedly and roaming about, in connection with the commission of offenses; therefore, committal to ever more strictly run homes or reform schools in the course of time	

Early emphasis on independence; parents' dwelling is increasingly considered a place to sleep only, not home	Also during one's youth, full integration in parents' home, whose dwelling is considered home
Early separation from parents' home withour creating one's own sphere of living; staying temporarily in the dwelling of acquaintances, in a dubious "milieu", with prostitutes, etc.	No separation from parents' home unless occupational training away from home or (non)military service; a "final" separation in the sense of becoming independent occurs only after marriage
In the following period, frequent changes of abode; no interest in a somewhat permanent dwelling but living as subtenant for short periods, company housing, or hostels for men or with acquaintances	Changes of place of abode are rare; if there are changes, they take place because of occupation or marriage; all changes are planned and well-ordered
Repeated temporary lack of place of residence in connection with roaming about and sleeping in the streets, in asylums, sheds, summerhouses, etc.	Always correct registration of place of residence, which is always used as such
After leaving home, an increasing tendency away from an immediate social environment to a more "anonymous," particularly large-city environment	
No social integration at place of abode; a change of abode means practically only a change of personal and material contacts, which are entirely interchangeable anyway	Manifold social integration in the local community through occupation, club memberships, acquaintances, family, and relatives; a change of place of abode is undesirable because of this integration
No interest in selecting place of abode or residential area according to certain points of view; acceptance of what is readily available or what is provided (e.g., by social welfare office), even a dwelling in "asocial" circumstances	Critical selection of place of abode and residential area with respect to place of work, (future) possibilities of education and training for one's children, and manifold social points of view (good area, neighborhood, atmosphere, leisure facilities, etc.); unsatisfactory circumstances are temporarily accepted, but with emphasized efforts to a personally satisfactory dwelling or environment
No interest in own dwelling and its furnishing; a dwelling is only a place to sleep, not home	Great interest in own sphere of living and efforts to provide dwelling with an individual character corresponding to one's own feeling of well-being - with a considerable expenditure of time; a dwelling is home

2.2.3 The Sphere of Performance

2.2.3.1 School

O-ideal-typical	*G-ideal-typical*
Negative performance at school due to lack of interest, laziness, idling, or frequent truancy	Interest in school and attempt to meet performance and behavior requirements
For this reason repetition of one or more grades in the *Grund-* or *Hauptschule* or going to a *Sonderschule* (see Part II, Sect. 2.3.2.1)	
No successful completion of school	Successful completion of the *Hauptschule* or attendance at a *weiterführende Schule* (see Part II, Sect. 2.3.2.1)
Frequent and persistent or temporarily continuous truancy, during this time roaming about, (petty) offenses (against property) and damage to property and attempts to cover up this behavior by sophisticated deceit and lies	No truancy or exceptional truancy, in no case persistent truancy and no concomitant behavior such as roaming about, deceit, and lies
Disturbing lessons by annoying (silly, boastful) behavior and constant unrest	Good cooperation and adequate behavior
Disobedience, rebellious and aggressive behavior toward teacher	Good relationship with teacher
Inconsiderate and brutal behavior toward fellow pupils leading to serious injury of others in fights	Holding back to some extent, also in fights to avoid any serious injuries
No interest in further education or training (at school)	Participation in further training and education (at school) or attempts to make up for lacking opportunities of education and training with evening classes or correspondence courses

2.2.3.2 Occupational Training

O-ideal-typical	*G-ideal-typical*
No interest in apprenticeship or training after finishing school	A specific occupational goal after finishing school; apprenticeship and training are regarded as a requirement

	for a satisfying occupation, occupation as an important element of life
No successful completion of apprenticeship or training; the possibility of earning money immediately as an unskilled or semiskilled worker is preferred to a sound training; for this reason, no apprenticeship is started or an apprenticeship is started, but not completed or apprenticeships (and occupation) are (repeatedly) changed without completion of any training	At least one completed apprenticeship or training as a sound foundation for later occupation; even if difficulties arise or chosen occupation is unsatisfactory, efforts to complete the apprenticeship, which is therefore not broken off
Reasons for breaking off an apprenticeship are: No inclination ("fed up"), no interest, arguments with superiors and fellow employees, wanting to earn more money, or losing job because of irregularities (poor work performance, stealing, etc.)	
Negative work performance, frequently staying away unexcused at apprenticeship, and truancy at vocational school	Positive work performance, interest in work, reliable and punctual completion of work tasks, regular attendance at vocational school
Frequent difficulties with master craftsman, superiors, and fellow employees	No serious difficulties with superiors and fellow employees or difficulties are always dealt with and solved
If difficulties arise, breaking off apprenticeship or giving notice and putting the blame on others (superiors, fellow employees, "circumstances")	If difficulties arise, blaming oneself as well and recognizing one's own share in problems
Apprenticeships started during stays in homes or prisons are not successfully completed either	
No interest in specialization or further training	Successful completion of additional training and specialization (e.g., in the form of courses) or attempt to make up for missed opportunities of training or education

2.2.3.3 Employment

O-ideal-typical	*G-ideal-typical*
The main purpose of occupation is to obtain money quickly and with as few efforts as possible	Preferring a slow but well-founded and secure upward occupational mobility as opposed to earning money quickly in the beginning without the possibility of upward mobility or occupational progress or career
Basic willingness to change jobs at any time in favor of supposedly better and easier ways to earn money without having obtained information on the actual circumstances	Exclusively jobs lasting several years
Preferring varied and independent activities without direct supervision or control and without any limits in time and space (i.e., as showman's helper and periodicals salesman or "independent" activities, e.g., "sales representative", or attempts to set up one's own business - which were unrealistic from the outset); in the course of time downward mobility with respect to lower occupational position and an increase of disordered activities in the form of temporary labor (without social insurance), etc.	Apart from the improvement of occupational position, the essentials are stability and security of job as well as a satisfying activity and a good atmosphere at work
Basic willingness to stay away from work unexcused, walk away from work, or give notice because of a minor difficulty, listlessness or momentary moods	One's own person and working capacity are considered indispensable for the company; thinking of poor work or staying away from work that "one couldn't do it" to the company, superiors, and fellow employees; coping with difficulties that arise
Frequent unplanned and spontaneous job changes without the prospect of a specific new job	Practically no job changes, if so, only upon careful consideration and after sure acceptance at a new job
No smooth transition between individual jobs but repeated long-term nonemployment, in some cases for several months, without any efforts to find a new job	Always smooth transitions between jobs; if, exceptionally, there is unemployment, it is not self-induced, and great efforts are made to find a new job even if it means (temporary) downward occupational mobility

Reasons for job changes are arguments with superiors or fellow employees or supposed (always only momentary and short-term) better earnings; in the course of occupational life frequent summary dismissals by employer because of poor work performance, arguments with fellow employees, etc.	Reasons for job changes are occupational progress and career as well as - also longterm - better earnings
Work attitude characterized by disinterest and listlessness leading to complaints about poor work performance, drunkenness, quarrelsomeness, and unreliability after a very short time	Work attitude characterized by a marked feeling of responsibility toward company, superiors, and fellow employees; a feeling of belonging to the company and willingness to bear responsibility
No interest in advanced occupational training; at best during stays in prison courses are taken for extraneous reasons and not applied later on	Considerable interest in occupational qualification, realized by successfully completing advanced training courses, etc.
Disordered financial circumstances; living from "hand to mouth"; squandering money as it comes in; many obligations to pay installments and huge debts	Solid and ordered financial circumstances; expenditures are planned and considered; savings agreements, life insurance, etc.; financial commitments are always limited and realistic with respect to their repayment
As a whole no provisions made, whether due to performing temporary labor, working for dubious companies without social insurance, or not providing for emergencies, e.g., by saving money	Extensive and sound provisions made: Besides the matter-of-course social insurance, private provisions by way of (life, liability) insurance, etc.

2.2.4 The Sphere of Leisure

2.2.4.1 Availability of Leisure Time

O-ideal-typical	*G-ideal-typical*
In the course of time, increasing and continuous extension of leisure time, mainly (also) at the expense of the sphere of performance, by staying away from work, tardiness at work, or giving up regular employment, accompanied by a total disorder in the course of a day (There is a shift: A day does not start until the afternoon and ends the next morning)	From childhood on, an increasing, considerable limitation of leisure time by many self-chosen, partially extremely performance-oriented commitments (overtime, second jobs, advanced training, helping at home, volunteer activities, etc.)

At the most an only temporary extension of leisure time at the expense of sleep or a certain limitation of leisure time after being released from prison; soon considerable extensions at the expense of the sphere of performance again	At the most an occasional extension of leisure time at the expense of sleep, never at the expense of the sphere of performance

2.2.4.2 Structure and Course of Leisure Activities

O-ideal-typical	*G-ideal-typical*
Leisure time is predominantly filled with activities with open and unpredictable courses; neither places nor time nor contact persons are known beforehand, and activities are neither planned nor prepared; these are „pub crawls," going to disreputable bars and going to meeting points of the criminality-prone "milieu", preferably the area of the train station, amusement arcades, and old-town areas of large cities, with corresponding contacts with socially conspicuous or delinquent persons, etc. and/or aimless driving around with mopeds, motorcycles and cars, constantly on the lookout for excitement, "adventure," etc. Leisure is determined to a large extent by "excesses" such as considerable alcohol consumption, uncontrolled spending, or violent arguments	Leisure time is increasingly determined by planned, systematically pursued, and/or formally organized leisure activities with definite courses from childhood on. Besides performance-oriented activities (extra jobs, continuing education, etc.), mainly regular sports, hobbies, or volunteer activities which are pursued with determination and considerable commitment
Also among leisure activities with surveyable courses inside certain limits, preferring activities involving a certain unrest, diversion, and commotion (e.g., going to the movies, to bars or discotheques)	Leisure activities with surveyable courses inside certain limits are mainly thought restful and relaxing; therefore preferring activities which are "leisurely" (e.g., reading, hiking, undertakings together with the family, etc.)
No commitment to or personal efforts for planned, systematically pursued, and/or formally organized leisure activities with definite courses; even if hobbies were pursued or opportunities of further education used during imprisonment, these activities are not continued after release from prison	No interest in leisure activities with entirely open and unpredictable courses; at the most, such leisure activities can occur during a phase of maturation; even then they are not predominant

2.2.4.3. Place of Leisure

O-ideal-typical	*G-ideal-typical*
Place of leisure is almost exclusively away from home; parents' or own dwelling is only a place to sleep, not a place for leisure activities	Place of leisure is preferably at home, where one's own, individually arranged sphere of living, being together with the family, and a certain "integration" are essential
Leisure activities at home are thought boring and are an exception	Leisure activities away from home are, as a whole, less important; such activities are limited to one or a few definite places and planned undertakings, often together with one's own family

2.2.5 The Sphere of Contacts

2.2.5.1 Given Contacts

O-ideal-typical	*G-ideal-typical*
Even during childhood, behavior and tactics lead to conflicts between persons rearing the subject, subsequently to disrupted relationships in the family, also among other family members	Even during childhood, membership of self in the family of orientation and responsibility for the family (suited to one's age) is recognized
No adjustment to the community of the family	Matter-of-course adjustment to the community of the family; being together with the family is almost a need
Rejection of or indifference toward family of orientation or according to one's own discretion or also to justify one's own behavior, changes between defaming the family and (especially for "asocial circumstances") entirely uncritical attitude toward the family (and circumstances) as well as an unlimited identification with individual members of the family and, if existent, their criminal practices	Protecting and defending the family of orientation and its reputation as well as shielding the family from the outside, even if there is no identification with the family
Early separation from parents and siblings and, in the period following, no close contacts with the family of orientation	After leaving home and external separation from family of orientation, relationships with the family and other relatives are more or less intensively maintained; strong ties to individual persons remain

In later years, (inconsiderate) exploitation of family of orientation in (financial) emergencies to one's own material advantage	Also in later years, holding together and reciprocal help are matter-of-course

2.2.5.2 Self-chosen Contacts with Friends and Acquaintances

O-ideal-typical	*G-ideal-typical*
Many superficial contacts with "buddies" and acquaintances but no true friends or strong ties with any particular person	Few friends and acquaintances; after leaving home, maintaining contact with the family of orientation or with individual family members (from now on as self-chosen contacts) and partially very strong ties
No interest in the individual personalities of contact persons; contacts serve to satisfy immediate needs and are utilitarian; individual contact persons are therefore entirely interchangeable on the corresponding level	Selection of one's acquaintances in view of the individual person and common, long-term interests, reliability, etc.; friendships last many years on the basis of a confidential relationship; a relatively small, stable group of acquaintances who are not interchangeable
Preferring "milieu" contacts with a casual group of "buddies" without any confidential relationship and with reciprocal overreaching; "tolerance" for and even insensitivity toward acquaintances and their peculiarities	No tendencies toward "milieu" contacts and rapid separation from "bad company," if it occurs at all (particularly during youth)

2.2.5.3 Sexual Contacts

O-ideal-typical	*G-ideal-typical*
As early as school age, first sexual intercourse with a much older, sexually conspicuous partner	First sexual intercourse as adolescent or adult with a socially inconspicuous partner of the same age
Frequent changes of sexual partners and frequent contacts with prostitutes	Limitation to one or a few sexual partners
Selection of sexual partners mainly according to "external" qualities; preferring these attributes to "inner" human qualities; important is the possibility of a sexual contact, not the individual personality; partners are therefore entirely interchangeable	Selection of sexual partners according to their individual personalities; partners are therefore not interchangeable; important are strong human ties, not purely sexual contacts

2.2.5.4 Own Family (of Procreation)

O-ideal-typical	*G-ideal-typical*
Corresponding to the basically negative attitude toward stable ties, lack of willingness to marry or if marriage, early on (as adolescent) and after only a few weeks of acquaintance or marriage during imprisonment without knowing one's partner well, frequently because of advantages (temporary leave, parole, etc.)	Basic willingness to undertake a lasting commitment and assume corresponding responsibility; marriage only after a prolonged acquaintance or engagement at an age when the obligations associated with marriage can be met on the basis of maturity and security of employment
Considerably younger, also socially conspicuous wife or (particularly in marriages contracted during imprisonment) considerably older partner	Socially inconspicuous wife of approximately the same age
Both parents bring children into the marriage or have to pay maintenance for a child not from the present marriage	No children with other partners before marriage
No (material) preparation for marriage; both partners bring debts into marriage; no security on the basis of regular employment; no dwelling, furniture etc.	Partners do not marry until a certain number of conditions are met and preparations made; apart from reciprocal affection, common interests etc., valuing that partner is accepted by the family; emphasizing material security of marriage by completing training for occupational and financial security, having a dwelling, etc.
Even after marriage, no change in behavior in the social spheres; both partners go their own ways; they have nothing in common; no responsibility for wife or children; own needs are more important than caring for the children for both partners; continuing the specific life-style with irregular work performance, extension of leisure time by spending one's - unstructured and "milieu"-oriented - leisure time	Marriage is an obvious turning point in life; one's own aspirations are limited in favor of the family; one's entire life is oriented toward the family; responsibility for partner and children is assumed and the family taken care of by corresponding efforts at work; leisure time is concentrated on the family and is spent together with the family; the corresponding group of acquaintances of the individual partners is limited fur-

away from home, including extramarital sexual contacts	ther or changes in favor of common (new) acquaintances
Divorce only a few months after marrying, in the wake of frequent, loud, violent, and public arguments (e.g., in front of the entire neighborhood) - especially after alcohol consumption	No serious disagreements between spouses, no serious arguments, particularly no violent ones, and no displaying of problems in front of third persons; rather, construction of a "bulwark" around the family

3 Comparisons in the Cross Section

3.1 Preliminary Remarks

The statistical evaluation of the distribution of characteristics and the description of the ideal-typical behavior patterns of the O- and G-subjects in the various social spheres provided important answers to questions such as: What is the behavior of recidivist offenders like? In what respects do recidivist offenders differ from the general population? General knowledge regarding these and similar, almost naive questions is of fundamental importance for any further kind of criminological conclusions. Only on the basis of such general knowledge can further facts, observations and findings be evaluated in a rough framework of "what can be expected." Such knowledge is still unsatisfactory, insofar as it is known *that* these characteristics are related with criminality but not *how* these characteristics "take effect" so that in the end criminality occurs.

An intensive analysis of all individual case investigations showed that, again and again, there were certain basic situations out of which the commission of the offense(s) was immediately comprehendible. The knowledge acquired in this way differs in quality from the mere finding *that* criminality is related with certain facts (see Sect. 1.2 above). It was important to "condense" this kind of knowledge from the individual case into general *rules*. For this purpose, basic situations or constellations were formed for which the commission of an offense was self-evident or for which the commission of an offense was completely unexpected (see Sect. 3.3 below). An important preliminary stage was the analysis of daily routines, which showed the interlocking among the various social spheres in a specific life pattern and was thus a first step on the way to an overall view in the cross section.

3.2 The Analysis of Daily Routines

A description of daily routines was made for one working day and for one day off (Sunday) during the period immediately preceding the offense (for the G-subjects during the period preceding the study). By thoroughly examining such a day, the interlocking between the various spheres in the cross section became apparent. An important result of this analysis was, for example, the criterion "expansion of leisure time" described above (see Part II, Sect. 2.4.2), which can be recognized only as a shift in the *daily* time budget.

The descriptions of daily routines were as detailed as possible to avoid leaving out seemingly unimportant periods. Therefore, for example, what the subjects did after working hours was recorded exactly. Here, it became apparent that many O-subjects went to one or more bars after work, i.e., *immediately* turned to their specific leisure contacts, activities, and places, even if they did go home later to change their clothes or perhaps eat. The G-subjects who indicated that they went home after work had regularly gone home immediately. In other words, there was no interval - of varying length - of unstructured leisure in between. In the individual case, the findings on how much *time was spent,* partially also the *order of occurrences,* could be used to determine how important individual facts were for the subjects. Though the time budget as such is only an external indicator of the importance of certain activities, this was also one way of elaborating the patterns of relevance (see Sect. 5 below) of the subjects: Activities which realize patterns of relevance always require a considerable amount of time. Frequently, general indications such as "staying at home in the evening" or "spending the entire weekend at the sports grounds" could be objectified or corrected.

The analysis of daily routines was not suitable for *generalizations.* It concentrated on meticulous descriptions of the individual courses and was a means to record preliminarily the *individual case* in the cross section - like the overview forms in the longitudinal section (see Sect. 4.2 below). Nonetheless, one general observation is worth mentioning. It was much easier for the G-subjects to report a *typical* course of a day, as they organized and structured their entire time (on Sundays and holidays as well) more systematically by fixed breaks in time and place (for instance meals). Several O-subjects, in contrast, were practically at a loss when asked such questions, as a typical course, i.e., one which can be anticipated and predicted, no (longer) corresponded to the reality of their life pattern, which was often almost entirely unstructured. For some O-subjects, a "working day" as such no longer existed. Thus, indications were more indefinite, unsure, and general: Such answers as "sometimes this way, sometimes another" or "it's also possible that" occurred frequently. Particularly for this reason, an accurate picture of *the* typical course could not be obtained.

As a whole, the analysis of daily routines was largely necessary to recognize the life patterns of the subjects and the specific interlocking among the various social spheres.

3.3 Criminorelevant Constellations and Criteria

3.3.1 Forming the Constellations

As was shown in the intensive individual case studies, the presence of individual facts as such was not necessarily relevant. Combined to form syndromes or constellations, however, they gained much greater causal importance than the sum of the individual facts. Thus, in some cases, such facts had no effect whatsoever with respect to criminality; in other cases, they fitted into further, more or less continuous social conspicuousness, where they could take full effect. In order to make general statements on these relationships - which were often extremely heterogeneous in the individual case - a further "condensing" was imperative. A comparison of individual characteristics or specific behavior patterns was insufficient. Instead, criteria were formed which could no longer be collected immediately, i.e., whose "presence" had to be determined for each individual subject by examining his social behavior in its entirety within the framework of the individual case studies.

It was necessary to progress toward such criteria, as the specific external circumstances in life often varied to such an extent that the number of subjects would have been extremely small for all attempts to operationalize strictly. In order to guarantee the comparability of the *importance* of the various circumstances in the subjects' lives, *relational concepts* had to be formed which expressed the behavior of the subject in its *relationship to his circumstances in life*. Thus, there was a systematic reason why it was impossible to operationalize. As assigning subjects to criteria was possible only with the knowledge of all individual case investigations, judgment *and* experience remained necessary to recognize, for example, whether there was any "neglect of the sphere of work and performance as well as of family and other social obligations" (see Sect. 3.3.3 below). Thus, the constellations formed in groping attempts had to be examined in view of their actual "presence" in the individual cases. This was quite an effort, as at least the overview forms (see Sect. 4.2 below), but usually the entire data had to be consulted for each individual subject.

The result of these efforts was a certain number of specific criteria for the O- and for the G-group. The *individual* criteria were still demonstrated by - very few - subjects of the other group; yet, in their *entirety*, they occurred exclusively for the O- *or* for the G-group. Only a relatively small number of O- or G-subjects exhibited *all* of the specific criteria. Therefore, various groups of criteria were formed (see GÖPPINGER 1970, pp. 88 ff.). In an examination of the material thus obtained, the following two constellations, where criminality seems to be the only "meaningful" consequence or where criminality is not to be expected, proved to "represent" the subjects best:

a. **The criminovalent constellation**

1. Neglect of the sphere of work and performance as well as of family and other social obligations
2. Deficient relationship to money and property
3. Unstructured leisure behavior
4. Absence of planning in life

b. **The criminoresistant constellation**

1. Fulfillment of social obligations
2. Adequate level of aspirations
3. Attachment to a well-ordered home (and family life)
4. Adequate relationship to money and property

3.3.2 Verifying the Constellations

The means of verifying the *actual* co-occurrence of several criteria forming a "meaningful" relationship with criminality in the sense of an inner logical consistency was once again the comparison of the O- and the G-subjects. It became strikingly apparent how wrong it is to conclude a danger of criminality immediately on the basis of certain kinds of conspicuousness not corresponding to certain "middle class" values. Obviously, there is a wide range of behavior patterns and conducts of life which contradict such value expectations. The specific life pattern of the O-subjects represented only a small part of this range. Precisely such judgments must be avoided if the relationships relevant to criminality are to be recognized.

Socially conspicuous behavior occurred for some G-subjects, expressed in a lack of willingness to adapt or in indifference or even inconsiderateness toward their families. Although these criteria were "present" in the same way as for the O-subjects, they were of no criminological importance if the subject's entire life pattern was marked, for example, by his pursuing an occupational career. This was no "absence of planning in life" and thus no *crimino*valent "constellation," whatever other "negative" effects it could have had. Similarly, some students in the G-group showed partially considerable conspicuousness in the spheres of performance, leisure, and contacts. Yet, on the one hand, the conspicuousness did not last long enough to seriously jeopardize planning in life; on the other, an adequate relationship to money and property usually remained. Here, again, there was no *crimino*valent constellation.

For the O-subjects, in contrast, a similar conspicuousness in the spheres of performance and leisure was often intensified in its importance by further criteria. The *neglect of social obligations,* in particular the complete *neglect of the sphere of performance,* which entails financial losses, has all the more serious effects if it occurs together with a *deficient relationship to money and property,* whereas economically sound behavior can bring some relief in such a situation. Finally, if *unstructured leisure behavior* constantly provides opportunities to spend money "unreasonably," the importance of the other criteria is strengthened in the direction of committing a (property or fraudulent) offense as the only possibility of maintaining the life-style underlying these criteria - certainly if there is an *absence of planning in life.* Such a life-style is possible without illegal means only if it is merely a temporary "dropping out" of the forms of life necessary to secure one's existence, a "dropping out," however, which remains integrated in a long-term framework of planning in life and thus allows one to contract debts temporarily. Here, the individual criteria join together to form *a constellation where the occurrences practically thrust an individual toward criminality.*

These two constellations are used at present in Applied Criminology (see Part IV) for two reasons. First, they are characterized by an *inner relationship* in the sense of a logical consistency with which criminality occurs out of a certain cross section of life. Second, they were also examined to see whether they were *actually present* for the subjects.

In this examination, the "presence" of the individual criteria merely meant a high degree of approximation, not the conceivable ideal form. Thus, for the individual subject, a more marked neglect of social obligations or an even more marked absence of planning in life than actually occurred was basically conceivable. However, the ideal form of the criteria can be viewed and presented only if they are related to specific circumstances in life. This is a consequence of the "relational" nature of these criteria, which makes it impossible to operationalize strictly. Thus, it is possible to conceive of the ideal type in its *pure* form only *within the relational framework of the actual circumstances in a subject's life.* The difference between ideal type and actual form lies in the conception of the purest "neglect" or the most absolute "absence" *conceivable* in the specific situation of the individual subject.

In the present study, this difference seemed to be indistinct, since it was actually very small for many O-subjects: Practically no further intensification seemed conceivable beyond the actual presence. Yet, here as well, the dual aspect of ideal-typical concepts should be kept in mind (see Sect. 1.3 above).

Consequently, no *general* limit could be given for the degree of approximation which determined whether a criterion was "present" or not. The attempts to present the content of the criteria somewhat more broadly (see Sect. 3.3.3 below) indicate how these decisions were made; yet they are necessarily of an exemplary nature. Therefore, the decision as to whether the individual criteria are "present" or not requires a certain degree of experience, similar to corresponding decisions in medical diagnostic procedures.

Determining whether the constellation occurred as a whole is an entirely different matter: There is only a clear yes or no. The *crimino*relevance of the constellation follows only from the concurrence of *all* criteria. Thus, it is entirely erroneous to speak of an approximation in the above sense if only three of the four individual criteria are at hand.

The verification thus conducted showed that the criminovalent constellation occurred for 60.5% of the O- and none of the G-subjects, the criminoresistant constellation for as many as 79.5% of the G-, but only a few (six) of the O-subjects. These O-subjects did not fit into the O-population at all. Their offenses were, for example, negligent homicide in a traffic accident, refusal to do alternative nonmilitary service, and fraudulent insolvency (the desperate attempt of an excellent artisan to save his business). These proportions confirm that the knowledge gained from experience and "condensed" in the constellations not only includes a relationship comprehendible in its inner logical consistency, but also can be considered a general rule. The inner logical consistency between the behavior underlying the criminovalent constellation and criminality became even more convincingly apparent in a separate examination of the O-subjects who had last committed a property or fraudulent offense (see Part II, Sects. 4.5 and 4.6): 81% of these subjects demonstrated the criminovalent constellation during the period immediately preceding the (property or fraudulent) offense.

It should be mentioned in this context that the constellations are a first attempt. In a continuation of corresponding research, more detailed pictures may well be expected, for example, differentiations according to specific groups of offenders or offenses, meaning that a considerably higher percentage of delinquency would be covered (see also Part IV, Sect. 1).

Points of reference for research concerning further constellations are provided by the *other criteria,* which emerged as criminorelevant but were not included in the constellations. These criteria are, among others, "attitudes" connected with a specific way of life. These attitudes are difficult to determine and cannot be ascertained directly but only on the basis of their specific importance in social behavior (see Part II, Sect. 3.4.4). They also express a relationship with circumstances in life, which becomes immediately apparent in concepts such as "inadequate level of aspirations". The following *O-specific* criteria emerged, which are not be understood as final: Inadequately high level of aspirations (60.5% O; .5% G), deficient sense of reality (74.5% O; 6.5% G), low tolerance for stress (77% O; 12% G), paradoxical expectation of adaptation (37% O; 2.5% G), demand to be free from any ties (70.5% O; 10% G), and considerable alcohol consumption (68.5% O; 4.5% G), which is of great criminological relevance, particularly because of its background effect. The following criteria were *G-specific:* Dedication to and satisfaction from work (91% G; 24% O), productive organization of leisure (82.5% G; 13% O), commitment to the affairs of persons and institutions (35.5% G; 3.5% O), willingness to adapt (45% G; 16.5% O), strong ties (93% G; 21% O), endurance and high tolerance for stress (45.5% G; 4% O), willingness to bear responsibility (61.5% G; 3.5% O), good sense of reality and self-control (57.5% G; 3% O), and planning in life and determination (61% G; 3.5% O).

3.3.3 The Content of the Criminorelevant Criteria

The individual criteria of the criminorelevant constellations and the other criteria cannot be operationalized strictly since they are relational concepts (see Sect. 3.3.1 above). Nonetheless, it is possible to sketch the content of a criterion by describing it in specific examples. This does not allow a simple assignment of cases to concepts: These "concretizations" still have to be related to the circumstances of the individual case. Thus, in the following presentation, indications such as "according to the situation of the subject", "adequately", "comparatively", etc. should always be supplemented in the reader's mind.

3.3.3.1 The Criteria of the Criminovalent Constellation

The criterion **neglect of the spheres of work and performance as well as of family and other social obligations** covers two different points: First, there are the *requirements related to performance* in the wider sense whose fulfillment is usually necessary to create the material and, in particular, financial foundation of life. Second, there are the social requirements whose fulfillment is necessary to be able to live together successfully in society and in particular in the family. A neglect of the spheres of work and performance was assumed if the subjects worked irregularly or did not work at all though they were basically able to (i. e., were not ill) and opportunities to work existed (which was usually the case during the period of the study) and if the subjects depended on the income from their work to support themselves (or their families). If the subjects were directly responsible for others (e. g., wife, children, or parents in need), this also meant a serious neglect of family and other social obligations (regarding "social obligations", see also Sect. 3.3.3.2 below).

For example, the subjects did not intend and were not willing to commit themselves to a long-term, regular job with the corresponding obligations and to fulfill them from the outset. They did not respect working hours, stayed away from work unexcused or on the pretext of being ill, and worked poorly. If they were not dismissed because of this, they gave up their jobs after a short time without any prospect of a new one. Periods of nonemployment followed, during which the subjects made no effort to find a new job. At best, they did temporary labor. As a rule, they also no longer helped to support the family in any way. The subjects used their meager income to satisfy their own needs or let themselves be supported by their families or wives without being prepared to do anything in return (e. g., assuming household duties).

A **deficient relationship to money and property** was judged by examining how the subjects handled their *own material assets,* i. e., mainly their money and property. Handling money and property of others was also taken into consideration, although, in this context, the relationship to "property" (of others) in the sense of the abstract object of legal protection was disregarded. Committing an offense against property alone was never decisive in determining a deficient relationship to money and property. It was relevant that the subjects lived "from hand to mouth," i.e., spent their *money* as it came in, and were in no way able to "budget" it. A deficient relationship to (their own) *property* was assumed if the subjects were not at all careful with their *own* property and did not look after their belongings.

With respect to a deficient relationship to their own material assets, it could be determined, for example, that the subjects concerned spent their entire weekly wages during the weekend, often on Friday evenings, e.g., by extending generous invitations to their "buddies," by paying for rounds in bars, by long taxi rides (in extreme cases all the way to the next large city where "something was going on"), or by going to bars or gambling without knowing what they would live on the next week. Even larger sums, for instance inheritances, were spent in the same way in a short time. Furthermore, there were huge installments to be paid on cars, television sets, furniture, etc., which were in no relation to the income the subjects could expect and were thus not paid or could not be paid from the start. On the whole, practically none of the subjects had any general idea of their financial situation, and almost none showed indications of planning their financial affairs. Practically no subject had ever saved an amount of money worth mentioning or had a savings account.

A deficient relationship to their own material assets was also shown, for example, in the way new furniture was treated. After a short time, it was damaged or even demolished. Necessary repairs - even smaller ones the subjects could have done themselves - were put off. Consequently, the damage became worse and the subjects had to buy new furniture (for which they usually could not pay). In extreme cases, the subjects did not wash their underwear and clothes but left them lying around and finally threw them out and bought new clothes. The subjects often left their belongings behind in pay lockers or rented rooms without bothering about them anymore or brought their last belongings to pawnshops with no intention of getting them back.

The subjects handled property of others, for example that of their employer or landlord, as negligently and carelessly as their own. This usually led to further problems and difficulties.

The most important indication of **unstructured leisure behavior** was leisure activities with entirely open courses, such as frequenting meeting places, spending time in the "milieu," or driving around aimlessly on the lookout for adventure and excitement. These activities took up the main part of leisure time; usually, the subjects extended leisure time at the expense of the sphere of performance, sometimes only at the expense of sleep.

It was characteristic of such leisure behavior that neither places, duration, nor possible contact persons could be mentioned specifically at the beginning of such a "leisure undertaking." Normally, there was a meeting place as starting point for further action; however, there was absolutely no planning or preparation, not even short-term planning geared to the coming evening. The subjects simply waited to see what possibilities would open up and then realized them more or less spontaneously. This normally meant at least a latent, often a rather acute willingness to indulge in "excesses", whether in the form of considerable alcohol consumption (e.g., in connection with frequenting several bars during the course of the evening - "pub crawls") or uncontrolled spending sprees (drinking up weekly wages, paying for rounds, long taxi rides, etc.), or in the form of quarrels or violent arguments. If a meeting place was not already a "notorious" bar, pub, or night club of the (large) city "milieu" - the sphere to which socially conspicuous and delinquent persons of all kinds feel attracted, where they find other people with a similar lifestyle and where they feel comfortable - such an undertaking almost regularly ended there.

An **absence of planning in life** was assumed if the subjects, on the basis of their previous behavior in the social spheres, did not look ahead with regard to the organization of their lives, did not make a continuous effort (in a long-term perspective) to achieve any specific aim, e.g., in view of occupation, and if, in their current behavior as well, no preparations for the future were apparent. This criterion did not stipulate that the subjects had detailed and specific ideas about their lives or even a more or less complete concept of life. However, momentary ideas for the future without specific indications of their realization were not sufficient to negate the criterion.

In the individual case, the absence of planning in life was expressed, for example, in the sphere of performance, where subjects repeatedly gave up their jobs thoughtlessly and spontaneously. This led to frequent job changes and was usually connected with downward occupational mobility. It could also be expressed in a marriage for which no preparations were made. This had to lead to (further) difficulties and problems alone because of a lack of material security - not to mention the short duration of acquaintance. Furthermore, the subjects had generally made no provisions for illness or other emergencies. It was shown repeatedly that the subjects had rarely thought about their past or their future. Thus, they had no specific (or realistic) ideas for the time after they would be released from prison and made no specific preparations in this respect. On the whole, the impression arose repeatedly that the subjects lived "for the moment" or "for the day," let themselves "drift" or "lived from day to day"; they were always open to any impulses from outside, to momentary feelings of like or dislike and to moods, etc., which they gave in to without any resistance.

3.3.3.2 The Criteria of the Criminoresistant Constellation

The criterion of **fulfillment of social obligations** cannot be described in a general way: Every individual is confronted with many social obligations of different natures in his specific environment, which, for example, go far beyond legally defined obligations. Social obligations are characterized, among others, by the necessity of showing a certain amount of consideration for others and a basic willingness to forego or at least curtail personal desires and amenities for the benefit of one's immediate environment. Fulfillment of social obligations was assumed if there was no indication that the subjects neglected any essential obligations in their specific environment.

Such essential obligations were, for example, supporting one's family (especially wife and children) or (financially) supporting parents or brothers and sisters in need, contributing toward household money at home, helping with household tasks or in the (parents') business, and neighborly help. Beyond the home and family, there were social obligations in other areas as well, for example, toward fellow employees and superiors at work, in the organization of leisure, and in contacts with friends and acquaintances. Social obligations cannot be defined comprehensively or presented in detail; yet they are characterized by the fact that the subjects clearly recognized corresponding expectations and demands of their environment and accepted them as self-evident. Typical in this context were statements such as "I couldn't have done that to my parents", "that goes without saying", "that was simply expected".

An **adequate level of aspirations** was shown in the subjects' realistic estimation of their own possibilities - i.e., an estimation which others would also basically agree with - to which their aspirations were geared. An adequate level of aspirations was usually accompanied by the subjects' being to a certain extent satisfied with their situation, even if they lived in rather modest circumstances. Here, high aspirations of the subjects toward themselves or toward aims in life must be strictly distinguished from an adequate level of aspirations. The one does not preclude the other. Insofar as the subjects' current aspirations were not higher than their current possibilities - despite high, not yet realizable aims in life - the criteria "adequate level of aspirations" applied.

It is remarkable that precisely the subjects with an adequate level of aspirations had less high aspirations for their lives and environment than would have been possible on the basis of their occupational performance and financial situation; in this respect, they often demonstrated a certain modesty.

Attachment to a well-ordered home (and family life) was determined if the subjects' homes, whether this meant their families of orientation or procreation or their own dwellings if they were single, were of immediate interest to them. A certain indication of the importance of home and family in the everyday lives of the subjects was the extent to which they spent their leisure time at home or with the family. In extreme cases, the subjects concentrated their entire leisure time on leisure at home or on being together with the family. As a rule, the impression arose that the subjects did not simply adjust to the orderliness of the home environment of necessity but that their "integration" in the home environment and in family life was a real need.

An **adequate relationship to money and property** was assumed if the subjects were able to "manage" and budget their money, i.e., had no huge debts they would probably not be able to pay back with their income, and if they handled their own property (or that of others) carefully, considerately, and gently.

But an (adequate) relationship to money and property was usually not limited to the absence of debts. The subjects often had (occasionally several) savings accounts, savings agreements with home building and loan associations, etc., to which they regularly transferred a certain amount of money. Purchases were made only after the advantages and disadvantages had been considered in depth, and they were aimed at obtaining the highest possible long-term value, i.e., were not made for the immediate present alone. That their own property was handled carefully was shown in the extreme by the subjects reserving a room "for guests" or "for Sundays." As a whole, the subjects showed that they wanted to conserve their own property and not impair other property.

3.3.3.3 Further Criminorelevant Criteria

O-specific Criteria

An *inadequately high level of aspirations* referred almost exclusively to the purely material aspirations of the subjects (such as high earnings, high standard of living in material respect) which were in no way related to the subjects' (economic) conditions, possibilities and (occupational) abilities or to their own contributions to social relations. As a rule, there was not even a basic willingness to meet the corresponding requirements by one's own (socially adequate) performance (i.e., by not committing offenses, not gambling, etc.) or by corresponding behavior in social relations.

The subjects were dissatisfied with any kind of work and pay, without realizing that those whose occupational position and standard of living the subjects desired were more highly qualified and performed much better than the subjects were prepared to do. Especially typical was that the inadequately high material aspirations were accompanied by rather meager immaterial aspirations in life.

A *deficient sense of reality* was assumed if the subjects were led by wishful thinking which was incongruous with their actual situation, abilities, and possibilities. Characteristically, the subjects had aims which were difficult and often impossible to achieve because they rejected any (temporary) sacrifices which, besides tenacious and continuous efforts, would have been necessary to reach these goals. Nonetheless, they often thought they would be able to realize these goals easily with a little luck.

This criterion was chiefly expressed in the desire to have a "dream job" with a high level of prestige and particularly high income; ideas from any sources were taken up without any critical distance. The subjects thought of (supposedly) independent occupations (e.g., "sales representative") or their own business ("self-employed"), wanting only the conveniences of the position, but not realizing the requirements and risks or the stresses and difficulties involved. A deficient sense of reality, however, could also be expressed with respect to human relations, for instance when the subjects did not see the difficulties which almost necessarily arose from their relationship with a certain woman or from having relationships with several women at the same time. The same uncritical attitude led the subjects to believe that everything would be fundamentally different after marrying, being released from prison, etc. It was almost characteristic of these subjects that they did not learn anything from previous setbacks when they tried to realize comparable desires or from the failures of similarly unrealistic plans, i.e., that they did not estimate their own possibilities more realistically. Usually, they blamed someone or something else.

A low tolerance for stress was mainly expressed in human relations, especially in the "normal" and usual requirements in everyday and working life: The subjects, for example, could take no criticism concerning their person, behavior, work performance, etc. and overreacted to a certain degree.

The subjects, for instance, stopped working because of a trifling argument with the master craftsmen, gave notice because of a minor complaint by superiors, or ran away from home after a banal argument with their parents. Some of them were unable to last a normal 8-hour working day, live up to specific performance requirements somewhat consistently, or remain at one job for a prolonged period (several months or even years). As a whole, it was characteristic that the subjects literally ran away from any kind of problem or stress situation and thus caused a further deterioration of their own situation.

A *paradoxical expectation of adaptation* was understood as the subjects' refusal to adapt to the environment in any way while expecting the environment to adapt to them. A certain indication of the presence of a paradoxical expectation of adaptation was the fact that the subjects blamed other aspects (people or "circumstances") for the situation they felt to be unsatisfactory - which nearly always occurred.

As a rule, these subjects - wherever they went in the course of their lives - always ran into problems with their environment, e.g., with their parents, schoolmates, fellow employees, teachers, or superiors, because of their behavior. According to the subjects, it was as obvious that *the others* were to blame for the supposed disadvantages in the manifold conflicts as it was that the subjects themselves were not even minimally to blame for the problem.

A *demand to be free from any ties* was assumed when the subjects tried to avoid any kind of obligations or adjustment in a certain area in order to remain - as they put it - "independent," "autonomous," and "free."

Generally, a demand to be free from any ties was expressed early on in a lack of adjustment to the family of orientation, and especially in an early separation from the parents' home. It continued in the form of an unstable sphere of abode (frequent changes, temporary places to sleep, "roaming about") and was also expressed in the spheres of leisure and contacts (no leisure activities connected with any kind of obligation, no stable contacts, particularly no marriage, or if marriage, no change of life-style and living as freely as before) as well as in the sphere of performance (resistance toward any kind of integration at the place of work). Usually, the subjects also exhibited a longing for adventure or for something to happen and looked for excitement and diversity. One extreme, for example, was the attempt to be accepted in the Foreign Legion (with respect to the desired "independence" and "freedom" certainly inappropriate); another extreme, roaming about without fixed abode and "loafing".

Of special criminological relevance, finally, was uncontrolled, excessive *alcohol consumption*. Relevant was not the acute effect of alcohol addiction or alcohol consumption as such, but the *background effect* of (regular) considerable alcohol consumption, which finally pervaded all social spheres and nearly always intensified the O-specific behavior patterns in the various social spheres.

Apart from the importance of alcohol during the time immediately preceding the offense and during the commission of the offense (see Part II, Sects. 4.5.2 and 4.6), there were criminologically essential effects of alcohol - for example, when alcohol tended to reinforce the neglect of human relations, to push leisure behavior in the direction of unpredictable courses, and to lead to (further) conspicuousness in the sphere of performance. At the same time, it was shown very clearly that, for a possible criminological relevance, the criterion could not be viewed in isolation, but only in relation to the specific circumstances in life and behavior patterns of the individual subject: While, for example, regular (and considerable) alcohol consumption during working hours is socially "customary" for a construction worker and therefore criminologically irrelevant, similar alcohol consumption on another job could lead to considerable difficulties and thus to a further neglect of the sphere of performance in a situation where the subjects are already only minimally willing to perform. This is particularly true if their remaining life pattern is marked by considerable social conspicuousness. The situation was similar in the other social spheres, where an existing disposition toward O-specific behavior patterns was always intensified by alcohol or where existing socially conspicuous behavior patterns became more persistent. A further example is leisure behavior with open courses, which were specific to the majority of the O-subjects, connected with the basic willingness to indulge in "excesses" of any kind. This behavior was almost necessarily accompanied by (excessive) alcohol consumption, which again pushed the subjects further toward leisure activities with entirely open courses. In contrast, a similar regular alcohol consumption among a group of "regulars" integrated in a partially structured leisure behavior was socially inconspicuous and criminologically irrelevant.

G-specific Criteria

The criterion *dedication to and satisfaction from work* was assumed if occupation and work were an essential element of the subjects' organization of life (also in relation to ideals) and in a certain sense served the self-realization of the subjects. In other words, occupation and work were not regarded simply as a job and an (exchangeable) source of money. The subjects were satisfied with their occupation and work, performed well, worked overtime, and often had a second job which also satisfied them. They demonstrated a marked feeling of responsibility at their work, felt attached to the company, and believed that they were more or less indispensable for the company.

A *productive organization of leisure* was assumed when the leisure time of the subjects was characterized by planned, systematically pursued, and/or formally organized, frequently performance-oriented leisure activities with definite, regular courses. Thus, there was a clear boundary between partially structured activities, which generally bring about a general mental and physical recuperation or, to a certain extent, easy entertainment and relaxation, and entirely unstructured activities with open courses (see Part II, Sects. 2.4.3.2 and 2.4.3.3). In detail, a productive organization of leisure could be expressed in overtime or second jobs, "moonlighting," helping at home, continuing education, volunteer activities, active sports, and (for some, particularly creative) hobbies.

A *commitment to the affairs of persons and institutions* was usually related to corresponding positions and functions in clubs, communities, and political, charity, or church organizations, often in the form of honorary posts or volunteer work. This commitment could be expressed in activities ranging from caring for children and old people, youth welfare work, and environmental protection to sports or various kinds of hobbies. These tasks were often a real purpose in life for the subjects. They were absorbed in these tasks, and their family occasionally receded somewhat into the background. In the extreme, these (often numerous and time-consuming) activities were even a strain on the family.

A *willingness to adapt* was assumed when the subjects were basically prepared to live up to requirements and expectations of others with respect to their own person and behavior (at least for the moment) if they thought the requirements and expectations reasonable. The subjects remained true to their principles - which was also demonstrated in the orientation of their lives. A willingness to adapt should not be confused with suggestibility, which is marked by a lack of resistance toward *all* kinds of influence. A willingness to adapt was the result of a certain tolerance, which again required certain firm principles or ideals.

An indication of this was, for example, that the subjects were willing to adapt initially to others at their jobs and among their friends and acquaintances, and realized that in the beginning, it was necessary to accept the way work was done at their jobs (for example, the subjects did their job without immediately fighting against orders opposite to their own ideas). It was characteristic that the subjects looked for another field which corresponded more to their nature and expectations and where they could realize their (firm) principles better if they could not integrate their own ideas and opinions in the course of time.

Strong ties meant that the subjects had at least one person who was important to them as an individual personality, whom they trusted, to whom they felt they belonged, and for whom they felt responsible. Such ties included, in particular, parents, later on friends, girlfriends, and especially wives (and children).

Endurance and a high tolerance for stress were not limited to immediate strains in specific situations. The criterion was mainly expressed in a particular commitment and corresponding achievements (in particular at work). Yet it could also relate to coping with one's lot. The subject also (actively) mastered considerable difficulties and blows of fortune. It was characteristic that they did not blame certain disadvantages, but took their lives into their own hands, dealt with the situation, or looked for socially inconspicuous alternatives (e.g., a satisfying hobby as compensation for a certain dissatisfaction with their occupation) without waiting for help from others - for instance, the government.

The criterion *willingness to bear responsibility* could be found in almost all social spheres. Characteristic was that the subjects recognized their responsibility at work, for their parents, their wives, their children, etc. and were prepared to carry it and forego their own expectations. This could be expressed in the form of a subject helping on his parents' farm, increased efforts at work to secure the financial situation of the family, spending leisure time together with wife and children while foregoing preferred leisure activities a subject had pursued alone, or assuming responsible positions in a company or honorary commitments in clubs. As a rule, the subjects also saw that they were responsible for themselves and their own lives and tried to solve problems by themselves.

A *good sense of reality and self-control* was assumed when it was apparent that the subjects estimated their own possibilities and abilities (for example in view of their occupational career) as well as their weaknesses and "problems" more or less realistically and were able to deal with them. They did not indulge in wishful thinking or try to base their lives on irrational expectations.

Planning in life and determination were shown in all social spheres by a very straightforward development in life, where, with respect to the social integration of the subject, any kind of sudden break was almost unimaginable. The subjects' behavior and previous development throughout the various social spheres were marked by realistic foresight and planning as well as by continuity and stability in pursuing certain aims. It became apparent that they were able to commit themselves to long-term goals, i.e., to forego something in the present in favor of these goals (interests or ideals) which had a higher value for them. It was also marked by provisions and specific measures for the future. Many of these subjects were to a certain extent ambitious, particularly regarding occupation; however, their lives could also be marked by an overall satisfaction with the situation and by a basic modesty.

3.3.4 Summary

The criminorelevant constellations are a central result of the present study. They are especially relevant in a twofold way. First, they are directly related to criminality, since the criminovalent constellation did not occur for any G-subject, but did for the majority (60.5%) of the O-subjects, (in the end) for even 81% of the O-subjects whose "last" offenses had been property or fraudulent offenses, while the criminoresistant constellation occurred for 79.5% of the G- but for only six (3%) - atypical - O-subjects. Second, the inner logical consistency with which the criminovalent constellation results in a development leading to the commission of offenses became apparent.

These two aspects indicate that the criminorelevant constellations and further criminorelevant criteria in the cross section of life constitute a decisive "condensing" of essential occurrences in the various social spheres. With respect to further criminovalent constellations, a more detailed differentiation according to types of offenders and offenses remains to be made. Nevertheless, these constellations are not useful for gaining "automatic" access to the phenomenon of criminality or to "exemplary life"; applying them directly in the sense of a simple subsumption of individual facts is impossible on the basis of their conceptual nature. The individual criteria of the constellation, as relational concepts, are related to the specific circumstances in a subject's life. Determining the presence of these criteria therefore requires extensive individual investigations into the social behavior of the individual subject. Otherwise, it would be impossible to speak of a "neglect" of social obligations or an "absence" of planning in life. Thus, the attempts to describe the content of the criteria can be understood only as examples, not as a catalog of characteristics in the sense of an operationalization.

4 Comparisons in the Longitudinal Section

4.1 Preliminary Remarks

By way of its immediate relationship in time with the offense, the cross section analysis offers a special access to criminal occurrences. Yet the cross section analysis is of no assistance in the essential question of the position of the offense in the longitudinal section of an offender's life: Is the "presence" (or "lack") of certain criteria or entire constellations immediately before the offense a "natural" result of an offender's *entire* development in life or is it a unique or perhaps temporary conspicuousness? Neither the statistical analysis of the distribution of characteristics (see Part II) nor the ideal-typical behavior patterns (see Sect. 2 above) are of any use in this respect, as they do not cover the interrelationship of occurrences in time.

In individual areas, a dynamic approach could supplement the statistical analysis. For example, a comparison between the O- and the G-subjects with similar basic situations showed that there was, as it were, a series of "switches" which were shifted in the sphere of performance, from school to occupational training to behavior at work (see Part II, Sect. 2.3). Many O-subjects who started off with an average performance at school could not keep up with the G-subjects in the following periods during which the sphere of performance was studied. Thus, a picture of *continuous* decline emerged. The statistical analysis, however, could not determine in particular whether the development in life of an individual subject was continuous or not.

Therefore, in the longitudinal section as well, it was essential to elaborate ideal-typical forms expressing the various positions of the offense in the longitudinal section of life (see Sect. 4.4 below). They were to be valid as general *rules* and related to the question of whether an offense was a logically consistent consequence in the development of a subject's life - beyond the purely chronological succession of characteristics or syndromes which were related to criminality.

A first preliminary stage was the creation of overview forms, which were still of a formal nature (see Sect. 4.2 below); yet not until "twin" pairs with comparable basic situations were compared was an important material step taken (see Sect. 4.3 below).

4.2 The Overview Forms

The 400 individual case investigations formed a nearly unlimited source of information, which would not have been accessible for processing if it had not been structured. For this reason, it was attempted to summarize concisely and schematically the information necessary to obtain a first rough overview of the development of a subject.

The design of the forms developed for this purpose made it possible to obtain rapidly a synoptic picture in the cross and the longitudinal section. This was facilitated by various special features in the graphic design of the forms. Intervals during which significant changes took place, such as stays in homes or reform schools, military service, or stays in prison, were noted in different colors throughout the forms. In this way, it was easy to classify interrelated facts according to time (see also the new systematization of Johanson 1981, who uses musical notation).

Although these forms were technical aids, studying them led to first indications of possible types of courses. It was immediately apparent, for example, that conspicuousness did not occur until late in the development of many O-subjects, while such indications filled the entire form during childhood for other O-subjects. It soon became apparent as well that, beyond their function of rough orientation, the forms could not lead to the recognition of *typical* courses, even if the graphic presentation were improved. The entries on the forms were necessarily as "abstract" as operationalized "characteristics" in statistical analysis; i.e., the actual *importance* could not be assessed in the individual case. Thus, from the forms of the G-subjects, similar to the statistical analysis, it became apparent that there was occasionally some "conspicuousness" in the social spheres corresponding to the conspicuousness of the O-subjects, without the consequence of (recidivist) criminality. It was impossible to proceed beyond these contradictory findings by means of the overview forms: The level of "condensing" which had been achieved by forming relational concepts (see Sect. 3.3.1 above) could not be achieved by this kind of graphic presentation.

4.3 "Twin" Pairs of O- and G-Subjects

4.3.1 Fundamental Importance

Considering the aim of the present study, i.e., to obtain knowledge of typical forms of courses, and the deficiencies of both the statistical analysis and the overview forms, the next step had to be the examination of differing developments in the lives of the O- and the G-subjects who started off with the *same* "circumstances," insofar as this is possible for two or more persons. In this way, an attempt was made, similar to the attempt to form criminorelevant constellations in the cross section, to find the "criteria" of the subjects which made it possible to understand why subjects with the "same" external circumstances developed in a different way. It seemed advisable to take basic circumstances which could be assumed not to be the result of the subjects' behavior. But where this was not the case, particularly because of the increasing age of the subjects, there were some considerable differences as well in the way subjects coped with situations in life - irrespective of the way these situations had come about. Such "basic situations" were, for example:

- Groups with comparable fates and difficulties involved
- Unfavorable conditions at home
- Physical disability

- Marked strains in the sphere of performance
- Particular forms of leisure and contact behavior

As mentioned above, this did not mean that the circumstances of the subjects concerned were identical but only that they were as similar as possible. Such comparisons had been made more or less implicitly during the entire investigations and evaluations. Furthermore, it was also attempted to form several "twin" pairs from the material of the individual case investigations for each of these "basic situations" (on the advantages of this procedure as compared with the usual kind of matching, see Part I, Sect. 4.3). In the following, one "twin" pair is roughly sketched for each of the basic situations. The presentation is exclusively limited to externally visible behavior patterns and the information provided by the subjects or other persons.

4.3.2 Presentation of "Twin" Pairs

4.3.2.1 Groups with Comparable Fates and Difficulties Involved

In this context, comparisons between refugee and expellee lots presented themselves, since many subjects of the O- and the G-group were concerned (see Part II, Sect. 2.1.2.2). The difficulties and problems involved were repeatedly emphasized, particularly by the O-subjects and their parents. Criminality in particular was often related to the strains involved in fleeing, staying in camps, and emergency housing, and the therefore frequent changes of schools or jobs, language problems, condition of being an outsider and, consequently, keeping bad company.

O-"twin" 1 (born in 1939) first grew up in Silesia. After his father died in the war, his mother earned a meager living for herself and her children by sewing. Since she did not work at home and often did not come back until late at night, the children were often left to themselves. The subject exploited this in all respects by playing truant, not doing his homework, and being constantly on the move. Even during childhood he repeatedly committed petty theft. Despite missing school often, he was able to complete school successfully and began an apprenticeship as a mechanic, but since the family emigrated to the Federal Republic of Germany in 1956, he was not able to finish his apprenticeship. The family arrived in A-village without any means and was taken in by relatives who helped tide them over the first difficulties. One year later, in the same village, the family found a three-room apartment, which they were able to furnish with the aid of the equalization of war burdens (*Lastenausgleich* by law).

According to the subject and his mother, their greatest problem had been that they had not been respected in the village, being refugees. The subject in particular had suffered because he had not been able to speak German and had difficulties learning it. He had been laughed at and ridiculed by children and adults alike because of his awkward German and had repeatedly been told that he should first learn German properly. When children had spotted him in the streets, they had shouted "refugee" and "Polack" after him. He had not been able to make any contacts and had been totally isolated. He had often told his mother that he was simply going to go back to Poland secretly.

According to the subject, he had not been able to continue his apprenticeship because of his difficulties with the language, and had therefore gone to work in a factory as an unskilled worker. But in the factory as well, there had always been difficulties between him and his fellow employees. They had ridiculed, insulted, and harassed him, and had simply called him "the Polack", which had occasionally led to brawls. What had bothered him most, however, was the fact that, since his mother had also worked in the factory, he had felt supervised. So he had looked for a new job.

During the examinations (in 1966), the subject said that he had felt like an outcast in the village. After some time, he had gotten to know someone of his age from Berlin who was also in not too good repute. They had gotten along very well, but he had become involved in his first offense with this friend, who had been a real "crook." They had forced open several vending machines, but had been caught very soon. On the way home from the trial he had met his friend from Berlin again. As they had needed money for the coming Easter holidays, they had planned their next burglary, which brought them DM 1000. Together with others, they had spent the money during the Easter holidays in bars.

After the subject was convicted and served his sentence, things continued more or less in the same way. The subject was involved in a whole series of burglaries, which finally led to a prison sentence of 3 years.

The subject mainly blamed his very difficult childhood and unpleasant youth. He said that he had always had to fend for himself, that he had had no father and that his mother had not been able to look after him. Particularly later on, as a refugee, he had not been able to establish any contacts or to complete his apprenticeship because of his difficulties with the language. He had not had anything, had not been able to build up anything, and had only been ridiculed and treated as an outsider. He was convinced that he would have developed differently, and in particular would not have committed any offenses, under normal and more favorable conditions.

G-"twin" 1 (born in 1939) grew up in Poland together with his three sisters and his parents. His father was missing in action, and his mother, who was illiterate, had to support the family by helping on a farm. In early 1945, the family temporarily escaped to Bohemia but went back home at the end of the war. In 1947 they were expelled for good. After stays in several camps, they found emergency housing in Thüringen toward the end of 1948. The mother worked almost day and night on a farm, and the children were left to themselves all day. This did not change when the family moved to relatives in Saxony in 1952. In Saxony they had only emergency housing again, and the mother had to work all day on a farm.

The subject first went to the *Volksschule* in Poland, then in Thüringen and Saxony for a total of 8 years. He had considerable difficulties with the language and, moreover, was not at all encouraged by his mother in school. She thought school unnecessary since she had never gone. Furthermore, the subject had a hard time with his schoolmates and was ridiculed as "Polack". Nevertheless, he went to school regularly and completed school successfully. According to the subject, he had never really been interested in school, but he had regarded it as his duty and had therefore done it.

After finishing school, the subject wanted to become a forester, but this was impossible for various reasons, so he started an apprenticeship as an automobile mechanic, which he successfully completed in 1958. After that he worked as a journeyman in his occupation.

In 1960, the family came to the Federal Republic of Germany and finally arrived in a small town in southern Germany after staying in several transit camps. The family lived poorly in a camp for 4 years until, finally, they obtained a public-assistance dwelling in a housing development. After their move, the subject worked only as an unskilled worker: His experience, mainly with mopeds and motorcycles, was considered insufficient at his new job.

According to the subject, being isolated as a refugee had been most difficult for him. During his first years in the West, he had established practically no contacts with people of his age, as he had lacked the basis for contacts, such as going to school together or belonging to a club. Moreover, his German had still sounded stilted and harsh, which had not helped establishing contacts with people of his own age. Especially the first 4 years, when they had lived in the somewhat notorious camp, had been unfavorable. Moreover, he had had no way of impressing people with clothes or money or anything else, since his family had been in financial difficulties after his mother became ill and he had to hand in all his earnings at home.

At the time of the study (in 1967), the subject had a job as a semiskilled worker in a certain position of trust, which he found satisfactory. He had found a large circle of acquaintances among his fellow employees. He had not taken his initial difficulties tragically. Asked expressly about the danger of criminality, the subject said that he could not imagine having kept bad company or even having become delinquent because of all his difficulties. He had committed a series of traffic offenses and received a few penalty notices, and he liked a drink from time to time and could then possibly be led to play pranks, though never such as would land him in jail. He really had everything he needed and was satisfied with his life. The subject was firmly convinced that he would never become delinquent. In the family, "everybody was decent," his mother had taught him manners. That just ran in the family. What had in the end prevented him from becoming delinquent, he could not say.

4.3.2.2 Unfavorable Conditions at Home

Among the numerous aspects which can be used to form "twins" out of structurally incomplete or functionally disrupted families (see Part II, Sect. 2.1.3.3), extremely negative circumstances in the family of orientation and general neglect were chosen.

The circumstances in the family of orientation of *O-"twin" 2* (born in 1943) were marked by continuous quarrels between his parents and could be termed "asocial" - according to coinciding information and findings. His father had worked as a quarrier for many years and was an invalid pensioner from 1958 on; he had a fatal accident in 1959. The mother was not employed; she ran the household and took care of the six children (another five children died shortly after they were born or during early childhood). In the opinion of the youth welfare office, rearing the children was too much for the mother, and they could do whatever they wanted. When the social worker came, the mother often did not know where her children were at the moment, whether they were at school, playing with friends, etc. She was also unable to keep the house in order and attached no importance to cleanliness. The children were dirty and had torn clothing; the dwelling was in a sorry state. Though the father earned decent wages, there was never enough money since he drank away a considerable amount of his wages and his wife could not budget. The father, according to the youth welfare office, was inconsiderate but no match for his wife in any respect; he drank more and more and had numerous affairs with other women, whom he occasionally brought home. He was usually drunk when he came home. There were continuous quarrels and rows about his drinking, also about the children or money, which often ended in violent fights between the parents. Irrespective of this, the mother always found a reason to pick a fight; she was feared in the entire village for her quarrelsomeness.

According to the subject, the members of the family had not had anything in common; they had all gone their own ways. Just as his parents had not paid any attention to him, he had not paid any attention to them. He had never been able to get along with his father or talk things over with him, and his mother had not been quite what she should have either. She had always been nagging, had been "explosive," and had always reproached the subject for things that had happened years before. In no way could he say that his relationship to his mother had been good.

In the course of time, the three older siblings of the subject were committed to homes because of various thefts, the two sisters additionally because of sexual conspicuousness. Both younger siblings grew up at home and demonstrated no serious conspicuousness. The subject himself had already been conspicuous at school: He often played truant, sometimes staying away from school for days or even weeks. According to the subject, this had been a "real habit" of his; he had simply preferred to "go for a walk" in the mornings. Sometimes he had been "on the move" until late at night and had roamed about in the woods or had - especially later on - spent a considerable amount of time in the nearest city. At home, no one had paid attention to this, just as no one had paid attention to whether he had done his homework, which had frequently not been the case.

Nonetheless, the subject completed the 8th grade of the *Volksschule* without having to repeat a year. The youth welfare office got involved with the subject for the first time when, at the age of 13, he lured a girl of his own age home and tried to have sexual intercourse with her against her will and when he - not yet criminally responsible - committed three thefts in rapid succession during the following period. According to the youth welfare office, the mother had lacked insight with respect to the negative development of her children and had always protected them, either denying the subject's offenses or blaming the other children in the village, saying they were lying. In this context, she threatened the social worker of the youth welfare office seriously several times, who refused to enter the house again without police protection.

According to the subject, he had not felt like starting an apprenticeship after finishing school and had therefore worked as an unskilled worker for a firm of builders and contractors. Since he did not like the work, he walked off the job after a few weeks. Similarly, he gave up another job as a harvester spontaneously after 2 weeks and stole a large sum of money from his employer as "compensation."

The years following 1958 were marked by his running away from homes, roaming about, being brought back to the home, attempting to work, and running away once again. In the meantime, he repeatedly committed theft and indecency with minors. After being released for good from the home, the subject committed various offenses against property and, apart from short periods of freedom, which lasted at the most a few months, was mainly imprisoned up to the time of the study (in 1966). He had no contact with his parents' home at all, neither with his siblings nor with his mother.

When asked about it, the subject said that he could now see that the circumstances at home had ruined his childhood. He had never known a real family life. Considering his childhood, his development was not surprising. Now he did not care anymore; he had closed that chapter of his life. Nevertheless, he was not isolated; he had a "home" and acquaintances around the train station and the old town, where he felt at ease and where he could always find someone to spend time with and talk to.

Similar circumstances prevailed in the family of orientation of *G-"twin" 2* (born in 1941). His mother was the third wife of his father, who had four children of previous marriages. His mother had not been married before but had two illegitimate children of different fathers, neither of whom was identified. The subject and another son came from the present marriage.

The economic circumstances of the family were always very difficult. The father did not earn much as a municipal worker, and the mother was not able to budget. According to the youth welfare office, the way the children were reared left much to be desired. Rearing the children was mainly the mother's concern. The children were mostly left to themselves and could do whatever they wanted. The youth welfare office had to caution the parents repeatedly to take care that their children went to school and were clean. Moreover, the youth welfare office also intervened repeatedly when the children came to school with bruises after being beaten by their parents - often for no specific reason. The parents did not recognize their faulty behavior. The parents also had frequent loud and violent arguments between themselves, especially when the father came home drunk and kicking up a racket - which happened often - or when the mother started a fight over some trifling matter, usually money. In later years, there were mainly serious and sometimes violent arguments between mother and stepchildren. In 1955, following such an argument, the father hanged himself.

After the father's suicide, circumstances at home deteriorated further. The mother did not look after the household and children at all; she was still considered difficult and extraordinarily quarrelsome and was generally avoided. The relation of the children to their (step)mother became even more difficult after the father's suicide, since they felt that she was to a certain extent responsible. The (step)children, all around the age of occupational training, went their own ways and eventually left home of their own incentive. Finally, the younger brother of the subject was committed to a reform school because he played truant and roamed about persistently.

Despite these very unfavorable external circumstances, the subject demonstrated no conspicuousness as a child. In the regular reports of the youth welfare office on the entire family, for example, it was always emphasized that the subject was also frequently dirty but that he went to school regularly, posed no difficulties, and, in contrast to his siblings, offered no reason for the youth welfare office to intervene. After the death of his father, the subject remained with his mother and began an apprenticeship as a mason after successfully completing the *Volksschule*. He completed the apprenticeship and passed the final examination.

During the investigations, the subject said that he was extremely proud of having worked for the same company for more than 10 years and of being, according to him, absolutely indispensable there. In the meantime, he was married and had two children. The family had taken in the subject's mother and took care of her. Neither he nor his mother had close contact with any of the remaining siblings. The mother was still difficult and often had arguments with the subject and his wife for no reason at all. This was not taken all too seriously by the subject and his wife. The subject himself could not say why he had not committed any offenses, like his younger brother, why he had not left home, like his siblings, or why he was the only child who had completed occupational training. He could not imagine leading any other life.

4.3.2.3 Physical Disability

Other basic situations which cannot be directly influenced by the person concerned are deformities, amputations, or the aftereffects of accidents, which some of the (O-)subjects indicated as the reason for difficulties and the onset of criminality (see Part II, Sect. 3.2).

According to the investigations, *O-"twin" 3* (born in 1941) demonstrated no conspicuousness until after the age of 19. After he had finished the *Volksschule*, he had completed an apprenticeship as a weaver and afterward practiced his occupation. He had spent his leisure time mainly at home or in the youth club; from time to time he had also gone to the movies with former schoolmates. After his parents got divorced when he was 17, he went to live with his aunt.

At the age of 20 he had a serious motorcycle accident, caused by one of his friends. His left leg had to be amputated. According to his aunt, the subject had first reacted calmly. He had never complained, and even after he had been discharged from the hospital and had been on sick-leave for half a year, there had been no difficulties. He had tried to move around on his crutches and had been surprisingly lively.

His company retrained him as a clerk and employed him when he was fit to work again since he could no longer work as a weaver. His new work represented a move up for him. He had no difficulties with his work and was able to buy a car with the insurance indemnity.

One evening, according to his aunt, he had come home entirely changed: He had positively broken down. He had sat at the table, crying bitterly. Finally, he had asked whether it was true that he was a cripple. She had explained that he would get a prosthesis and would be able to walk again, but he would not calm down. He had just been visiting a friend. The two of them had been talking about the upcoming call-up for military service, and the subject had said that he would surely be able to do some kind of military service. His friend had answered laughingly that he was a cripple and that they would surely not take him. The subject had then attacked his friend and beaten him so violently that his friend's parents had almost called the police. The friendship had been more or less destroyed. According to his aunt, this was simply one example. After the incident, the subject had changed markedly and had become very sensitive. He had met with very few of his former schoolmates and had no longer gone to the youth club. He had often cried and would not be consoled. While the two of them had got along very well earlier, there had suddenly been friction between them. He had pushed her away from him, saying she was only his aunt, what did she want.

During the following period, the subject spent less and less time at home. He went out to drink in the evening, often immediately after work, and slowly acquired a corresponding circle of acquaintances. His aunt fought against this, but could not assert herself. It was of no use when she simply did not give him any money; he let the others pay for him. During the following period, brawls frequently occurred. Whenever the others made fun of his leg when they were drunk, he repeatedly beat them blindly with his crutches.

A few weeks after the subject could and did start working again, he committed his first offense, a joint rape, together with his new acquaintances, under the influence of alcohol. The sentence was suspended. After a short period of pretrial detention, the subject was taken into a church home, through the interventions of the village pastor. There, however, he soon ran into difficulties because of his drinking and had to leave. He went back to his aunt, where he immediately started meeting his old acquaintances and drinking again. Only 3 days after his return, he caused a serious car accident and absconded from the scene of the accident.

G-"twin" 3 (born in 1942) also exhibited no conspicuousness before his accident. He had grown up at his parent's home and had gone to a *Gymnasium* up to the *Mittlere Reife*. He was a loner but had good contacts with his schoolmates. He spent most of his leisure time at home. He was totally absorbed in his hobby, model-making, and was firmly resolved to go to a school for precision-mechanical engineering.

When he was 17, an explosion tore off his right hand while a friend and he were experimenting with a rocket. His arm had to be amputated.

After the accident, he was at a loss regarding his occupational future. What had interested him and what had been the content of his life was now out of the question as an occupation. According to the subject, the conflicts after his accident had been very difficult. His life had changed entirely. He had had to give up many things he had taken for granted before. But he had been aware from the outset that everything had depended on his getting a good and secure job. Therefore, he had done everything to build up a future in the occupational respect. Since the only possibility for him had been an office job, he had more or less reluctantly and perforce let himself be persuaded to pursue a career in the intermediate administrative service. However, no suitable apprenticeship could be found near his home. Therefore, he first went to commercial school for a year. By the time he started occupational training, he was already 20 years old. He successfully completed the 3-year training and became a civil servant.

According to his parents, the subject had been more isolated and had lived more seriously than his friends after his accident. The distance between them had also increased because of his occupation. The subject himself said that he would never have thought of keeping "irresponsible" company at the time or distracting himself with alcohol. He would never have let himself be carried away in this respect by external influences.

4.3.2.4 Marked Strains in the Sphere of Performance

There are many points of view according to which "twins" can be formed with respect to marked strains in the sphere of performance. Particularly in this context, characteristic "switches" became apparent in the statistical analysis (see Part II, Sect. 2.3). A pair of "twins" was chosen who exhibited marked difficulties, both in apprenticeship and vocational school, that led to comparable reactions but were dealt with very differently.

According to his information, it was *O-"twin" 4*'s (born in 1943) own wish to start an apprenticeship as a plumber after completing the *Volksschule*. However, he could not find satisfaction in his work. The master craftsman was often drunk and left the apprentices to themselves. Yet the subject did not make any special efforts of his own; he had always had - as he said - other things on his mind and had always been up to all kinds of tricks. He often played truant from vocational school and received a bad report. Since his father would have called him to account, he simply put the report on the table at home and left. He had been tired of the whole story and had decided to "go abroad." He went to see a former schoolmate who had recently been fired from his apprenticeship. The friend immediately agreed to go along. They hitchhiked into the next large city, where they spent two nights, sleeping at the train station. Then they stole two bicycles and camping equipment and moved on. When they had neither money nor food left, they broke into a kiosk. With the alcohol, cigarettes, chocolate, and the little money they found there, they were able to keep above water for a few days. They were picked up by the police 5 days later.

After the subject came back, his parents organized a new apprenticeship. The prison sentence for juveniles was suspended on probation. The subject went on meeting his former schoolmate and finally got into a group of juveniles with whom he committed an armed robbery. During his 4-year term in prison he completed his apprenticeship, but he did not last long in his occupation after being released and soon committed offenses again.

According to the information, *G-"twin" 4* (born in 1944) was dissatisfied with his commercial training. Originally, he wanted to become an artist, but his stepfather had refused because of the high costs involved. His next wish, to become a cook, was rejected by his mother because he would have had to live away from home. Finally he decided in favor of an apprenticeship in the commercial sector. The subject did not like his employer, however, who exploited him. When he protested against constantly having to do overtime, a vehement argument ensued. He did not have the courage to change or break off his apprenticeship. In the end, he took his final examinations, which he initially thought he had passed. It turned out, however, that the education board did not acknowledge the compensation of a poor grade in German by a good one in geography. First he thought he would simply have to repeat his German examination, but then was informed that he had to repeat the entire theoretical examination.

The subject indicated that he had largely been on his own in this situation. He had not been able to talk about it with his parents. They had not been interested. When he had been informed of the decision of the education board, he had lost his head and had run away. With the DM 270 he had had, he had bought a train ticket to Rome and had gone on to Naples from there. In the beginning, he had slept in hotels; when he had run out of money he had hitchhiked and slept outside. He had roamed about Italy for nearly 4 weeks. He had never stolen anything during this period. When he had not had any money left at all and had not even been able to get his suitcase from the luggage deposit, he had simply gone to the train station and offered to work as a porter. He had usually gotten a decent tip. Then he had been able to buy something to eat and get his suitcase back. Naturally, at the train station, he had got to know others who had also been roaming about and who had finagled to get whatever they had needed. Yet he had never thought of going along with them. He had been too afraid. He could not guarantee that he would not have "gone astray" even more in the course of time if he had had nothing left to do but steal. But he had simply got enough of this way of life; he had been homesick and had seen to it that he got home as quickly as possible. His only incorrectness had been that he had told the consulate in Florence that his money had been stolen. He had been given DM 10 to buy something to eat and a train ticket to Basel. From Basel, he had hitchhiked and walked home.

At home there had been no difficulties; his mother had been glad that he had come back. He then looked for a new job and repeated the examination after some time. At the time of the study (in 1967), he was still working in his original occupation and was taking an additional course as a programmer. No offenses were known up to that time.

4.3.2.5 Particular Forms of Leisure and Contact Behavior

An example of a differing development on the basis of the "same" external circumstances and situations in the sphere of contacts and leisure is belonging to a group of juveniles who commit offenses together.

According to the investigations, *O-"twin" 5* (born in 1946) did not complete an apprenticeship after leaving school but worked as an unskilled worker for the same company for 6 years.

Shortly after leaving school, he became a member of a group of 16- to 20-year-olds which called itself the "vampire gang". Its mark was a red scarf. Initially, the group was rather harmless; its members loitered on street corners, played small pranks, etc. without committing any serious offenses. Later on, an "extra gang" split off. The members of this group, which was more or less a motorcycle gang, were somewhat older; the subject was around 18 at the time. The gang's marks were a leather jacket, a helmet, a black scarf, and tattooed arms. In the beginning, the main activities of the group were roaring through the streets on mopeds and motorcycles, making a racket, and annoying people. The group then set up "statutes" and defined the "purpose" of the club as sitting around in bars, drinking, and playing pranks (meaning brawls, damage to property, etc.). The group, including the subject, committed a series of burglaries and damage to property, taking along steel rods and blackjacks. The subject provoked brawls and was finally reported to the police for unlawful entry after the group violently disturbed a dancing lesson.

The subject's confession within the framework of the police inquiries contributed essentially toward breaking up the group; nonetheless - according to the subject - the police interrogation and particularly the trial had not impressed him at all. The prison sentence for juveniles was suspended on probation. The subject soon became a member of another gang, which committed a series of burglaries. Among these, the gang broke into 40 cars.

Asked about it during the investigations (in 1967), the subject said that he was not thinking of changing his life-style; this was a highly interesting kind of leisure activity, anything else was an "awful bore" and "square."

During his apprenticeship, *G-"twin" 5* (born in 1945) also started visiting hoodlum bars, where jukeboxes made a racket and where something was always going on. Some of his "buddies" had already been convicted and imprisoned several times. Besides, as a member of a rock-and-roll band, he was on the move a lot and got to know the entire surrounding area. A lot of "rabble" had gotten together during the performances, and there had often been rows. In the course of time, a real gang of 16- to 20-year-old hoodlums developed. They met in "bars" and drank together, and at some point somebody would come up with an idea for something to do. For example, some of them knew how to handle vending machines, and the subject - according to his own opinion later on - had been stupid enough to go along with everything. After 6 months, a whole series of thefts from vending machines had occurred. He had always depended on the others and had gone along with the crowd. If you were right in the middle of things and 50 people were saying yes to bad things, you couldn't be against them. He had just gone along and had not thought anything about it. They had been a clique, and, when the clique had done something, he had gone along because he would have felt an outsider if he had not. The clique and solidarity had been more important than anything else at that time.

The whole affair finally came out, and the leader of the clique was sentenced to 1 year in prison for juveniles, the subject to 2 weeks of detention for juveniles. The detention had made a deep impression on him, and he had realized that he had not really been on the "right track." He had met juveniles who had been in pretrial detention and had been real "criminals." The whole thing had been somewhat shocking for him and had intimidated him. In time, he had become more sensible by himself. But he believed that everything could have turned out differently if his father had not intervened. His father had been a support for him during that time. After his detention, his father had gone out with him three or four times and had taken a look at the people he had been spending his leisure time with. His father had made a selection and determined with whom he could spend time and with whom he could not, and he had obeyed or rather had had to obey. If he had not, his parents would have sent him to his uncle in the countryside. There would have been no entertainment or fun there, so he had "taken it easier." The subject still met members of the gang or people with previous convictions later on since he preferred places where rock-and-roll music was played. There had also often been brawls, but he had never taken sides or gotten involved in them. This was really possible, all it needed was a little willpower.

At the time of the study (1969), the subject was married and, as far as could be determined, had not been involved with the police in the meantime.

4.3.3 Summary

In the foregoing comparisons, the more or less obvious purpose was to elaborate the (criminologically) essential differences between the groups of the study. Of necessity, it was only minimally expressed that there were also *transitions* between the behavior patterns of the O- and the G-subjects. The examination of the G-subjects' delinquency alone showed that some of the G-subjects previously convicted for "classic" offenses had shown obvious conspicuousness, mainly in the spheres of leisure and contacts. Yet this conspicuousness, as well as that of the "twins" presented here, remained rather sporadic (see Part II, Sect. 4.7.2). The statistical analysis offered a certain impression of these transitions as well: Serious "strains" also occurred occasionally in the G-group. This was mainly the case for given circumstances, especially in the family of orientation, which initially affected both groups to an equal extent.

The foregoing "twin" comparisons carried on in this direction. In contrast to the statistical analysis, the comparison took into consideration not characteristics but "situations" for which it could be assumed that "switches" which were *decisive* for the lives of the subjects were shifted. Especially with respect to the differing reactions of the subjects to such situations, the question arose as to whether the causal importance of external facts, even if they accumulated and came to a head in crisis-like situations, would not have to be relativized in the end in favor of other "internal facts," such as the fundamental attitudes of the subjects in connection with certain patterns of relevance and a corresponding value orientation (see Sect. 5 below). In the foregoing cases, the question was which criteria led to recidivist criminality for the O-subjects but not for the G-subjects, though, in light of all existing knowledge of "external facts," such a development would have been "comprehendible" for the G-subjects as well.

For the further examination of these questions, a differentiated examination of the longitudinal section of life offered itself to determine certain processes in the development in life which occurred regularly in relationship with delinquency and, on the basis of the visible facts of development in life, to draw conclusions concerning "attitudes," the content of which was described in content in the criminorelevant constellations and criteria (see Sect. 3.3 above). For this purpose, an interlocking analysis of the cross and the longitudinal section of life was necessary (see Sect. 6 below).

4.4 The Position of the Offense in the Longitudinal Section of Life

4.4.1 Fundamental Importance

The foregoing "twin" pairs do not allow for making any statements on the longitudinal section of life of the subjects for two reasons: On the one hand, they represent only a few individual cases, and on the other hand, their presentation is limited to a single segment of the longitudinal section - though a particularly important one for the subjects concerned.

To make any statement on the position of the offense in the *entire longitudinal section of life,* it must be attempted to trace the courses of criminal developments whose outcome, (recidivist) criminality, either follows with an inner logical consistency from the continuity of the previous development in life or constitutes a break in the development in life (or also an intermediate form which can be described qualitatively). These courses were the aim of the efforts toward "condensing" knowledge from experience *in the longitudinal section,* as were the criminorelevant constellations *in the cross section.*

In no way, however, was the aim a complete typology taking into account the entire spectrum of delinquency. Contrary to the constellations in the cross section of life, which presented extreme (ideal) pictures of a broad range of the subjects of *both* groups of the study, a differentiation of types of positions of the offense in the longitudinal section was limited to a certain extent by the manner of selecting the O- and the G-group (see Part I, Sect. 1). The selection criterion for the O-group consciously aimed at marked criminality. Therefore, it was expected that a majority of the O-subjects would show a development in life into which repeated offenses would fit more or less naturally and that only a few subjects, some of them among the 47 previously convicted G-subjects, some among the (atypical) O-subjects, would demonstrate forms where offenses do occur, though not in a lasting, persistent way.

Therefore, the following description is open insofar as intermediate forms between the two extremes, the "continuous development toward criminality" and "criminality as a sudden event" are not given full treatment. There is room both for further differentiation inside the forms and for new forms. Conspicuous behavior and criminality due to mental impairment, for example, are not covered. Moreover, the position of offenses committed by negligence in the longitudinal (and the cross) section is not considered, though it should be possible in principle to subdivide them according to corresponding criminological criteria based on experience.

4.4.2 The Continuous Development Toward Criminality Beginning During Early Youth

The presentation of the continuous development toward criminality beginning during early youth necessarily overlaps with the examination of the cross section and the statistical analysis. This type of course is characterized by the earliest possible and most marked behavior patterns of the "ideal-typical" O-subject. Therefore, it is unnecessary to repeat *all* possibly relevant facts (for details, see GÖPPINGER 1980, pp. 313 ff.).

Nonetheless, in the examination of the longitudinal section, it becomes apparent once again that the importance of individual facts can vary considerably. Thus, on the one hand, there are the syndromes which indicate a high probability of criminal development and, to this extent, are distinct alarm signals for a possible prophylaxis. On the other hand, there are individual facts which *also* occur frequently in a continuous development toward criminality, but which are too unspecific in their effect and can be compensated for in many other ways. The latter holds particularly for circumstances which are *far removed* from the offense, materially and in time. Yet this says nothing about the importance of these circumstances *in the individual case.*

Decisive for a continuous development toward criminality are the (complementary) developments in the spheres of performance and leisure. A continuous development toward criminality often begins at preschool age: The subjects run away from home and roam about. Later on, at school, there is conspicuous, often aggressive behavior toward schoolmates and teachers and persistent truancy, which is usually used for roaming about aimlessly and which is often covered up by clever lies and deceit. During occupational training and employment, the tendency *to avoid all requirements of performance and order* continues: Leisure time is extended not only at the expense of sleep, but also at the expense of the sphere of performance. Leisure activities which take place away from home, are (unproductive and) unstructured, and have entirely open courses predominate. This - in a form in keeping with the subjects' age - corresponds to the earlier roaming about at preschool and school age. Significantly enough, these facts form the heart of the criminovalent constellation. From this central point, even the most serious conspicuousness in the spheres of abode and contacts is easily comprehendible: Efforts to actively avoid any family supervision during childhood or to exploit a lack of supervision in all respects, which, apart from other conspicuousness, can lead to stays in homes; leaving parents' home at an extremely early age irrespective of committals to homes; a repeated lack of abode; the lack of strong ties (first) in given *and* (later) in self-chosen contacts; instead frequently changing, noncommittal acquaintances made for short-term, utilitarian purposes as well as a one-sided exploitation of parents and other relatives.

The inner *dynamics* of the continuous development toward criminality becomes apparent in particular when the presence of the individual criteria of the criminovalent constellation are traced back in time. Here, a differentiated analysis of the last offenses yielded useful information (see Part II, Sect. 4.6). The typical unstructured leisure behavior with entirely open courses can continue for a relatively long time if leisure time is extended only at the expense of sleep. As long as the sphere of performance remains at least fairly intact, the subjects still have the means to keep up this kind of leisure organization, though, as a rule, at the expense of other obligations. However, it is quite natural that, alone because of the need for rest and sleep, the extension of leisure time affects the sphere of performance at some point in time. Unexcused absences from work, flagging work performance, and frequent job changes with intervals of nonemployment cause each other reciprocally and affect the sphere of leisure: More time becomes available. If the subject continues pursuing the same leisure activities, which are usually rather expensive, the situation comes to a dramatic head. Everything practically forces the subject to obtain the means he needs but does not have for lack of employment by committing an offense (against property). At the same time, the requirements for an offense are already at hand, on the basis of the specific situation in the leisure activities mentioned and the typical contacts involved. Thus, in the continuous development toward criminality, there is a total collapse of the structuring of all social spheres, including the sphere of abode, immediately before the offense.

Yet the inner dynamics of the development cannot be traced back indefinitely in the sense of an immediately comprehendible inner logical consistency. The farther back one goes, the more frequently situations occur which (still) offer various possibilities of development and which also apply to an increasing number of G-subjects. Here, the ideal-typical examination of the continuous development toward criminality must be limited to determining *that* such situations occur without being able to find a conclusive inner logical consistency.

This type must be clearly differentiated from earlier, purely tautologous attempts to explain criminality by a "propensity" toward criminality. In the continuous development toward criminality, there are criteria of *social* behavior of the offenders in the context of their social relationships which are ideal-typically "condensed," but which can be gained from experience in the individual case - though not fully operationalized - *without* criminality itself being of any importance. The corresponding behavior patterns and "attitudes" can thus be presented without any reference to definitions of offenses or concepts relevant to criminal law.

Such a development cannot not be continued indefinitely. Well-founded statements on the further development of the subjects during the next decades are not yet possible; they cannot be made until the follow-up study has been completed.

The following is an *example* of a continuous development toward criminality beginning during early youth:

A. was born in 1942 in M-city as the second youngest of his mother's eight children. Two of his older siblings were illegitimate, and one child had been brought into the marriage by his mother. The father had worked for years as a semiskilled milling machine operator in one company but was repeatedly ill for longer periods of time. The household and rearing of the children were the mother's responsibility. The marriage was rather unhappy. In the beginning, the parents had many arguments (also in connection with his father's drinking), but later on they just lived alongside one another. The economic circumstances were always inadequate, but the mother always kept the apartment in order and saw to it that the children were fairly clean.

Child rearing was inconsistent, ranging from hitting the children to exaggerated protection. Particularly the mother closed her eyes to what the subject did and excused herself by saying that she had not been able to keep track of her many children; she had not known where or with whom her children were at any given moment or what they had been doing.

The subject started going to school in 1948 and attended the *Volksschule* for 8 years. His performance was always barely adequate. He had to repeat the second grade. Later on, the teachers stretched a point and let him go on to the next grade. He frequently failed to do his homework or did it carelessly, all the more so since it was not checked at home. He often played truant, frequently for several days at a time - usually together with his younger brother. The two of them roamed about the streets of the city. Usually, the parents did not notice this, and the teacher "knew" the two in this respect and no longer required excuses in the higher grades, since he was simply told brazen lies and received no support from the parents. During leisure time as well, the subject spent his time roaming the streets with his brother. He was expelled from several clubs (athletics, trick cycling, town band) after a short time because he was always up to no good and did not get along with the others, which made constructive cooperation impossible. In the summer of 1955, the subject and older acquaintances of his repeatedly went to see a mentally disturbed neighbor, about 40 years old. He repeatedly had sexual intercourse with her and afterward stole small sums of money in her apartment. Because of this and his truancy, the youth welfare office ordered supervision (of morally endangered minors). This brought about no fundamental improvement.

After finishing school in spring 1956, the subject found a job as an unskilled worker in a furniture factory with the help of his father. He gave up the job after 3 weeks. At another job, he no longer showed up after 5 weeks. Finally, in August 1956, he found a job as an unskilled worker in a shoe factory, where he stayed - except for frequent unexcused absences (usually in connection with roaming about and committing offenses) - until May 1958. While he initially paid for his board at home, he refused to do so later on and used his wages for his almost daily visits to bars. In addition, he spent most of his leisure time at the movies with his younger brother and some acquaintances of his age or driving around aimlessly with mopeds and motorcycles. He committed several offenses in this connection: During the summer of 1956 he repeatedly stole motorcycles together with others, drove around on them without a license, and caused several accidents including damage to the stolen vehicles. In three cases the juvenile court ordered juvenile detention.

In the spring of 1957, the subject and two acquaintances of his age agreed to go to Hamburg together and to emigrate "to Texas" from there. In order to obtain the necessary money, they planned to rob a grocery. However, since a customer happened to pass by, they did not. The following night they committed two burglaries of the offices of their employers. Since they found only a small amount of money, they gave up their plans to emigrate. In the summer of 1957 they broke into basements together twice; in December 1957 more thefts followed, in connection with roaming about for several days. During the second attempt to emigrate together, the subject and his "buddies" obtained the necessary money by visiting an aunt on the way to Hamburg and stealing DM 500 from her.

After the subject again missed several days of work because of this, he was dismissed. During the following months, he worked for no more than a few weeks, and finally, in July 1958, correctional education was ordered, and the subject was committed to the reform school in O-city. During the first few weeks, the subject escaped repeatedly and went back home. He committed several offenses against property on the way, among these, embezzlement of the money of two fellow inmates with whom he had escaped and who had given him money to buy tickets. In the course of time, he adjusted to the home and the group and was willing and handy at work. Therefore, the reform school tried letting him do an apprenticeship as a butcher. The apprenticeship failed after a few weeks because he showed no interest and constantly played truant at vocational school. He then worked on the farm of the home. In May 1960 he was given a job as a farm worker. On the farm he had contact with the family, behaved himself, and mainly spent his leisure time at home. Then, his father, who had retired in the meantime, urged him to come back home so that (as the father said) "there would be some money." The subject was released from correctional education in October 1960 and went back to his parents.

During the following period, the subject was still under supervision, being on probation from an 8-month prison sentence for juveniles for the offenses of 1957/58. Although he did not work regularly at first and spent the whole day in bars, his parents refused to cooperate with the probation officer. Up to the summer of 1961, the subject spent several weeks or only several days at nine different jobs. He sometimes went for weeks between jobs without spending any time looking for one. When, following two sentences for bodily injury and a traffic offense, a revocation of probation was impending, he left home with the support of his parents and roamed about for 4 months with no fixed abode. He supported himself by working as a showman's helper or temporary laborer, as well as by committing minor offenses against property. He slept wherever he was working at the time or in sheds, at the train station, etc. In the fall of 1961 he ran into a police check and served his 8-month prison sentence for juveniles.

When he was released in June 1962, he went back to his parents. After a few short-term jobs, he worked for a warehouse for almost a year in 1963/64. He lost the job because he had embezzled goods and sold them. He held eight different jobs as an unskilled worker, mason's assistant, coal carrier, codriver, etc. up to his last term in prison (1966). He again often stayed away from work unexcused or on the pretext of being ill (often after spending the night drinking). Between jobs, he did not work at all for several weeks, partially living on welfare, partially letting himself be supported by his parents. In the summer of 1965, he and an acquaintance temporarily worked as "self-employed underground engineers", which meant digging ditches and laying tiles. Since their work was mainly unsatisfactory, the customers paid accordingly less. Moreover, the subject got into difficulties with the tax authorities because he did not pay taxes, which made him give up his business. He no longer worked regularly up to the time he was arrested.

Besides paying damages for several traffic accidents, which he did only partially, and paying board irregularly, he spent his money mainly in bars, where he often paid for his buddies and for any woman who was there. He also spent a considerable amount of money on long taxi rides to the nearest large city in connection with visits to bars, etc. He was always on the move during his leisure time, usually in (what he called) "*remmidemmi*" bars, where something was always going on, where there were girls, and where he sometimes performed as a fire-eater. According to his mother, the subject frequently came home drunk three times a day, slept for a few hours and then went back to the bar. He never had enough money and (in his opinion) was unable to budget. He always had debts, since he bought cars and television sets, which he destroyed when he was drunk. He usually used up his weekly pay in the course of the weekend; once when he received a DM 600 tax refund, he spent the entire amount in one evening in bars. Furthermore, he also had debts because he had to maintain two illegitimate children of different women, with whom he had temporarily lived together at his parents' place. His relationship with his parents fluctuated. While he sometimes supported his parents, they repeatedly called the police when he threatened them when he was drunk. In July 1965, the subject and his father had a violent argument. His father fled by the window and broke his foot. While the subject was serving a 4-week sentence because of this, he demolished his cell. For the rest, his criminal record showed a total of 17 offenses during the period from his 8-month prison sentence for juveniles (1962) to his last imprisonment (spring 1966): Besides traffic offenses (driving without a license, drunken driving, unauthorized use, and hit-and-run driving), there were offenses in connection with alcohol consumption (among others insults, threats, bodily injury, and coercion of and resistance to police officers) and various burglaries, as well as a joint check fraud against his employer. The subject had repeatedly been sentenced to fines and short sentences in prison. At the time of the study, he was serving a sentence of 1 year and 3 months for the offenses he had last committed.

4.4.3 The Development Toward Criminality Beginning During Adolescence or the Early Years of Adulthood

Although the concept of the development toward criminality is more related to the entire development in life, it can also be applied to a development where conspicuous social behavior starts in early adulthood and where, as a consequence, increasingly persistent criminality occurs. The statistical analysis showed some considerable differences between the early and the late delinquents (O_1- and O_2-subjects), greater ones in the family of orientation, smaller ones in spheres which become more relevant the older the subjects (for a summary, see Part II, Sect. 5). The fact that there were many O-subjects who, from the external *appearance* of their social behavior, were practically as inconspicuous as the G-subjects for a long time does not mean that there can be no development finally leading to recidivist criminality.

In the *individual case studies* there were sufficient indications that these subjects remained to a large extent inconspicuous at school age and at the age of occupational training as long as they were integrated in a strong system of order, usually the family of orientation, and that they remained socially integrated for a prolonged time because of favorable external circumstances in the spheres of performance, leisure, and contacts. Yet, to the degree to which the social integration *given* in the normal course of phases in life can be exchanged by *self-chosen* contacts, leisure activities, and jobs (or job changes), the subjects created the free area with respect to requirements of performance and order characteristic of a continuous development toward criminality beginning during early youth.

Thus, despite the relatively late onset of externally visible conspicuousness, it is a comprehendible development, simply with a different emphasis as regards age on given circumstances and the subjects' own, active creation of a life pattern. In the cross section immediately before the offense, these differences have practically disappeared. There is the same inner logical consistency of a development which comes to a drastic head mainly with the collapse of the sphere of performance.

On the basis of the observation of the subjects after the present study, there are certain indications that the related life-style continues in a marked form for subjects with a rather late onset of a development toward criminality. Detailed information, however, will not be available until the follow-up study has been completed.

An *example* follows of a development toward criminality beginning during adolescence or the early years of adulthood:

B. was born in 1941 in A-city as an illegitimate child. His father was a member of the *Wehrmacht*, his mother worked. Because of this, and also because of the war, the subject spent his early childhood with a foster mother in C-city. She had a small farm, and the subject never suffered want, during or after the war. He first went to kindergarten and then to school in 1947. In the first few grades, he was an average pupil since he was not particularly interested in school and preferred helping on the farm to doing his homework. In 1948, his parents, who had found a spacious apartment in D-city, a large city in southern Germany, took him back. The economic circumstances at home were well ordered. His mother no longer worked and could devote herself entirely to him. The subject had a good relationship with his parents; he posed no serious difficulties. After he went to live with his parents he attended school in D-city. He was more interested in school than before and completed the *Volksschule* with good grades. During his childhood and at school age, he spent his leisure time mainly with other children, playing soccer, etc., in addition to helping on the farm. From 1950 on, he also took part regularly in the group evenings of the YMCA, went hiking, and was an enthusiastic and active soccer player. Toward the end of school, he became a member of a sports club, working out once a week and playing on Saturdays. For some time he was also a member of the boxing club. However, he got into an argument there and left.

After completing school, he started an apprenticeship as a waiter, which - according to him - was great fun. He usually worked from 9 a.m. to 2 p.m. and from 6 p.m. to 9 p.m., weekends as well. In the afternoons and on his days off, he usually roamed about the city or, in the summertime, went to the swimming pool. In the evenings, he said, he had regularly met fellow employees with whom he had gone to several bars. Alone due to the change in his daily routine, his soccer enthusiasm decreased, but his other interests also changed. According to him, he had practically not missed any dances from the age of 18 on and had gotten to know every bar in D-city.

During occupational training, he spent 8 weeks a year taking courses at a school of hotel administration. The school was very strict; however, B. had no more problems there than at his job. Toward the end of his apprenticeship, he first got into an argument with a fellow waiter, then with his employer about tips and almost lost his job. However, he managed to complete his apprenticeship in April 1958 with very good results.

Because of the tension between him and his boss, he gave notice immediately after completing his apprenticeship and started to work for a renowned hotel in D-city. Since he wanted to get to know other hotels as well, he gave up the job at the end of 1958. He could not get a job right away and therefore helped out in four seasonal places for several weeks each, with interruptions in between. With the assistance of his parents, he found a seasonal job beginning April 1, 1959, as a waiter in E-city. After the end of the season, in October 1959, he came back to his parents, worked in various places in D-city as a temporary waiter, and finally found a new job in F-city from the middle of December 1959 on by way of a trade journal.

He worked for only a few months in F-city, and then went to another hotel in G-city because he did not earn enough. He was judged positively and usually earned good wages wherever he worked. As he himself said, he needed diversity. In the middle of August 1960, he gave up his job in G-city. He had saved about DM 2000 and wanted to "relax." To do so, he went to Hamburg with a fellow employee, and they had fun for a few days spending their money in bars and with prostitutes. At the end of August 1960, the subject came home to his parents more or less "stone-broke." First, there were vehement arguments because of his behavior, but in the end his parents supported him. His father helped him get a job as a waiter in another also rather renowned hotel in D-city. After only 6 weeks, he spontaneously gave up the job when he was reprimanded for an unexcused absence from work.

During his various jobs away from home, he had usually lived in rooms in the hotels, but had sometimes rented apartments. During his leisure time, however, he was never at home. He was always on the move, with acquaintances or alone, in bars and at dances. As he said, he had known "scores" of girls and had become intimate with them rather quickly. Especially in the old town of D-city (with many notorious bars and establishments), he had been known all over and had behaved, according to him, as if a few thousand marks more or less would have made no difference. Since he had come back from Hamburg, he had spent practically all his evenings in the old town meeting his "buddies" and acquaintances and having fun. Since the whole affair had been relatively expensive, they had - according to B. - naturally talked about how to get money easily. Offenses had been planned and partially carried out by the others. When he had no longer had a job, it had become "kind of acute" for him. He had thought about "making money" as a sales representative; but that had not worked out either. One evening, he was sitting in the X-bar of D-city with two "buddies" and the wife of one of them. As the three of them needed money urgently, they decided to "pull something." One night early in November 1960, they tried unsuccessfully to break into the pharmacy where the wife of his "buddy" worked. After this failed, they met in the X-bar again to make further plans. Finally, they decided to rob a bank messenger in H-city, an opportunity which a "buddy" who had worked for the bank had told the subject of. The following Friday, they went to have a look at the surroundings and watched the bank messenger. The next Friday, the four of them went to H-city in a rented car, but had to give up their plans since the messenger was accompanied by another man. Afterward, they went on to Frankfurt the same afternoon to rob a prostitute the subject knew from earlier visits. They decided to rob her late at night in her apartment so that she would have enough money. They spent the evening in various bars. When the subject contacted the woman after midnight to go to her apartment the way they had planned, he no longer had enough money, and they had to give up this project as well. The following Monday, they went to Frankfurt again. In the meantime, they were entirely "broke"; his "buddy" had to pay for the gas with uncovered checks, and the subject had to find some excuse to borrow the money for the prostitute from his parents. The offense was now committed as planned: While the subject went to the apartment with the prostitute, the other three waited below in the car. When the subject left the apartment, he tried to knock out the prostitute with ether, but she screamed, which her pimp heard. There was a short fight. The subject managed to escape and got his "buddies". The three of them went back to the apartment, where they hurriedly gathered some money and jewelry. Since the prostitute had called the police in the meantime, they were apprehended in Frankfurt.

The subject was sentenced to 3 years and 6 months in prison, of which he served 2 years and 6 months. After being released in May 1963, he went back to his parents in D-city for a few days. As they urged him to start working, he left home again and found a temporary place to stay with a woman he had recently gotten to know. According to him, he had had to recuperate from having been in prison and had spent 6 weeks "vacationing": He spent his time in the bars of the old town. When the probation officer also urged him to start working, he helped out as a bar mixer in various bars of D-city, partially only for the sake of form. Usually, he was dissatisfied with something or other after a short time and gave up the job. From another female acquaintance he heard of a job in a hotel in I-city. Without the probation officer knowing about it, he went to I-city with his new acquaintance and worked in the hotel. He and his acquaintance soon broke up. Then he got into an argument with his employer, gave up his job, and was back in D-city after 5 weeks. There he supported himself by helping out as a waiter and bartender and finally went to K-city in the summer of 1964 since he wanted to "see something new."

In K-city he worked as a bartender in a restaurant of good repute in a position of trust for about half a year. After a fight with a fellow worker, he was fired on the spot; he was sentenced to 1 month in prison for bodily injury. Later on, it appeared that he had embezzled about DM 3000. In order to avoid being reported to the police, he had to promise to pay the DM 3000 back. After losing the job and serving the month in prison, he worked as a sales representative for a short time only; otherwise, he was not regularly employed. Instead, he lived off the woman he was "engaged" to, a 20-year-old barmaid, who bore him a child in August 1965. Since they were both in financial straits, the woman no longer worked as a barmaid but as a prostitute after her pregnancy. According to him, and also according to the police investigations, he had had several other prostitutes whom he had taken money from. He had had a lot of spare time during this period. As a rule, he had met his girls and had gone to a café or the movies with them. Almost every day, he had gone to the movies two or three times. He had seen almost all the movies, some of them several times. When he had been at the movies, he had often not known which movie had been playing. He had also usually had girls with him since (as he said) the "relations with young ladies could be encouraged in an excellent way" in movie theaters (i.e., he tried to get them to be his "girlfriends" and then his prostitutes). He had had his own special tactics. In the evenings, he had gone to bars and talked with his many acquaintances. There had been certain bars where he had spent most of his time. He had often made his rounds in the evenings and had always met someone he knew. From time to time, he had had to check on his girls. This employment had been rather lucrative. He had managed the girls' entire money since they would have spent it all right away if they had been given the opportunity. Considering his visits to bars and taverns, he had naturally needed a great deal of money for himself.

From January 1966 on, B. spent almost 6 months in pretrial detention for procuring; at trial, however, he was acquitted for lack of proof. Only 2 days after his release, he forced a 21-year-old countergirl he had got to know in a notorious bar in K-city to work as a prostitute. Because of the rape and the serious bodily injury he committed in this connection, he was again brought before the judge. These proceedings had to be stayed as well, since the victim retracted her statement. According to the subject, K-city had become too "hot" for him in the meantime. Therefore, he had preferred to go into temporary hiding in Zürich, also because of the threatening revocation of probation. In the fall of 1966, the subject was arrested at the border on his way back to Germany and served the remaining year of his sentence.

4.4.4 Criminality as a Sudden Event

If the ideal type of the continuous development toward criminality is the extreme where (recidivist) criminality is the "comprehendible" result of a subject's development in life, then criminality as a sudden event is the opposite extreme (see Sect. 4.4.1 above). For criminality as a sudden event, the offense or the violation of a legal norm constitutes a *break* in a development in life - it comes "out of a clear blue sky." Here again, the particularities of the conception of ideal types (see Sect. 1.3 above) must be emphasized. It cannot be precluded that, for a specific individual case, there were certain indications in the entire previous behavior of the offender which would rule out a purely "coincidental" occurrence of the offense. Thus, such a case can certainly be "explained" or "understood" from a psycho(patho)logical perspective; yet criminality is unexpected (and not to be expected in the future) according to the specifically *criminological* criteria presented here.

For the (ideal) extreme of "criminality as a sudden event," it must be initially assumed that there are no indications or tendencies in a subject's social development which are connected with criminality. Thus, as a rule, there is social inconspicuousness or even total social integration. The offense or its consequences are a break in the social continuity of the life of an offender. Apart from his one-time offense, an offender exhibiting criminality as a sudden event is and remains socially inconspicuous provided he is not torn out of his social integration by the legal punishment of the offense.

An *example* follows of criminality as a sudden event:

C. (born in 1946) spent his childhood with his mother and brother, who was 5 years older and also illegitimate, in the household of his grandmother in W-city. Since his mother worked as a kitchen helper, he was essentially reared by his grandparents, with whom he had an extremely warm relationship. In 1955, his mother married a trucker, and initially lived with him at the grandparents' house. Two years later, parents and children moved to a rented apartment at the other end of W-city. Although his mother no longer worked and could devote herself entirely to the children, the separation from their grandparents was very difficult for the children. When the parents started quarreling frequently because of the stepfather's excessive alcohol consumption, the good relationship between children and stepfather suffered. Particularly the subject dissociated himself from his parents and secluded himself in a certain sense. Yet there were never any problems rearing the subject; he was never beaten and was considered an extremely well-behaved child.

There were no difficulties at school either: The subject was an average pupil (the change of schools after the move posed no problems), played truant at the most two or three times during his entire school education, and completed the *Volksschule* with good grades. He spent his leisure time with schoolmates and children from the neighborhood. Since the subject no longer felt at ease at home after they moved, not least because of the arguments between his parents, he spent most of his afternoons at his grandparents' house, with his mother's knowledge. From the age of 9 on, he regularly took part in the workouts at a soccer club. From the age of 11 on, he earned additional pocket money by helping in a grocery store, where he helped stock the shelves for about one hour every evening. He was allowed to keep the money. Thus he could spend money for himself independently. As he could not manage both working and playing soccer, he gave up soccer.

After completing the *Volksschule,* he did not know what to do and therefore decided to go to a secondary commercial school. Here again, he was a relatively good pupil, only stenography posed some difficulties. Beginning during the last few grades of the *Volksschule,* he had regularly helped out in a home for the aged during the weekends and holidays. For some time, he continued working in the grocery store, but later on he concentrated on his work in the home. Unexpectedly, after 2 years of commercial school, he had the opportunity to do practical training and then to work fully in the home and live there, an opportunity he immediately seized. He liked his work very much and was entirely absorbed in it, all the more since he got along very well with the people in the home, the management of the home, and his fellow employees. He even spent most of his leisure time together with the people in the home. In the course of time, the subject became the "right hand" of the director. The subject had some female acquaintances during this time. However, they were not very important for him: His purpose in life was the home.

As living in the home did not appeal to him in the long run, he tried to find an apartment nearby, and, with the assistance of the director of the home, he found one with two rooms in the house of the couple O. There was a good neighborly relationship between the subject and the O.'s, who were about 20 years older. The subject occasionally helped the husband in renovating the house. The husband also encouraged the subject to become a member of the local marksmen's association, where he regularly worked on his pistol shooting once a week.

In the course of time, it turned out that the couple often quarreled, especially when the husband came home drunk at night. On these occasions, O. had beaten up his wife more than once, abusing her and accusing her (incorrectly) of having rented the apartment to C. in order to have a young lover. The subject always tried to stay out of these quarrels, all the more so since he was good friends with O. when O. was sober.

One night, when the subject had already gone to bed, he heard O., who was drunk, knocking on the door, clamoring for his wife to open the door. Since she did not react, O. came to the window of the ground-floor apartment and pounded on it, abusing C. and telling him to open the door at once, he was going to put an end to this; first he was going to give it to his wife, then to C. According to his indications, the subject was terribly afraid. He went to the door, opened it and was pushed aside by O., who was much stronger than C. O. stormed up the stairs and immediately started beating his wife. When she began to scream, the subject called the police, telling them to come at once, O. was killing his wife. As the woman was still screaming and O. was still ranting and beating her, C. did not wait for the police to come but got his pistol from his closet, went to the staircase, and shouted upstairs: "You bastard, leave her alone!". When O. heard this, he let his wife be and came thundering down the stairs. The subject raised his pistol, aimed, and shot (as he said) "again and again - until the magazine was empty." O. fell, slid down a few steps and lay halfway down the stairs, critically injured. The subject threw the pistol away, rushed to his room, took the receiver, which he had not put back before, and shouted that he had shot O. Then he collapsed, crying, and was arrested by the police shortly afterward. He was sentenced to 3 years in prison for a minor case of attempted manslaughter.

4.4.5 Criminality in the Course of Personality Maturation

The continuous development toward criminality, where there is an entirely continuous development in life to criminality, and criminality as a sudden event, where there is a full and sudden break in a previously ordered development in life, can be considered the two ideal-typical extremes of a continuum expressing the "expectedness" of criminality. "Criminality in the course of personality maturation" has a position midway between the two: The conditions or factors concerned are neither continuously effective nor sudden or unique, but *temporary*. Temporary should not be understood in the formal sense of a duration which can be expressed (or estimated) as a specific length in time. It is related to a stage in the development of a person which can be accompanied by considerable difficulties and distinguished relatively well as "development specific". The subjects are most seriously conspicuous in the *sphere of leisure,* which occasionally gains paramount relevance during this stage of development. The conspicuousness in the sphere of leisure, particularly in connection with corresponding contacts and alcohol or drug consumption, creates the situations out of which offenses can be committed, even if this does not correspond to the "attitudes" of the subjects.

Partly because of the shock of the offenses as such, partly due to the impression made by the punishment or by other social effects of the offense, and partly as a consequence of a consolidation of the subject's system of values or after the completion of biological maturation processes, the social conspicuousness disappears (often abruptly), and the subjects no longer commit any offenses. In contrast to a continuous development toward criminality, there is usually no criminovalent constellation with criminality in the course of personality maturation. As a rule, requirements in the sphere of performance are still met at least minimally. Also, the sphere of abode is normally inconspicuous, without this being due to a social adjustment forced upon the subject from outside.

In contrast to social inconspicuousness in the case of a (late) development toward criminality, there is no discrepancy between the integration in an ordered family framework earlier and the socially conspicuous life pattern later (see Sect. 4.4. above). The subsequent social (re)integration of the subject, with the changes corresponding to stage of development, picks up the thread of an earlier life pattern.

An *example* follows of criminality in the course of personality maturation:

D. (born in 1946 in R-city) came from an ordered and well-to-do home. His father was an engineer who had worked his way up to manager of a large company in Mecklenburg after the war. In 1953, the family escaped to the Federal Republic of Germany and came to S-city, where the father was employed by a large electrical firm. During the following years, the mother worked full time in an office. During the day, the subject was supervised by his sister, who was 6 years older. He got along with her very well, but she had him under control. The parents attached importance to rearing their children well, and made an effort to create a positive atmosphere at home. Although the father was very strict, the children had a relationship of confidence with him and their mother.

The subject had first gone to school in Mecklenburg. Because of their escape, he had some initial difficulties in school but managed to get over them during the following years. From then on, he obtained very good results and got a good final report. Afterward, he went to a school for occupational orientation, which he completed around Easter 1962 with a good final report.

He was very clever with his hands and wanted to become a radio mechanic. Since he had only gone to the *Volksschule*, the employment office was not able to find him an apprenticeship. So he went from shop to shop, offering to work as an apprentice. Finally he was employed by the company Z. in S-city for a trial period and then as an apprentice. He was very enthusiastic and could soon work quite independently because of his knowledge.

He had obtained this knowledge through his hobby. He was particularly interested in technical things, read a lot about them, and had furnished his room as a workshop, where he spent every spare minute he had. For the rest, he spent his leisure time reading (particularly Edgar Wallace detective stories) and listening to music, another hobby of him. His collection of jazz and particularly Elvis Presley and other rock-and-roll musicians was his pride. At the age of 15, he became interested in motor sports. His father gave him a moped, and he drove around on it a lot. Earlier, in the spring of 1961, he had been ordered by the juvenile court to do 12 hours of public service work because he had driven around with the moped of a friend without a permit.

After the subject started his apprenticeship, and particularly after his sister married in 1962, he was no longer strictly supervised and often went out in the evenings with other apprentices and friends from school, especially to the movies. In the course of time, he got into a group of boys and girls of his age who met frequently in the weekend house of the parents of one of them. First, they only listened to rock-and-roll records and danced. Then, older boys and girls, who had already been convicted for offenses against property, started to come. Frequently, individual groups committed theft together, taking the loot along (especially cigarettes and alcoholic beverages) and giving it away. In October 1962, the subject also took part in such an excursion, together with two others: First they went to a club house, broke open the shutters, and entered. While the other two searched the house for things to steal, the subject stood around doing nothing, not really daring to join in. Since they did not find anything other than pretzels, sugar cubes, and a gas cooker, they left empty-handed. Almost one week later, the subject, again at the instigation of someone else, broke into a summerhouse. The two of them found two bottles of schnapps, which they practically emptied. When his friend was overpowered by sleep and could not be woken up, the subject, who had not had as much schnapps as his friend, felt that he could not leave him behind and reach safety alone. So he waited. Finally, he and his friend, who was still asleep, were surprised and arrested by the police.

Their son's offenses were a great shock for his parents. The subject was repentant and followed the orders of his parents without any resistance. One consequence, for example, was that the subject had to be at home regularly at 7 p.m. on the dot. The juvenile court sentenced the subject to 4 units of work of 6 hours each.

Afterward, up to the time of the study (1969), the subject had been convicted only once, when, at the age of 19, he was caught with a "souped up" moped. After the offenses of 1962, the subject had completely separated from the group and later joined a motor sport club, where he spent most of his weekends. For the rest, he usually stayed at home in the evenings and listened to music or spent the time with his girlfriend. He completed his apprenticeship and continued working in his occupation.

4.4.6 Criminality Despite No Other Social Conspicuousness

There were only a few cases of "criminality as a sudden event" in the present study, which was not surprising, considering the selection criteria for the O-subjects (see Part I, Sect. 2.2). This is also true for criminality despite no other social conspicuousness. It occurs, as does "criminality as a sudden event," mainly for subjects who commit offenses, but for whom the criteria elaborated here do not apply in their entirety. The social inconspicuousness exhibited in this context, when regarded in isolation, provides as incomplete a picture of the offender in the context of his social relationships as it does for criminality as a sudden event. Yet there is an obvious distinction between the two types. While a unique, extraordinary extreme situation occurs, and the offense is an entirely unexpected break in the continuity of life with criminality as a sudden event (see Sect. 4.4.2.3 above), moving (occasionally) in a certain borderland of criminality belongs to the usual life-style of the offender exhibiting criminality despite no other social conspicuousness. The possibility of breaking the law is at least accepted, and the expected advantages of doing so are directly intended. In this respect, there is certainly an "instrumentally rational" connection between the offense and the offender's development in life or conduct of life. This is expressed in particular in the patterns of relevance and the value orientation (see Sect. 5 below), where there are distinct differences from nondelinquent subjects.

An *example* follows of criminality despite no other social conspicuousness:

E. (born in 1939) grew up in his parents' home together with his brother, who was 2 years older. After his parents got divorced, his mother started working again and could no longer devote enough of her time to the children. So, at the age of 12, the subject was sent to his grandparents, while his brother went to live with an uncle. The grandparents had a large, prospering textile company. The subject regularly helped out in the company, and was clever at it. He received DM 10 a week pocket money for his help, which he made do with. The subject was an extremely well-behaved child. His grandparents were very proud of him; relatives and acquaintances were almost envious. According to his grandmother, E. let himself be positively influenced by her. The subject, like his grandparents, was religious and went to church regularly.

While he was living with his mother, he had gone to the *Gymnasium* after 4 years of the *Volksschule*. There, however, he was only an average pupil and had to repeat one year. Since he also was not promoted to the 10th grade, he left the *Gymnasium*. He also gave up an apprenticeship as a retailer after about 3 months, since the activity did not interest him. On the advice of his grandfather, he went to commercial school for a year, which he completed successfully. As he had decided to become an interpreter, he went to a private language school, a boarding school, and his grandparents paid school fees and board. After almost a year, he left the school without a degree and worked as a trainee in a publishing house.

The subject still lived at his grandparents' house. He mainly spent his leisure time at home watching television, listening to the radio, and mainly reading. He was particularly interested in detective stories and parapsychology, but also in philosophy. Furthermore, he took care of the bookkeeping of his grandparents' business, which he always conducted very correctly according to his grandparents. Yet he consistently refused to take over the business of his grandparents, which, according to them, he should have done.

Early in 1960 he let himself be lured away from his job in the publishing company by an acquaintance and became a free lance for a real estate agent. In view of the profit margin of the owner of the business, he was no longer satisfied with his income after some time and became independent in the spring of 1962. With the intention of being active as a real estate and financial broker, he rented an office and called the business *Industrieberatung E.* (Industrial Investment Consulting E.). Since he did not have any cash to speak of, he first tried to get his grandparents to take out a mortgage on their property. This was impossible since the property was already heavily mortgaged. So he contacted a wealthy old woman, Mrs. Z., whom he had gotten to know while working for the real estate agent. With his dexterous, polite appearance and his supposed business efficiency, he succeeded in convincing her that she could obtain comparably high profits by investing in his company. She granted him a loan of DM 30000. During the following period, he acted as a real estate agent by answering newspaper advertisements of people who wanted to sell their property. In some cases, he bought the property himself and sold it at a profit; in other cases, he convinced the owners that they needed his services to sell their property. He obtained the necessary capital through new loans and investments by Mrs. Z., who only needed a profitable investment and did not depend on the profits for her living. Thus, at the end of every quarter, E. supplied her with a convincing statement showing her current capital and her (very high) profits, which were (supposedly) reinvested.

In 1963, since the business was flourishing, E.'s cousin, who was 5 years older, entered the firm. He had been working as an insurance salesman. The business was renamed *E. & V. BauGmbH* (E. & V. Construction Ltd.), the necessary capital again being provided by Mrs. Z. The *BauGmbH* was moved to a new office and a secretary employed. The *BauGmbH* was also solely concerned with real estate and financial services; no construction projects were ever carried out. Mrs. Z. was treated as politely as ever; she was repeatedly invited out during the weekends and driven about, and E. showed her the various projects the *BauGmbH* was supposedly carrying out.

With the income from the company, E. and his cousin could afford a relatively high standard of living. They occasionally had several cars, went to expensive restaurants and discotheques, and joined the tennis and golf clubs. After E. had had several girlfriends, he married the daughter of an engineer in 1965 and moved to a large apartment with her.

When, in the fall of 1965, Mrs. Z. wanted some of her profit paid out for the first time, it became apparent that she had been duped for years. She had provided a total of almost DM 500000. Her sole "security," which she had gotten only after insisting on it, was E.'s notarized will, according to which he was single and Mrs. Z. his only heir. In the police investigations, it turned out that E. and V., besides having conducted correct transactions, had amassed a considerable fortune by repeated fraudulent manipulations, particularly when their partners were inexperienced. According to the police, this sum also amounted to about DM 500000. While V. was able to avoid being apprehended by leaving the country with part of the money, presumably almost DM 100000 in cash, E. was sentenced to 2 years and 6 months in prison for repeated fraud, dishonest dealings, and forgery of documents.

4.4.7 Summary

The foregoing types do not constitute an exhaustive typology. From the point of view of the position of the offense in the longitudinal section of life, two (ideal-typical) extreme cases can be distinguished: In the "continuous development toward criminality," increasing social conspicuousness finally leads to a criminovalent constellation and, with an immediately comprehendible inner logical consistency, to an offense. The counterpart to this type is "criminality as a sudden event," where the offense constitutes an (entirely) unexpected break in the previously entirely inconspicuous continuity in an offender's life. Between these two "pure" extremes, there are several intermediate types. In the "development toward criminality beginning during adolescence or the early years of adulthood," external social conspicuousness does not appear as long as the subject is still under the influence of a strong social system of order, or as long as there are favorable external circumstances in various social spheres. Later on, however, the subjects' conspicuousness becomes so marked that, immediately before the offense, there is no longer any difference between the cross section of the subjects with an early development toward criminality and that of the subjects with a late one.

In "criminality in the course of personality maturation," social conspicuousness does not affect all the social spheres (in the cross section), nor does it persist (in the longitudinal section); usually, there is a full social (re)integration when this stage of life has been completed.

Finally, "criminality despite no other social conspicuousness" is a type to which - as with "criminality as a sudden event" - the O-specific criteria do not apply. Yet while for "criminality as a sudden event," the offense is the result of a unique, extraordinary extreme situation and a fully unexpected break in the continuity of life, moving in the borderland of criminality does belong to the usual life-style in "criminality despite no other social conspicuousness."

It should be noted that the differentiation between the various positions of the offense in the longitudinal section of life is made solely on the basis of criteria of *social* behavior, without the fact or kind of delinquency having any importance in determining even this differentiation. This does not mean that a criminological examination of (current and previous) offenses, not only in view of their position in the longitudinal section of life, but also with respect to how an offense was committed and how it developed, is not a useful supplementation of the *assessment of an individual case* on the basis of social behavior (see Part II, Sect. 4.5; see GÖPPINGER 1980, pp. 687 ff.). However, the mere fact of recidivist criminality does not necessarily indicate a "development toward criminality." In order to distinguish it, for example, from a "criminal period" within the framework of personality maturation, criteria of social behavior alone are decisive.

Finally, it should be mentioned that what was true for the "application" of the criteria of the cross section also applied to that of the positions of the offense in the longitudinal section. Usually, the specific circumstances of the individual case did not correspond exactly to one of the described types. Classification could take place only on the basis of a (more or less) rough approximation to a certain type. Occasionally, it was impossible to make a classification, and, furthermore, there were transitions between the types.

Thus, the social conspicuousness (and criminality) of a subject which initially appeared as "criminality in the course of personality maturation" occasionally led to a development whose course was similar to that of a (late) "development toward criminality," for example, through a pronounced influence of people from the "milieu." Furthermore, a short phase of criminality appeared occasionally in adolescence or very early adulthood. Similar to criminality in the course of personality maturation, there was no consistent social conspicuousness and criminality. This phase abated after a short period of time: It seemed to be criminality in the course of personality maturation shifted in time.

5 Patterns of Relevance and Value Orientation

The knowledge of the longitudinal and the cross section of the lives of (recidivist) offenders rests mainly upon a comprehensive investigation of the *socially* relevant behavior of the subjects in the various spheres. In the statistical analysis and even more so in the formation of ideal types, it became apparent that the gap between the O- and the G-specific characteristics and criteria as well as the criminorelevant constellations and positions of the offense in the longitudinal section cannot be understood from the perspective of (external) social behavior alone. It is possible to gain access to the differences between the O- and the G-group by considering not only the mere presence of facts, circumstances, or characteristics, but also, beyond the external behavior of the subjects, the underlying "attitudes" (see Part II, Sect. 3.4.4) which enable certain situations to develop or which lead the subjects to react differently to certain situations in life.

It is often forgotten that the behavior of a person is also the expression of personality traits: Social behavior is always based on the individual personality and its specific attitudes. These attitudes, on the other hand, easily reveal relationships with the personality of the subject. Therefore, seemingly purely external facts as such are of further importance, and their position in the life of an individual becomes apparent in an overall examination (see, for example, Sect. 4.3.2 above).

The following results on these attitudes and personality traits were not elaborated by way of the usual test-diagnostic procedures. The latter could not distinguish sufficiently between the O- and the G-group (see Part II, Sect. 3.4.3.3). This is not surprising, considering that psychic characteristics are value neutral and therefore allow any direction of social behavior for (almost) any decision. Thus, the specific attitudes characterizing the O- and the G-subjects in relation to their circumstances in life could not be psycho(patho)logically assessed in the immediate situation of the examination itself. They could only be revealed in the examination of behavior patterns occurring time and again in the longitudinal section (see Part II, Sect. 3.4.4).

As explained for the individual criteria of the criminorelevant constellations and for further criteria (see Sect. 3.3.3 above), these criteria express a relationship with circumstances in life. This is apparent in concepts such as an "inadequately high level of aspirations." As a whole, however, they are of a more formal nature. The strength of these criteria lies precisely in the comparability of the lacking, the paradoxical, the inadequate attitudes in *each individual case*. Despite their relationship with circumstances in life, these criteria (necessarily) abstract to a certain degree from the organization of life from the point of view of content. Thus, for example, the concept "deficient sense of reality" can cover differing forms of individual realities which are not adequately controlled.

The examination of the **patterns of relevance** was an attempt to penetrate better into the personality-specific area by way of the specific content of life. We expected to see whether there were differences between the O- and the G-subjects with respect to which objects, needs, and purposes in life the subjects' intentions were most concentrated on. Patterns of relevance "are the relationships with persons, objects, and locations which are of particular importance for an individual in everyday life, which he cultivates most, neglects last, and endeavors to maintain or obtain under any circumstances" (GÖPPINGER 1980, p. 325; trans.). They reveal the "fundamental intentions of a personality," and they may well be, at least partially, "the expression of a complex of effects deep in the (biomental) personality, which leads to certain behavior patterns. Generally, they have a marked personal note; occasionally, they can even characterize a personality. Correspondingly, there are numerous variants with respect to content; the kinds of patterns of relevance of a person and their reciprocal relationships vary considerably as well. This also holds for the intensity of their effect, which ranges from a relatively loose relationship to a keen interest, an urge, or even an irresistible attraction emanating from the object of a pattern of relevance, which is best compared to the helplessness of addiction" (GÖPPINGER 1980, p. 325; trans.).

Essentially, there are two kinds of patterns of relevance: On the one hand, patterns of relevance can be the expression of *basic intentions,* which belong to the "vital sphere." Usually, these intentions are not essential needs in life (e.g., eating, drinking, sleeping), but in exceptional cases, for example in times of need, they can become highly relevant - as understood in this context. Far more frequently, however, this kind of pattern of relevance is related, for instance, to motoric agitation and is expressed in a need for physical exercise and activity, especially outdoors ("out in the fresh air" - "nothing holds him at home"), or in a constant search for diversion and a permanent need for activity. As a rule, such patterns of relevance can be determined practically throughout the entire life of a subject.

On the other hand, patterns of relevance can be expressed in very particular and marked *interests.* These patterns of relevance are more purposive and are related to the object of interest in a material sense. This relationship can be aimed at certain locations or things but also at cultural events, persons, or one specific person. However, not all interests of a person *take effect* in the sense of a pattern of relevance; an interest cannot be regarded as a pattern of relevance unless it influences a person's general organization of life in a decisive way. Patterns of relevance which are expressed in marked interests usually change in the course of time, shift to other areas, and are influenced to a certain extent by a person's environment. Particularly for juveniles, it is often difficult to differentiate between these patterns of relevance, which are more marked by the external offer - for instance contact persons and the general company of a subject or also current trends - and their "actual" and therefore lasting patterns of relevance, which can often be determined only very roughly.

It soon appeared that statements could certainly be made on the "*relevant*" and, no less important, the "*nonrelevant*" according to this definition within the framework of in-depth individual case studies. To a certain extent, the descriptions of daily routines (see Sect. 3.2 above) were informative - though merely insofar as the way time is organized is an external measure of preferences. However, it was not possible to arrive at statements that were general *and* at the same time specific. Patterns of relevance can be realized or expressed in many different ways. Therefore, the same thing became apparent here as in the social spheres for specific facts and characteristics: It was practically impossible to elaborate *specific* patterns of relevance for the O- and the G-subjects. Therefore, the patterns of relevance as such are, for the time being, *criminologically unspecific.*

Nonetheless, it is very well possible to see, with the knowledge of the *remaining* circumstances in life *within the framework of an individual case study,* that a certain pattern of relevance (e.g., alcohol, a passion for driving, or the "milieu") considerably contributes toward a "danger" of criminality. In this respect, determining the patterns of relevance is of great importance for prophylaxis, prediction, and interventions. But general rules as valid as the criminorelevant constellations and further criminorelevant criteria (see Sect. 3.3 above) are sought in vain - for the present.

Nevertheless, to present a few aspects, it is striking that many O-subjects felt attracted to the "milieu," to the noisy environment of pubs and bars and the corresponding activities and contacts. While work was acceptable at best as a way to earn money, a life-style oriented to definite categories of order was entirely irrelevant. In contrast, occupation (activity *and* job) and family were particularly relevant to the G-subjects. Yet these rather general indications were to be expected on the basis of the results in the social spheres.

It proved to be even more difficult to penetrate into the values guiding the subjects and influencing their behavior. Basically, persons could be much more extensively comprehended in the context of their social relationships than they have been to date if it were possible to gain access to their *system of values*. The system of values "is the foundation or at least the decisive background of the self-evident everyday decisions and behavior patterns of an individual, usually without his being aware of it as such. Thus, on the one hand, the personality is embedded in the system of values; on the other, the personality envelops the system of values. In no way do the same values and norms which become accessible in the course of a person's development in life become relevant in the same way" (GÖPPINGER 1980, p. 326; trans.).

For methodological reasons, however, the system of values cannot be investigated directly by empirical means. At best, it is possible to gain some access to the **value orientation** of a person. However, this poses even more problems than determining the patterns of relevance, which are much easier to understand and to elaborate from the longitudinal and the cross section of life. The value orientation is carried by abstract principles, which can become decisive for the action of an individual in the most differing everyday (and unique) situations.

The relationship between patterns of relevance and value orientation is not such that the value orientation is realized in the patterns of relevance. Often enough, patterns of relevance (or a certain pattern of relevance) *prevent* an individual from acting in agreement with his value orientation. In this sense, patterns of relevance are important in their own right.

For the same reason, it is erroneous to conclude *directly* a corresponding value orientation on the basis of a specific organization of social behavior. If the value orientation is to be introduced as an independent element of the examination, one must reckon with the value orientation *deviating* from what is actually realized. Thus, there are very strict limits to empirical access. Some findings, however, merit attention.

It was occasionally revealing to see to what extent the O-subjects accepted as natural the incorrectness, trickery, or lack of comradeship and solidarity of their "buddies" without their relationship suffering because of it. The G-subjects, in contrast, broke off a relationship if anything of this kind occurred. It was striking how the G-subjects, particularly those living in adverse circumstances, repeatedly stated "I could never have done that to my family", "there was no question of my doing so", "that just wasn't possible", etc., to express that criminality was simply impossible on the basis of their value orientation, irrespective of their circumstances, as poor as they may have been.

Yet these are only attempts to gain access to the value orientation of the subjects. To a large extent, the subjects do not express or reflect on their value orientation and are usually not (consciously) aware of it in everyday life. As a *general* impression, it can be stated that the sometimes marked "positive" value orientation (oriented to a socially integrated life) of the G-subjects was *not* mirrored by a "negative" value orientation of the same intensity of the O-subjects. What differed was the object of a more or less express value orientation. There were not exclusively agreeing or exclusively disagreeing concepts in both groups for the same "values": The values of one group were in some cases simply not part of the concepts of the other group. On the other hand, the O-subjects *fully developed their actions according to definite guiding principles (that they were aware of)* - which gives a life pattern its continuity - less frequently than the G-subjects. What remained were immediate incentives and short-term utilitarian reasons orienting personal and material relationships, which were expressed in the erratic and changing lives of the O-subjects.

As for the patterns of relevance, no general rules comparable to the criteria of the longitudinal and the cross section of life could be gained from experience for the value orientation. Since it is very closely related to the personality, it has its own importance alongside the longitudinal and cross section criteria in the study of the individual offender in the context of his social relationships.

Particularly with respect to prophylaxis, prediction, and interventions *in the individual case*, the value orientation is of utmost importance (within the framework of an applied criminology, see Part IV). The gap between patterns of relevance and value orientation is of special diagnostic interest and forms a starting point for possible interventions. Thus, for example, for criminality in the course of personality maturation (see Sect. 4.4.5 above), there is often a considerable discrepancy between the socially conspicuous behavior and current patterns of relevance on the one hand and the value orientation on the other, which basically aims at socially inconspicuous or even integrated behavior (see GÖPPINGER 1980, p. 327).

6 Summary: The Unity of the Offender in the Context of His Social Relationships

The steps of evaluation in Part III were aimed at "condensing" the wealth of information from the individual case studies in such a way that it would be possible to make generalizations and yet to preserve the proximity to reality of the individual case studies. The ultimate objective was to obtain a complex, overall view of the offender in the context of his social relationships.

On the basis of the various "ideal-typical" behavior patterns in the individual social spheres and stages of life (see Sect. 2 above), which were presented first, these findings were "condensed" in various directions. One direction was the examination of the *cross section of life* spanning the various spheres (see Sect. 3.3 above), which resulted in the criminorelevant constellations (and further criminorelevant criteria). Whenever these constellations occurred - they were to a high degree characteristic of both groups of subjects - the absence (or presence) of criminality became immediately comprehendible.

Another direction of "condensing" led to the various "positions of the offense in the *longitudinal section of life*" (see Sect. 4.4 above). One extreme, the "continuous development toward criminality", was a development whereby the criminovalent criteria became the more marked and practically "forced" the subject to commit an offense the closer in time to criminality. The counterpart to this extreme was "criminality as a sudden event", where there was no indication that an offense would be committed. In other words, offenses were committed "out of a clear blue sky." Between these two extremes there were other positions of the offense with varying degrees of social conspicuousness.

Once again, it must be emphasized - as for the criminorelevant constellations - that these criteria are not definitive. On the contrary, they are open, insofar as only a few intermediate positions between the two extremes were presented. Moreover, a number of other offenses committed with intent, offenses in connection with mental disorders, and offenses committed by negligence have not (yet) been taken into consideration.

For the purpose of a complex view of the offender in the context of his social relationships, the criteria of the longitudinal and the cross section do not suffice. Though the relationship between these two dimensions became in part apparent - the criminovalent constellation, for example, usually occurs in an (ideal-typical) continuous development toward criminality - additional criteria are necessary to gain a third dimension regarding the intentions of a personality. This gap in the complex view of the offender in the context of his social relationships was closed by taking into consideration the patterns of relevance and the value orientation (see Sect. 5 above). They substantiate the examination of the longitudinal and the cross section in a general way as well: If, for example, a classification on the basis of external criteria is uncertain or borderline, as in a differentiation between temporary conspicuousness during a stage of development or maturation on the one hand and the beginning of a continuous development toward criminality on the other, the patterns of relevance and value orientation can be essential. Not until one sees the more or less constant "attitudes" of a personality behind the subject's social behavior can the continuity of a development toward criminality, for example, be understood: Unfavorable circumstances take full effect *and* opportunities to return to or continue a socially inconspicuous life-style are not seized. Only the consideration of the intentions deeply rooted in the personality enables one in the end to comprehend the loss of structuring in all spheres in the life-style typical of the majority of the O-subjects.

Therefore, a sound opinion of whether a person's social behavior fully corresponds to his basic intentions or whether there are discrepancies can be given only on the basis of a complex study of the longitudinal and the cross section of life on the one hand and of the patterns of relevance and value orientation on the other.

Yet these rules are not comparable in their generality to those used in the examination of the position of the offense in the longitudinal section and the examination of the cross section. Thus, the patterns of relevance and the value orientation are important mainly as a supplementary instrument for the *assessment of the individual case.*

The difficulty of arriving at *generalizations* from experience also shows that the complex view of the offender in the context of his social relationships cannot be presented in *a general way*. The interlocking of knowledge in the three dimensions of the "*Criminological Triad*" - the cross section of life, the position of the offense in the longitudinal section of life, and the patterns of relevance and value orientation - can become apparent only *in the specific, individual case.*

The specifically criminological criteria elaborated here are particularly suited for application to individual cases. However, certain peculiarities deriving from the conceptions must be considered (regarding the methodology in detail, see GÖPPINGER 1985). An "application" of, for example, the criminovalent constellation in the sense of a simple subsumption of the individual case under the conception is impossible. The individual criteria of the constellation are related to specific circumstances in life, and comprehension of these requires investigations into the entire life pattern of a subject if the "presence" of the criminovalent constellation is to be determined in the individual case. Moreover, this "presence" can be meant only in a certain way. If the rules gained from experience are exaggerated with respect to ideal types, as is the case for the criminorelevant criteria and the continuous development toward criminality, they apply in their pure form only in extreme cases. This circumstance in particular makes it possible to determine the measure of approximation to or deviation from the "ideal" form. In this way, the ideal types formed in the longitudinal and the cross section of life become the system of reference in the comparative analysis of individual cases based on ideal types from a *methodological* point of view. Together with the individual examination of the patterns of relevance and the value orientation, they serve the complex criminological assessment of the individual offender in the context of his social relationships.

IV Applied Criminology – The Method and Criteria of Criminological Diagnosis and Prognosis

1 Importance and Range

1.1 The Aim of Applied Criminology

The *aim* of Applied Criminology as it is understood here is to utilize directly the knowledge of the criminological research presented above in practice and in specific individual cases. The instruments elaborated for this purpose have been tested in many cases and have proved successful in practice. Object and criteria of assessment were described in 1971 in the first edition of my book *Kriminologie* (4th edn., GÖPPINGER 1980) and were presented to the public in a systematic form in 1975 (GÖPPINGER 1976). Since then, more than 10 years of experience have been gathered in applying the method to the criminological assessment of offenders. Thus, the procedure has been constantly improved: Its use has been simplified, and its reliability and validity have been tested by various persons, also in practice. Nonetheless, the method has to be developed further, like any subject matter which is directly concerned with the reality of life.

The following is an introduction to the method of the comparative analysis of individual cases based on ideal types and the system of reference of the criminological triad **in practice.** The method is an aid to *criminological* assessment and judgment of individual cases, i.e., individual offenders in the context of their social relationships, on the basis of one's own special knowhow and without any expert knowledge in the fields of psychology or psychiatry. In this way, it is possible to make a criminological diagnosis and prognosis and thus to acquire the foundation to choose and apply specifically the measures indicated in an individual case from a preventive point of view. These include sanctions with their manifold possibilities to punish and influence a person, and other interventions of a prophylactic and, in the widest sense, therapeutic nature.

The criminological assessment of an individual case is of importance in practice wherever persons *in connection with criminality* are to be assessed differentiatedly. Yet the method of the comparative analysis of individual cases based on ideal types facilitates not only access to "offenders" in the context of their social relationships but *also* to persons *who have not yet been convicted.* The analysis points out elements of danger or dangerous developments in individual social spheres or in the life pattern and entire orientation in life of a person before any offenses have been committed. If these elements or developments continue consistently, they usually lead to criminality at some point in time. Consequently, this method is not only of immediate practical importance for the *administration of criminal law* and those active in this field, in particular lawyers and social workers, but also for the field of *general public welfare,* in particular that of youth welfare.

The limited framework of this book rules out a comprehensive and entirely unified presentation of Applied Criminology. Nevertheless, the systematics of the procedure in an individual case assessment can be presented as a whole. For the (material) criteria of assessment, however, the presentation in Part III is referred to repeatedly. The reader who wishes to obtain a first impression of the procedure and to become familiar with the essential criteria of analysis and assessment should therefore first turn to the unified presentation and assessment of a case (see Case A., Appendix). The Appendix contains cross-references pointing to the general and systematic presentation of the method and criteria of the comparative analysis of individual cases based on ideal types.

That the presentation offers only a rough outline is not the only reason why the present chapter cannot be a "tutorial" in the traditional sense: In particular, wherever assessments and evaluations, not simple classifications, are to be made, (criminological) experience is required. This experience cannot be taught or learned but only acquired through practice. Those who come from practice can and should bring their own experience into the investigations and bring it to bear in the assessment of an individual case - oriented to the systematic procedure and the empirically valid criteria of assessment. On the basis of our impressions to date, working with this method - as soon as one is familiar with it - requires no additional expenditure of time in the majority of cases relevant to practice (see Preliminary Remark, Appendix).

1.2 The Special Nature of the Comparative Analysis of Individual Cases Based on Ideal Types

The method of the comparative analysis of individual cases based on ideal types is an independent criminological approach. It does not refer (or no longer refers) back to the special models and approaches concerning analysis, appraisal, and explanation of the sciences related to criminology, such as sociology, psychology, or psychiatry. From the perspective of these sciences, a person *who has been convicted for an offense* appears in a mere (usually very small) segment of the entire spectrum of their interest, and he is - fragmentarily - assessed and analyzed only from certain points of view, i.e., those relevant to the specific science (see GÖPPINGER 1980, pp. 7 ff.). In contrast, the object of scientific interest in basic criminological research is the complex unity of the individual *who has been convicted for an offense,* i.e., the offender in the context of his social relationships. This research is the foundation of the method *and* the (material) criteria of assessment. Therefore, the method and content of this approach enable one to make specifically *criminological,* i.e., relevant and valid, statements about the offender in the context of his social relationships relevant to the fact of criminality. Consequently, in the procedure presented here, only those points are taken into consideration which distinguish (recidivist) offenders from the general population and are therefore specific to the question of criminality.

The **starting point** for this criminological approach is constituted by relatively easily assessable, mainly externally recognizable *behavior and reaction patterns in the present and past everyday life* of a subject. To enable those without psychological or psychiatric training to use this method, genuinely psychological and psychiatric points of view and areas were left out. Consequently, application of this method cannot replace either the psychiatric or the psychological expert when there are indications of mental abnormality or when differentiated psychological questions arise, particularly in connection with juveniles. For the majority of the problems and questions in daily practice which require a more or less thorough consideration of the personality of the (psychologically inconspicuous, "normal") offender, however, the method presented here fully suffices to criminologically assess an individual case.

The **measure** of the specific behavior of a subject consists of various forms of *ideal types* (regarding their development, see Part III, Sect. 1.3). These ideal types reflect criminologically relevant behavior patterns, circumstances, and developments, as it were in their purest form. They are a special kind of abstraction: The conception shows the characteristic core of a real manifestation by disregarding anything (else) which is regularly more or less simultaneously connected with the manifestation in real life. Thus, an ideal type is always an extreme which occurs at best exceptionally in reality. Normally, there is a varying distance between the real occurrence and the ideal type. If a yardstick were used to determine the distinctness of a real manifestation, its outermost mark would be the ideal type. Consequently, when measuring factually existing circumstances with an ideal type, the real occurrence can only *approximate* the ideal type or show *tendencies* toward one or the other direction of the ideal-typical extreme forms. This means that the individual case to be assessed can be related to the ideal type only by comparison, not by deduction or subsumption.

The ideal-typical criteria of assessment used here are not a number of characteristics whose "presence" or "absence" can simply be checked and "ticked off" in turn. On the contrary: *In each individual case,* a qualitative estimation and judgment must be made as to whether and, if so, to what degree the specific behavior of a subject approaches the ideal type, and as to which facts this classification and estimation should be based on (for details, see Sect. 2.2.1.1 below).

The **assessment** of the individual subject by means of the various forms of ideal types takes place in two stages. First, the specific behavior of a subject in the *longitudinal section of life,* i. e., from his childhood up to the time of the study or his last offense (see Sect. 2.2.1.1 below), is compared with the ideal-typical behavior of (recidivist) offenders on the one hand and that of the (socially inconspicuous and noncriminal) general population on the other. Between these extreme poles of criminorelevant behavior - in the sense of a danger of criminality or a particular resistance to criminality - one obtains an individual *profile* of each subject. In the examination of the *cross section of life* (see Sect. 2.2.2 below), the behavior of a subject during a relatively short period of time preceding the offense is related to specific criminorelevant criteria. Finally, a subject's *patterns of relevance* (see Sect. 2.2.3 below) are used to determine the interests and intentions which are important in everyday life and deeply rooted in the personality and to gain access to his *value orientation,* which functions as a decisive background.

Delinquency plays a role on this level merely insofar as it is regarded as a fact (which is not taken into consideration for the time being, but which is the reason for the criminological assessment). The sphere of delinquency (see Sect. 2.2.1.2 below) is also analyzed by means of purely descriptive criteria. At this stage, the sphere of delinquency is not yet directly related to a subject's remaining social spheres and his development in life.

Not until the *second stage* of the assessment of an offender in the context of his social relationships (see Sect. 2.3 below) is his delinquency related to his general social behavior. The points of reference for this complex assessment are the criteria of the **Criminological Triad:** Proceeding from various (ideal-typical) *positions of the offense in the longitudinal section of life* and the *criminorelevant constellations in the cross section of life,* under consideration of the *patterns of relevance* and the *value orientation* of the offender to be assessed, one attempts - retrospectively - to make statements on the relationship between a specific offense, possibly also previous offenses, and an offender's general social behavior. In particular, it is determined whether and to what degree of logical consistency the offense developed out of the social behavior and the life pattern of the offender.

A glance at the criteria of analysis and assessment shows how decisive the interplay between the various perspectives and the complex approach is: The *individual* criteria - being individual facts - can occur for any number of persons who are altogether noncriminal and to a large degree socially integrated. It is the *interplay* between a large number of certain individual aspects which is essential for the *criminological relevance,* and thus for the importance of these points of view. Therefore, for the *validity of the method presented,* it is of decisive importance to *collect data systematically,* to **evaluate consistently and systematically all criteria and aspects of analysis,** and to **gain a complex** view which brings these individual aspects together by means of the criteria of reference of the criminological triad.

1.3 Capability and Limits

If it becomes apparent that a certain social behavior has led to an offense consistently (see, in particular, The Continuous Development Toward Criminality Beginning During Early Youth, Sect. 2.3.2.1 below), it is also possible to reach a **prognostic conclusion,** in the sense that, *as a rule,* a specific individual will commit further offenses in the foreseeable future if his basic intentions, attitudes, and behavior patterns, his life pattern and life-style, and the circumstances and conditions in his social environment do not change (to any significant extent). Initially, the foundation of such a statement is simply the determination of certain (constant or recurring) behavior patterns of a subject in the various social spheres, certain developments, or even mere individual facts and circumstances in his general social behavior. Decisive for the conclusion is that these characteristics - as rules gained from experience - are precisely the ones which precede or accompany criminality. Insofar as the offense is a "consistent" consequence of social behavior at all, the logical consistency can only become apparent if there is a close relationship in time between the behavior patterns and the offense. The further back one proceeds in the life of an offender, the more frequently one finds situations where alternative developments were still possible or where the subject was still able to decide between alternative behavior patterns and developments, and the less one is able to derive the offense "consistently" from these earlier behavior patterns.

Here, it must suffice to determine that these behavior patterns occur for the subject concerned and correspond to the behavior of recidivist offenders without immediately recognizing their direct relationship with criminality.

Consequently, the comparative analysis of individual cases based on ideal types cannot give a genetic or even causal explanation in the strict sense which would ultimately trace delinquency back to certain factors of socialization, (genuine) personality structure, or personality development. Thus, the method does not aim at making any statements on who (e.g., a subject's parents) or what (e.g., his poor socioeconomic circumstances) might be responsible for the development of delinquency. This is both appropriate and necessary if the method is to be a useful practical instrument, considering the extent to which the manifold causal explanations of criminality contradict each other. Furthermore, finding a "cause" of a specific offense or of criminality, such as a certain infantile disorder, would generally add nothing with respect to the tasks of criminal law occurring in practice [This is not so in (analytic) psychotherapy; concerning treatment in general, see Sect. 2.4.2 below].

Yet, assuming a logical consistency between social behavior and offense does not mean that the development is inevitable (see Part III, Sect. 1.3). This is shown in the opposite direction, i.e., in criminality as a sudden event, where offenses are committed entirely unexpectedly, out of a socially inconspicuous life pattern (see Sect. 2.3.2.5 below). But in a continuous development toward criminality as well, an offense is *not absolutely inevitable.* Though it is a truism, it must be emphasized again and again: In empirical science, it has never been possible to determine courses of behavior definitely programmed by certain factors; consequently, no prognosis is absolutely certain. For example, there may be unforeseen changes in external circumstances (such as an inheritance which enables a subject to keep up an expensive life-style without having to earn money by working), or unexpected changes in the personal sphere (such as a strong relationship with a socially integrated partner or a religious experience - which may occur occasionally).

The *diagnosis* made on the basis of the method of the comparative analysis of individual cases based on ideal types is not an end in itself. Like a medical diagnosis, a criminological diagnosis goes hand in hand with a *prognosis* and treatment or intervention. As in medicine, a diagnosis may well be correct even though the prognosis was incorrect. Furthermore, in medicine, a diagnosis implies a certain therapy, and the expected effect of the therapy is included in the prognosis. Here, the situation is similar: The criminological prognosis is not made on the basis of unchanging circumstances but always takes into account the effect of a possible intervention following an offense as well. Therefore, considerations concerning prognosis and actual possibilities of influencing the subject are closely related in legal practice.

Even though the emphasis of the criminological assessment lies on diagnostic (and implied prognostic) statements, it also provides *indications* for **specific possibilities of intervention in the individual case,** an important point in practice. In this respect, the special nature of the comparative analysis of individual cases based on ideal types is brought to bear in particular. Because the individual case is not subsumed under headings but compared with ideal-typical criteria, *its special nature* *not only remains but is even specifically elaborated.* Even in cases where there is no relationship in the sense of a logical consistency between general social behavior and offense, where the individual case deviates considerably from the O-ideal-typical picture or does not correspond to it at all, there are, as a rule, many indications for effective interventions. The comparative analysis of individual cases based on ideal types facilitates in particular not only the elaboration of the special (criminologically relevant) "weak points" in the behavior of the individual concerned but also the recognition of his (criminologically relevant) "strong points." Often, the knowledge of a certain "strong" or "weak point" suffices to achieve an adequate decision in the individual case, for example, by means of an appropriate court order. Even in difficult cases, particularly of subjects who, over a prolonged period, exhibit recurring behavior patterns leading to offenses, the criminological diagnosis can show the points of reference for specific interventions.

A criminological statement made on the basis of the method of the comparative analysis of individual cases based on ideal types reaches its limits where - for a minority of offenders - a successful intervention is not conceivable without special *therapeutic* measures in the strict sense (e.g., psychological or psychiatric ones). The criminological assessment of an offender in the context of his social relationships, however, also enables one to find indications of "weak points" in the personality of the offender by means of his "special aspects," especially his "internal aspects" (see Sect. 2.3.3 below). Yet how these criminologically relevant "weak points" are to be approached in the individual case from the point of view of *therapy*, and which measures ought to be taken, cannot be decided on the basis of a criminological diagnosis alone. This decision requires the methods and approaches - whether traditional or yet to be developed - of the sciences related to criminology, in particular psychology. It is the task of these sciences to use their own instruments to tackle the (personality-specific) problematic points of offenders which become apparent within the framework of the criminological assessment by means of the method presented here (see also Sect. 2.4.2 below).

The immanent **limits of criminological diagnosis** result from the special nature of the comparative analysis of individual cases based on ideal types. Seen in retrospect and from an external point of view, there is a degree of logical consistency between behavior patterns and attitudes on the one hand and most offenses on the other which makes them "comprehendible." Yet such relationships do not occur for all offenses or kinds of offenses. In principle, all offenses related to *mental abnormality* cannot be assessed with the instruments presented here. Yet, the fact that an offense cannot be understood with the aid of criminological analysis, i.e., that it does not "come out," indicates a mental abnormality - e.g., for the judge concerned with the case - and an expert can be called upon if necessary. To this degree, a criminological analysis is certainly useful in this context as well.

Though there may well be a relationship between *offenses committed by negligence* and life pattern or social conspicuousness, this relationship has not yet been sufficiently elaborated and differentiated. Thus, for the time being, a criminological analysis is limited largely to offenses committed with intent.

Property and fraudulent offenses constitute the center of the spectrum of offenses committed with intent. Criminological analysis is tailored to these offenses, and the relationship between general social behavior and most of these offenses is immediately comprehendible. For *violent offenses* in the strict sense and most *sexual offenses,* it is extremely revealing in the criminological analysis to determine whether or not a subject exhibits serious social conspicuousness. The criminological analysis is unable to make a diagnostic (and prognostic) statement only if such offenses, for example sexual offenses, are entirely isolated from the remaining complex of life of the subject.

With criminality *despite no other social conspicuousness,* there is no particular conspicuousness in general social behavior. Yet, to evaluate the offender, it is important to determine that an offense was committed out of social inconspicuousness; in such cases, it is possible - even if there is a general inconspicuousness in the longitudinal and the cross section of life - to make significant statements for the reaction according to criminal law: If it is possible to assess the patterns of relevance, i.e., the interests and intentions deeply rooted in the personality (see Sect. 2.2.3.1 below), as well as the attitudes and value orientation of the offender (see Sect. 2.2.3.2 below) which determine his everyday behavior, significant knowledge and insights can be gained with respect to his criminality (see Sect. 2.3.2.4 below).

Though the (material) criteria of assessment were elaborated on the basis of male offenders and the general male population, there are no fundamental reasons which would preclude applying the present method to *female offenders.* First impressions from a corresponding study show that the criteria of assessment have to be modified merely insofar as there are some special aspects in the life pattern of women which may be due to their traditional role in social life. However, there are no valid results yet in this respect.

2 The Criminological Assessment of Individual Cases

2.1 Collecting the Necessary Information

The foundation of the assessment of the offender in the context of his social relationships consists of comprehensive and differentiated information on his development in life and his life pattern, as well as on his integration in his social environment. Although, in principle, as detailed information as possible should be aimed at, one should not simply collect a large amount of more or less random information. The investigations must be limited to collecting facts and impressions (based on circumstances) concerning the behavior of the subject in various situations in life and in the various social spheres and on developments in these social spheres, as well as - at least within certain limits - knowledge of the social environment of the subject relevant to the later analysis.

Within the framework of the investigations, one attempts to trace back the essence of the development in life of a subject from his childhood to the present. In principle, the more recent or close to the offense the facts, the more detailed and differentiated the investigations should be.

One should basically try to obtain as precise and truthful information as possible for each relevant question in the development of a subject's life. This is not always possible. Yet precisely because of the large number of individual facts collected in the course of the investigation, which fit together like the pieces of a mosaic, so to speak, to form a picture of the offender in the context of his social relationships, it can be acceptable to do without one or the other fact if the effort to collect it can no longer be justified. Equally, a not entirely convincing statement can be accepted if the picture as a whole is already largely defined by the multitude of other facts.

In judging whether the collected facts are reliable and true, one must pay special attention to the extent to which certain indications are consistent and agree with the corresponding indications from other sources. Besides a general experience of life, a certain criminological experience is often necessary. It would be positively wrong to collect data according to a certain criminological theory. It would be equally wrong to let oneself be led by one's own notion or basic idea of the development of a subject up to the offense: Only facts which would "match" the theory or idea would be collected. In the end, the theory or notion would be confirmed but the *real* picture of the subject lost.

2.1.1 The Criminological Exploration of the Subject

The focal point of the collection of criminologically relevant facts and circumstances is the direct *exploration of the subject*. Carrying out the exploration correctly requires being familiar with the specific points of view of the criminological assessment of individual cases as well as the individual criteria of the analysis. The aim is to assess the offender in the context of his social relationships as *objectively* as possible and to obtain *systematic* knowledge of all *relevant* criteria of analysis in the individual case by means of the appropriate questions.

As opposed to the form of most interviews, which are merely concerned with obtaining the (subjective) data and information offered by the interviewee (the "in-depth interview" is an exception), the exploration also requires one's own **judgment of this information** and the *correct assessment of a subject.* Thus, the exploration differs from the interview in its purpose and in the specialist knowledge necessary to conduct it. While a person who has mastered the technique of interviewing is able to conduct skillful interviews in many areas, it is precisely a corresponding specialized knowledge which is necessary in an exploration.

In a criminological exploration, one cannot limit oneself to obtaining information from the subject on the various social spheres by asking corresponding questions. One must examine this information to see to what extent it is important for the criminological assessment of the offender in the context of his social relationships. At the same time, the subject's answers offer some indications as to the direction in which one should continue to obtain additional (relevant) information on a certain group of problems and on certain criteria of analysis. Thus, in a skillful criminological exploration, as in a psychiatric or psychological exploration, a constant analysis must be made "of what is assessed and observed during the exploration; at the same time, one should attempt to reduce the complex impressions and, subsequently, to make a synthesis of the individual facts to form an overall picture of a subject. Each question is based on the result of the previous question and is developed and worded step by step" (GÖPPINGER 1980, pp. 118ff.; trans.) against the background of the general knowledge of Applied Criminology. Therefore, theories of criminality or one's own ideas of relationships with offenses must remain entirely unconsidered.

The details of the techniques used in an exploration or interview are not discussed here. Only a few points are referred to which relate to the special nature of a criminological exploration.

A criminological exploration generally takes place in a **conversation** between subject and investigator. It can also be conducted by a number of investigators together.

To conduct as comprehensive and complete an investigation as possible, it is advisable to explore the subject *several times, at least twice,* and on more than one day. It is also advisable to make a short criminological analysis on the basis of the information collected in the first session. Usually, there are open or contradictory points or divergences between the information provided by the subject and that in the records. These points can be clarified in the following session.

The exploration is basically conducted in a **conversation** which should be as **casual** as possible and develop "organically": One should change from one (criminologically relevant) topic to another, touch one sphere of life, then another, and thus give the subject the opportunity to express himself in more detail on certain topics, to explain on his own initiative (what is criminologically relevant), to present his behavior, to describe certain situations in life, etc. One should therefore attempt to win the subject for a lively response.

Though the various social spheres and criteria of analysis must be checked *mentally* during the discussion to see whether the data are complete, it would be harmful and incorrect to ask questions about each separate social sphere systematically or even to "check off" the criteria of analysis and points of view in a certain order in the individual social spheres. On the contrary, the casual situation of the discussion should also be supported by the **way questions are asked.** Essentially, *simple, even naive and open questions* should be asked (i.e., questions which do not imply a certain answer) which prompt the subject to tell as much as possible about himself. Such questions might be: What did you do then?; What was that like?; How did that happen?; What's that?; What happened then? etc.

Finally, it is especially important to insist on obtaining as **detailed and precise information** as possible. While this is self-evident in practice in those fields which are of immediate importance in one's daily work (e.g., information on the elements of the offense for a criminal court judge), the impression often arises that one is satisfied surprisingly quickly with superficial and generalized answers in other fields, for example those relevant here (Example: "Did you complete an apprenticeship?" - "Yes." - No further questions, though there is reason enough to doubt it. Or: "What did you do last year during your leisure time?" - "I went for walks and picked berries." ...?).

One must be particularly careful with *supposedly clear concepts* and estimations as well: "Temporary work" or "going to a bar" can differ considerably in meaning, for example in view of structure, course, and formal requirements. Equally, one can have an entirely different idea of concepts such as "friend", "buddy", "bride", and "girlfriend" than a subject has.

Generally, although one is continuously classifying and checking the information collected (in one's mind), one must absolutely avoid *classifying the subject prematurely* and trying to find a justification of the classification by asking further specific questions. Otherwise, one runs the risk of pressing the subject into a framework and obscuring the particular aspects which each case has and which are important for the analysis.

As a rule, the exploration can be facilitated by certain **aids.** In particular, it can be conducted economically from the point of view of time: Even for short personal records (e.g., those of juveniles), it is useful to elaborate a brief *skeleton of essential dates in the life of a subject* (e.g., date of birth, dates the subject first went to school, completed school, started and completed an apprenticeship, did military or alternative nonmilitary service, started and left jobs, moved, etc., and also important dates in the spheres of leisure and contacts). This allows oneself and the subject, who is usually unable (like most people) to produce the exact dates in his life spontaneously, a better orientation.

Usually, this skeleton makes it possible to cover all social spheres for *certain intervals.* Intervals can be delimited by the duration of a job at a certain company, by the period the subject lived at a certain place or by the time the subject was together with a certain person (e.g., "during your first marriage"). In this way, for example, the subject can remember what he did after work during a period more easily than when questions are based on largely abstract dates. (Example: "What did you do during the weekends in May 1976?" Better: "What did you do during the weekends when you were working for X. and lived with your girlfriend Y.?")

A quite clear picture of an offender and his life pattern can often be gained by means of a *description of daily routines* (see also Part III, Sect. 3.2). Besides the day an offense was committed, a recent day can also be useful to obtain as up-to-date a picture as possible of his life; a comparison of daily routines during various intervals of a subject's life can be advisable as well. Such descriptions of daily routines, for example for a "typical" working day and a "typical" day the subject did not work (e.g., a Saturday or a day the subject stayed away from work unexcused), offer revealing indications of a subject's entire life-style, of the things which are of particular importance in his everyday life, of his interests, etc. At the same time, such a description offers points of reference for further questions. This requires, however, that the subject is urged to describe what he does in detail. A description of a daily routine limited to determining that a subject worked during the day and went to "have a beer" after work is entirely unprofitable. More details are necessary, for example on the situation after work: Tell me what you do after work. What exactly do you do when you leave the workshop? Do you go straight home? Is there a specific bar you go to after work? Whom do you meet there? What happens then? And then? Are you still together with the same people? And what happens then? Which bars do you go to in the course of an evening? What do you do in each bar? How many beers do you have? etc.

With some experience, one should be able to *picture the investigated social spheres* and the specific situations and courses. If this is impossible, further information must be collected. The efforts to gain access to the subject in the various situations in life and social spheres in this way are much more helpful in the assessment of the offender in the context of his social relationships than the simple collection of - possibly also relevant - facts. Even with an almost infinite number of individual indications and facts, the actual circumstances in life cannot be accessed and remain vague until one succeeds in picturing the situations and circumstances on the basis of the facts.

The attempt to put oneself in a subject's place and to see oneself and one's own personality in the situation of the subject and his personality must be clearly distinguished from the above efforts. This should be avoided by all means, as it is virtually impossible to put oneself in another person's place. If one tries to do so, one always experiences oneself, one's own perceptions, and one's own reactions in the corresponding situations, not the experiences and perceptions of the other, who alone is concerned. Any lapse into such subjective interviewing involves the danger of incorrect and therefore useless data and can render the entire criminological assessment worthless.

2.1.2 Further Sources of Information

Besides the criminological exploration, the contents of **records** on the subject (e.g., case records, prison records, records on execution of sentence, records of the youth welfare office) are of particular importance. The knowledge gained by means of these two methods of data collection can be supplemented by direct **investigations of the social environment** - if possible in terms of time and if actually necessary. These investigations can include a visit to the wife or parents of a subject by the (juvenile) court assistant, information provided by other persons who reared the subject, by schools and employers, and by friends, and other persons with whom a subject had contact. Here again, one must take care that facts, not assumptions or interpretations of the persons interviewed, are collected.

Particularly the *combination* of various sources of information enables one to obtain a comprehensive, relatively reliable, and fairly objective assessment of an offender in the context of his social relationships. In this way, the inherent weaknesses and shortcomings of each method of investigation are compensated to a large extent. The record analyses, for example, provide information only on much too narrowly defined circumstances of a subject's life. In many individual questions on a subject's development in life, however, they are an effective corrective for the interviews, particularly since a subject's (or other person's) power of recollection may not suffice for a precise reconstruction, especially if exact indications of time are important. On the other hand, interviews (and on-the-spot investigations) in the social environment of a subject can be much more informative than the exploration of the subject himself or the record analysis, particularly when "soft" data and circumstances (e.g., the "real" reason for leaving a job, the relationship of the subject with a certain person) and estimations are concerned. Moreover, interviews with other persons offer a further perspective - independent of the perspectives of the subject and the person compiling the record - on a subject's social reality, which can only be investigated fragmentarily in any case.

The *special natures* and *weaknesses* of the many methods of investigation and perspectives, which only do justice to the complexity of the object when they are added together, must be taken into consideration - insofar as their relevance to the criminological individual case analysis is concerned (see also Part I, Sect. 3.2). Basically, no kind of source may be given preference in view of reliability and degree of truth.

2.2 Data Analysis

The assessment of the offender in the context of his social relationships and thus the criminological diagnosis (see Sect. 2.3 below) are ultimately a question of the relationship between a development in life and general social behavior on the one hand and delinquency, in particular a subject's last offense, on the other (see Sect. 2.3 below). This *last offense* is usually the final point of the development to be analyzed and, at the same time, forms the *point of reference in time* to which the entire analysis is oriented. Central to the analysis is a subject's general behavior in the various social spheres.

The *object of the analysis* is basically the *behavior of a subject when he is not imprisoned* (extramural behavior). If there is a long interval between the last offense and imprisonment (or the time of the assessment), the analysis also covers this interval, not only in view of the further behavior of the subject in the various social spheres, but also in view of offenses committed during this period - if there were any. Earlier or current periods of imprisonment remain unconsidered at first; in a later stage of the analysis, they are also taken into account against the background of the overall assessment of extramural behavior (see Sect. 2.3.4 below).

2.2.1 Analysis of the Longitudinal Section of Life

2.2.1.1 Analysis of General Social Behavior

In the first part of the analysis, a subject's *general social behavior* and - separately - his *delinquency* are examined in the longitudinal section from his childhood up to his last offense. For this purpose, the subject's **general social behavior** is assigned to the various social spheres and analyzed. There are the *sphere of abode*, the *sphere of performance*, the *sphere of leisure*, the *sphere of contacts*, if applicable including the *sphere of the family of procreation*, and behavior in connection with *child rearing* during childhood and (early) youth.

The relevant **criteria of assessment** consist of the ideal-typically "condensed" behavior in the various social spheres (see Part III, Sect. 2.2): At the one extreme, there is the ideal-typical behavior of recidivist offenders - **"O-ideal-typical behavior"**, at the other extreme, the ideal-typical behavior of socially and criminally inconspicuous people from the general population - **"G-ideal-typical behavior".**

The subject's real behavior patterns in the various social spheres are *related* to these ideal-typical forms *in a certain way:* His behavior can sometimes tend more toward the one pole, sometimes more toward the other. Corresponding to the special nature of the conception of ideal types (see Part III, Sect. 1.3), examining the specific behavior of each subject can determine only a more or less pronounced **approximation** of the real occurrences to the ideal type or **tendencies** in one or the other direction of ideal-typical form (see Case A., Appendix). In the synopsis presented above (Part III, Sect. 2.2), it is not the *particular* behavior pattern which must be considered "ideal-typical" but the *entire* behavior in the corresponding social sphere: Besides, it is logically impossible for all of the behavior patterns noted in either column to occur in an individual case; some of them exclude each other or represent alternatives.

In the analysis of an individual case, the behavior of a subject is examined systematically on the basis of the behavior patterns presented in the synopsis. By comparing a subject's actual behavior with the ideal-typical behavior, it is possible to determine, both in and beyond the various spheres, *developments and basic tendencies* pointing in a certain direction in a subject's *entire life pattern*. It can also be possible to elaborate *individual phases* in the life of a subject where his behavior deviates from his behavior before with regard to intensity and tendency. Although such *changes in behavior* are often first observed in one social sphere alone, a thorough examination can show changes in other spheres as well, whether immediately before, simultaneously, or afterward. This frequently leads to first indications for later considerations concerning interventions.

In reality, a subject's behavior patterns only rarely point to the O-ideal-typical pole alone. Even recidivist offenders with a large number of offenses and convictions can demonstrate a number of individual behavior patterns which correspond to or tend toward the behavior of the inconspicuous general population (see Case A., Appendix). Conversely, a (largely) socially inconspicuous person can exhibit one or the other behavior pattern belonging more to the ideal-typical behavior of recidivist offenders (i.e., to the O-ideal-typical pole). Normally, these "different" behavior patterns are largely isolated and rarely characterize an entire social sphere.

The **result** of the analysis of the longitudinal section is a **differentiated longitudinal profile of an individual subject** which is *specific* to the subject in several respects: On the one hand, the profile characterizes the subject with respect to the degree of *approximation* of his individual specific behavior patterns to the corresponding ideal-typical pole. On the other hand, it sketches *outlines in the various social spheres* and creates a *picture of the entire longitudinal section* which integrates all social spheres.

2.2.1.2 Analysis of the Sphere of Delinquency

The analysis of the sphere of delinquency is entirely separated from the previous one of general social behavior. The analysis of delinquency covers a subject's last offense and his previous registered and nonregistered offenses, as well as "offenses" committed before the age of criminal responsibility.

Practically everyone has committed **"offenses"** during childhood, though they rarely come to the knowledge of the police. In view of later criminality, these "offenses" can be entirely or largely unimportant; yet they can also be first signs of an increasingly persistent delinquency. This can often be determined only *in retrospect,* against the background of later delinquency, when there were first precursors of later offenses during childhood. This can be of importance for the current assessment of the juvenile or the adult, particularly in view of a reinforcement of criminality in the sphere of delinquency.

The analysis of (registered and nonregistered) **offenses** at the age of responsibility is not limited to a presentation of normative definitions of offenses or of groups of offenses. On the contrary, it is oriented to points of view which describe the appearance of the modalities of the offense, i.e., the way the offense came about, the planning of the offense, the way the offender participated in the offense, the procedure in the offense, the reaction after the offense, etc. The integration of the offense in the offender's general situation in life is of special importance (see below). These points of view enable one to **gain access to the individual offense.** However, not every aspect is significant in every offense, and their importance varies from case to case according to the interplay of the various modalities of the offense. (For example, a differentiated plan to commit the offense can point to an increased purposefulness in a property offense, while this is not necessarily so in the homicide of a specific victim out of a conflict situation which has been smoldering for a prolonged period.)

The following comparison offers certain *indications* of which forms of individual modalities usually point to an increased or decreased purposefulness in the commission of offenses:

Modalities which point more to an **increased purposefulness** *in the commission of offenses:*	*Modalities which point more to a* **decreased purposefulness** *in the commission of offenses:*
The Way the Offense Came About/The Decision to Commit an Offense	
Decision to commit offense on the basis of sober consideration	Decision to commit offense under the influence of considerable alcohol consumption, extraordinary mood, or conflict situation, or under the influence of the participants or other persons
The Planning of the Offense	
Careful planning of the offense (preparation, victim, object of offense, procedure, alternative procedures, particular safety measures, etc.) and the consequences of the offense (measures to suppress evidence, turning loot to account, etc.)	No planning in the actual sense, spontaneously seizing "good" or "tempting" opportunities
The Participation in the Offense	
After considering the advantages and disadvantages, committing the offense alone or together with others	Committing the offense alone or together with others more or less by chance
The Procedure in the Offense	
Proceeding according to a plan determined in advance; if others participate, a division of functions; a differentiated, sophisticated or brash procedure; completing the offense or attempting to complete it with all available means, even if the situation of the offense changes unexpectedly, and if need be by using violence heedlessly against persons - this was planned in advance or decided after quickly judging the situation	Largely unconsidered procedure; naive, partially even simple procedure; the offender stumbles into the offense and from one step to another in the procedure of the offense; if the offense is committed jointly, there is reciprocal stimulation and encouragement in the sense of group dynamics; the offense can develop its own dynamics in another connection as well (victim puts up defense, instruments in the offense), which cause the offender to lose con-

	trol; if unforeseen difficulties arise, the offense is more likely not committed; a contribution of the victim in the sense of a facilitation or forcing of the offense

Behavior after the Offense

Leaving the place where the offense was committed in a well-considered or planned way; taking special measures to conceal the offense and suppress evidence; in property and fraudulent offenses, turning the loot to account according to a plan (selling it, giving it away for a certain purpose)	Largely unconsidered, precipitate flight or unsuited, naive hiding place; in property and fraudulent offenses, hoarding the loot uselessly in a hiding place, leaving it lying about carelessly, or giving it away without any obvious advantage

For a comprehensive access to the offense, a subject's **general situation in life,** in particular in the context of the time of the offense, must be considered in addition to these modalities (for examples, see Part II, Sect. 4.6). Here, the interplay between a certain behavior in everyday life and a certain life pattern on the one hand and the occurrence of the offense on the other often becomes apparent.

If a subject has committed *several* or even *numerous offenses* (or "offenses"), it is not absolutely necessary to assess each individual offense on the basis of the above criteria. Instead, on the basis of these criteria, one should attempt to find **aspects which the offenses have in common or which differ between them** and **tendencies in the development of the sphere of delinquency** in view of the modalities of the offenses, from "offenses" during childhood up to the last offense. In this way, one can state how a subject's last offense fits into his entire delinquency, for example whether it is more or less unconnected and isolated from other offenses or whether it is an almost consistent development from earlier offenses.

To recognize such superordinate points of view, it is essential to free oneself of a normative judgment and describe and recognize the (external) appearances of the offenses, here even more so than in the analysis of the individual offenses: Thus, normatively different offenses may well be *similar,* insofar as they exhibit largely *uniform courses of occurrences* for a specific offender or developed out of *comparable situations in life.*

Tendencies in development in the sphere of delinquency can be observed in particular if there are more and more modalities which indicate an increasing purposefulness in the commission of offenses: A change from simply seizing opportunities to steal or defraud to planned burglaries or large-scale, sophisticated fraud, an increasing value of the damages in fraudulent offenses, a sophistication of the procedure or the use of violence against people in the commission of an offense for the first time as well as a change from committing the offense alone to committing it jointly or vice versa for well-considered reasons (better chances of success, danger of being discovered, necessity of sharing loot, etc.), or an increasing routine in finding and recognizing "good" opportunities as well as an increasing range of action to commit offenses are good indications of a further reinforcement of criminality.

Besides individual phases during which a subject committed offenses relatively frequently, an increasing or decreasing *duration of intervals during which a subject did not commit or was not punished for any offenses* offers further indications of changes in the sphere of delinquency.

Despite the differentiated assessment of a subject's offenses, the analysis of the sphere of delinquency does **not have any independent importance** for immediate conclusions as regards diagnosis, prognosis, and interventions. On the contrary, the offenses must be *related to the subject's behavior in the remaining social spheres*; only against this background is it possible to make any well-founded statement on the importance of the individual offense and of delinquency as a whole in the life of an offender (see Sect. 2.3.2 below).

2.2.2 Analysis of the Cross Section of Life

The *cross section of the life* of a subject *before he committed his last offense* is central to the second part of the analysis. Though his behavior as a whole, and therefore also that immediately preceding the offense, was the object of the analysis of the longitudinal section, it is examined separately from another perspective in the cross section analysis: The *measure* for this analysis are the *criminorelevant criteria* (see Part III, Sect. 3.3), i.e., the following *O-criteria* (which basically involve a danger of criminality) and *G-criteria* (which are basically more likely to prevent criminality):

O-criteria
Neglect of the sphere of work and performance as well as of family and other social obligations
Deficient relationship to money and property
Unstructured organization of leisure
Absence of planning in life
Inadequately high level of aspirations
Deficient sense of reality
Low tolerance for stress
Paradoxical expectation of adaptation
Demand to be free from any ties
Uncontrolled and excessive alcohol consumption

G-Criteria
Fulfillment of social obligations
Adequate level of aspirations
Attachment to a well-ordered home (and family life)

Adequate relationship to money and property
Dedication to and satisfaction from work
Productive organization of leisure
Commitment to the affairs of persons and institutions
Willingness to adapt
Strong ties
Endurance and a high tolerance for stress
Willingness to bear responsibility
Good sense of reality and self-control
Planning in life and determination

As opposed to the ideal-typical behavior in the longitudinal section, the immediate *relationship* in time must be taken into account for the *crimino*relevant criteria: The starting point for the analysis of the cross section is the period preceding the last offense. The precise length of this interval cannot be determined in general terms. Essentially, it depends on how long the life pattern lasted out of which the offense developed. In some cases, this can be merely a few days or weeks, in others, several months (see also Case A., Appendix). The examination of each criminorelevant criterion not only relates to the interval of the cross section but also traces back the criterion to see *how long* it has occurred before this interval. It must also be examined whether the criterion has already occurred at some earlier time or has repeatedly occurred *temporarily* and whether there has been any relationship with the commission of offenses.

The **criminorelevant criteria** abstract from individual behavior patterns. Therefore, they cannot be determined directly, but only on the basis of a comprehensive examination of various behavior patterns. Some of them describe attitudes which are not limited to an individual social sphere but are expressed in various spheres and related with a subject's general life pattern. Some of them concentrate on general tendencies in the individual social spheres which can be determined on the basis of a subject's everyday behavior. The "presence" or "absence" of the criteria can be judged only if **the specific behavior of a subject is related to the specific circumstances of his life** and is regarded inside this framework. The relational character of the criteria (see also Part III, Sect. 3.3.1) becomes immediately apparent, for example, in the concept "inadequately high level of aspirations": It cannot be generally determined - for example on the basis of the average income of the general population - from what point on a level of aspirations must be regarded as inadequately high. It depends on which level of aspirations is still suited to the specific situation of a subject's life. For example, the aspiration of consuming two packs of cigarettes and several bottles of beer a day or even of having a car, besides having to support oneself and pay for a roof over one's head, is inadequate for a pensioner or an apprentice with at the most DM 600 a month at his disposal but adequate for someone with DM 2000 a month.

Since, therefore, the specific personal situation is decisive, the criteria cannot be defined in an abstract and generally valid way but can at best be explained in the form of examples and indications (see Part III, Sect. 3.3.3) to show the behavior patterns on the basis of which the presence of a criterion can be concluded. These examples, however, may not lead one to disregard the fact that the criteria must be related to the specific circumstances of the individual case. Externally identical behavior can correspond to a criterion in some cases, but not in others: In the examination of a "fulfillment of social obligations," for example, it always depends on the persons to whom such obligations exist. Thus, a certain behavior in a family whose members go their own ways without regard to the others cannot be regarded as a neglect of social obligations toward the family for *this* specific family, while the same behavior can be such a neglect in a family with a strong social cohesion.

The **result** of the analysis of the cross section must be a clear statement on **which** of the **O-** and **G-criteria** are present during the interval of the cross section and **how far** the underlying behavior patterns can be traced back in time. As in the analysis of the longitudinal section, a subject rarely demonstrates *all* O- or *all* G-criteria; usually, he exhibits several criteria pointing in one direction and only a few or none pointing in the other.

2.2.3 Patterns of Relevance and Value Orientation

2.2.3.1 Patterns of Relevance

The third part of the analysis attempts to assess, by way of a subject's *patterns of relevance,* the characteristic interests and determining basic intentions which characterize and form his behavior and conduct of life in particular (see Part III, Sect. 5).

The *basis* for this analysis is once again a subject's *general social behavior in everyday life.* After the largely descriptive analysis of behavior in the longitudinal section and the cross section analysis, the interests and basic intentions which determined and determine a subject most during his entire life (or only during a certain period of his life) are now central. At this stage, their criminologically relevant effects are disregarded (see Sect. 2.3.1.3 below). At this point, the analysis merely attempts to gain access to the personality-specific area of the subject by way of his general social behavior without using psychological concepts or models.

The *tool* used for this purpose is the analysis of the **patterns of relevance.** The patterns of relevance do not form a unified system of concepts; on the contrary, they are a framework for the analysis of personality-specific interests and intentions. This framework must be understood in a heuristic way and is not entirely defined in view of its content. The patterns of relevance point to particularly important and specific segments of life or spheres of activity of a person and, simultaneously, show a direction of orientation in life which is not immediately phenomenologically accessible and of which the individual is often unaware. If they are correspondingly intense, several patterns of relevance together or even one pattern of relevance alone can become so important as to determine a subject's orientation in life.

However, at least at this point in time, *no* rules as generally valid as the criminorelevant criteria (see Part III, Sect. 5) can be given for the – criminological –

direction of effect of certain patterns of relevance. Patterns of relevance can be filled with purposes in life which involve a danger of criminality (e.g., driving around aimlessly while being willing to run great risks in traffic, possibly with a vehicle stolen for this purpose and without a driver's license) or with purposes which are "neutral" or prevent criminality to a certain extent (e.g., satisfying one's passion for driving by becoming a trucker). This is not surprising, considering that there are mental or psychological characteristics behind the behavior expressing patterns of relevance which are value free per se and can take effect in one or the other direction. Particularly since patterns of relevance which have been realized in behavior involving a danger of criminality can also be realized in a socially adequate way, they are of considerable importance in *considerations concerning prophylaxis and interventions or therapy* (see Sects. 2.3.3 and 2.4.2 below).

To **gain access to a subject's patterns of relevance** within the framework of the analysis of a specific individual case, it is useful to examine the life of the subject to see whether similar tendencies underlie his behavior or certain behavior patterns in one or more social spheres and whether these tendencies have appeared constantly in the life of the subject, have appeared repeatedly, become more pronounced, etc. Marked patterns of relevance can be found particularly in an in-depth examination of the spheres of leisure and contacts, since the relevant developments in life are often expressed most clearly in these two spheres. Furthermore, a subject's attitude and dedication to his work can provide useful indications. The analysis of a "typical" day of a subject can also offer some insights: It is easy to determine what orients the organization of his everyday life, which preferences in time he has, what guides and attracts him, what he concentrates on, and what he "bypasses."

The **result** of the efforts to assess what is relevant to an individual subject in this way usually consists of **several patterns of relevance** (exceptionally only one particularly relevant pattern) which can be determined throughout the life of the subject in a more or less pronounced form. It should be noted whether certain basic intentions (which rarely change) underlie each pattern of relevance or whether particular interests (which are more likely to change) are concerned (see Part III, Sect. 5)

Some additional points of view must be taken into consideration: For example, patterns of relevance can exist alongside each other - in varying intensity - though they are in a certain sense conflicting. This can be a first indication of possibilities to intervene for the purpose of resocialization. This is also true when, in the course of time, the importance of various patterns of relevance has shifted or when the organization of a certain pattern of relevance has changed (for example, if a pattern of relevance is first expressed more in socially conspicuous behavior patterns involving a danger of criminality and later on shifts more in the direction of socially inconspicuous and accepted or tolerated behavior patterns or vice versa).

Finally, in view of later interventions, it can be of great importance to state what has **not** been **relevant** in the life of a subject yet can be almost absolutely necessary for a socially inconspicuous life, such as working regularly and continuously (see also Sect. 2.3.3 below).

2.2.3.2 *Value Orientation*

In the criminological individual case analysis, the attempt to gain access to the values which guide the subject and which enter his behavior is limited from the outset (see Part III, Sect. 5). One must make do with obtaining a certain impression of a subject's **value orientation** and thus indications of his attitudes and his concept of life. Essentially, it is a question of *which abstract principles and values have been decisive for the actions of a subject in various everyday (or extraordinary) situations.*

In the individual case to be assessed, efforts will have to remain limited to reaching certain conclusions with respect to the value orientation on the basis of certain *statements:* For example, it can be useful to note how a subject speaks of his work, parents, wife, or children; to a certain extent, it is possible to determine whether they are important to him, whether he assumes responsibility in this respect, etc. Such statements, however, should always be examined to see whether they have been realized *in the social life* of the subject. Only rarely does a subject generally reject current social values in his statements though there is often a certain discrepancy between the concept of values (he indicates) and his behavior, of which he is not necessarily aware.

Irrespective of the concept of values a subject *expresses,* it is generally more useful in the analysis of the value orientation to examine the life of the subject and ask the following general questions: Are the actions of a subject *shaped* by certain guiding principles which impart some stability to his life pattern, or are there largely personal and material interests oriented to immediate urges and short-term utilitarian motives, expressed, for example, in an erratic and changing life? Is the value orientation of a subject only "hedonistic," does it follow the "pleasure principle"?

Despite great efforts, it can be impossible to find a value orientation for some subjects. Such a vacuum can occur, on occasion, for the patterns of relevance as well. In such cases, one has to accept the fact that there is nothing to be found, particularly to avoid the danger of reading false values (or patterns of relevance) into a vacuum.

The **result** of an analysis of the value orientation is therefore necessarily based on *isolated and rough impressions.* However, these impressions show at least certain tendencies as to whether there are any values relevant to and important for a subject at all and whether they offer any indications for specific interventions or whether his value orientation stands in the way of a socially sound and noncriminal life.

2.3 The Criminological Diagnosis

The *findings* of the analysis of the investigations must now be brought together *to form a comprehensive picture of the offender in the context of his social relationships as a unity* and to make a *diagnosis* of the individual offender in the context of his social relationships on the basis of the criteria of reference of the Criminological Triad (see also Sect. 1.2 above). Although this step is based exclusively on the findings of the previous analysis, it is not simply the sum of the points of view of analysis up to this point; it goes further in two respects: On the one hand, the findings of the various perspectives concentrating on one segment of the life of a subject are seen in relation to the findings of the remaining perspectives. In this way, the importance and weight of individual points in the life of a subject as a whole can be estimated. On the other hand, *a subject's delinquency is related to his social development and his life pattern.* Here, a subject's individual development in life is compared with certain (ideal-typical) pictures describing various forms of relationships between general social behavior and delinquency.

Subsequently, the "*special aspects*" are extracted from the host of facts processed up to then and presented (see Sect. 2.3.3 below). These are the aspects which are characteristic of an individual offender, his behavior, life-style, and orientation in life, which could be distinguished in the analysis of his life and which are of importance particularly for prognosis and interventions. Central are a subject's - criminologically relevant - "weak" and "strong points," but also his social intertwinement and the - criminologically relevant - external influences of his environment.

This leads to a **differentiated criminological diagnosis.** It is a solid foundation for conclusions concerning a *prognosis* tailored to the *individual subject* (see Sect. 2.4.1 below). At the same time, it leads to specific criminologically important indications for promising *interventions* in the sense of resocialization (see Sect. 2.4.2 below).

If there is a prolonged period between the last offense, i. e., the time the diagnosis relates to, and the time of the criminological assessment - whether the criminal proceedings do not take place until months or years after the offense or whether the subject has been imprisoned for a prolonged period in the meantime - the further behavior of the subject is also observed against the background of the knowledge of his life pattern and development up to the time of the last offense. Of particular interest are any changes in his behavior and his basic orientation in life since the time he committed the offense.

2.3.1 Criteria of Reference of the Criminological Triad

In the preceding analysis (see Sect. 2.2 above), a subject's social behavior is separated into various spheres and examined from various perspectives. This means that the unity of a subject's life is artificially divided - a necessary step for the purpose of analysis. These aspects must be brought together again to form a unified picture if one is to judge which position delinquency occupies in the entire life of an individual offender. The *aid* and *measure* for the classification of an individual offender are the criteria of reference of the **Criminological Triad.** On the basis of these criteria, it is possible to gain a complex and yet uniform, as it were three-dimensional, *overall picture of the offender in the context of his social relationships.* These criteria are the various forms of the *position of the offense in the longitudinal section of life* (see Sect. 2.3.1.1 below) and the *criminorelevant constellations* spanning the various social spheres in the cross section of life (see Sect. 2.3.1.2 below); the *patterns of relevance* and the *value orientation* (see Sect. 2.3.1.3 below) help complete the picture.

The criteria of the Criminological Triad complement each other and, at the same time, interlock in such a way that the *differing forms of the three criteria of reference,* particularly those of the longitudinal and the cross section of life, fit together and form *certain* - criminorelevant - *pictures of delinquency in the development in life.* In this way, certain forms of developments in life can be distinguished: Criminality is either the result of a continuous development in life with an inner logical consistency - the one extreme - or a break in the continuity of life - the other extreme - or an intermediate form between the two extremes which can be described in a qualitative way. Each of these forms is marked by the characteristic nature of the behavior in the longitudinal section of life, which is complemented by a certain cross section as well as certain patterns of relevance and a corresponding value orientation (see Sect. 2.3.2 below).

2.3.1.1 The Position of the Offense in the Longitudinal Section of Life

The starting point for the various courses of developments in the longitudinal section is the ideal-typical behavior in the various social spheres, which is the foundation of the analysis of the longitudinal section (see Sect. 2.2.1 above). The various *positions of the offense in the longitudinal section of life* each appear in a characteristic way in this respect: They are characterized by a maximum of pronounced tendencies toward O-ideal-typical behavior ("the development toward criminality" - see Part III, Sects. 4.4.2 and 4.4.3) or by a maximum of pronounced tendencies toward G-ideal-typical behavior ("criminality as a sudden event" - see Part III, Sect. 4.4.4) during a subject's entire development in life and throughout all social spheres. Or they are characterized by the fact that the tendencies point to the one (O-) and/or the other (G-)pole in varying intensity or that they are limited to a certain phase or certain individual social spheres (e.g., "criminality in the course of personality maturation" - see Part III, Sect. 4.4.5). Thus, these courses differ in the degree of continuity and logical consistency with which a development in life and related specific social behavior lead to an offense. They form the decisive measure for deciding what position an offender's last offense(s) and delinquency as a whole have in the development of his life. At the same time, the various positions of the offense in the longitudinal section serve as a skeleton for classifying the remaining criteria of reference of the Criminological Triad - the criminorelevant constellations and the patterns of relevance and value orientation - for pragmatic reasons. Finally, the unification of all three perspectives leads to characteristic combinations.

2.3.1.2 The Criminorelevant Constellations

The question of a logical consistency of delinquency becomes even more marked in the evaluation of the analysis of the *cross section of life* than in the examination of the longitudinal section of life. This analysis gives a most up-to-date impression of the life-style and life pattern of a subject - related to the time preceding the last offense - and thus supplements the knowledge obtained in the examination of the longitudinal section.

A maximum of logical consistency occurs when the O- and G-criteria examined in the analysis of the cross section do not simply occur at random, i.e., when several specific criteria occur together to form constellations which are indicators of criminality of far greater significance than the individual criteria. The *criminorelevant constellations* are such combinations of criteria (see Part III, Sect. 3.3).

The **criminovalent constellation** (see Part III, Sect. 3.3.2) means that there is a great *danger of criminality* for the subject concerned. Decisive for the importance of the constellation is the concurrence of all four criteria of the constellation:

1. Neglect of the sphere of work and performance as well as of family and social obligations
2. Deficient relationship to money and property
3. Unstructured leisure behavior
4. Absence of planning in life

Only when the criteria concur does the inner relationship in the sense of a logical consistency with which delinquency results out of a certain cross section of life become immediately apparent; for *this* criminorelevant constellation in particular, it is the consistency of the development of delinquency in the form of property and fraudulent offenses (see Part III, Sect. 3.3.2).

Consequently, in the specific *individual case to be assessed, all four criteria must be present during the period preceding the last offense*. Otherwise, the criminovalent constellation cannot be assumed as a whole and its specific importance considered. The *duration of the presence* of the entire constellation varies considerably, from a few weeks to several months (see, for example, Case A., Appendix, Sect. 4.1). Likewise, the individual criteria of the constellation can be traced back in time for a varying amount of time and have occurred for years as individual criteria (see Sect. 2.2.2 above). However, it is decisive that all four criteria concur; only then can the *constellation* be assumed to be present. If, in contrast, only three (or two) of the four criteria occur, the constellation is not "approximately" present; it *is not present at all* (see, for example, Case A., Appendix, Sect. 4.1).

The same is true for the **criminoresistant constellation,** which indicates a particular resistance to criminality (offenses committed with intent). Its importance also stands and falls with the *concurrence of all four criteria:*

1. Fulfillment of social obligations
2. Adequate level of aspirations
3. Attachment to a well-ordered home (and family life)
4. Adequate relationship to money and property

However, the criminoresistant constellation is no absolute guarantee against delinquency; this becomes apparent with "criminality as a sudden event" in particular, where an offense occurs despite the presence of a criminoresistant constellation (see Sect. 2.3.2.5 below). Similarly, the criminovalent constellation does not always of absolute necessity go together with (property or fraudulent) delinquency, though the absence of criminality is improbable, particularly when the corresponding life-style has been kept up for a prolonged period. Therefore, both constellations must be seen against the background of the other criteria of reference of the criminological triad, and they only gain their specific importance in this context. Thus, in particular, they should not be regarded in isolation or as a kind of prediction table.

2.3.1.3 Patterns of Relevance and Value Orientation

The diagnostic classification of the offender in the context of his social relationships according to the various forms of developments in life and the positions of delinquency in these developments is based mainly on the examination of the cross and the longitudinal section. But the classification is *substantiated additionally* by taking into consideration the **patterns of relevance** (possibly also the value orientation - see below). This "third dimension" is of special importance particularly within the framework of interventions for an individual offender but is also significant for the diagnostic classification. Only when a subject's intentions as well as the characteristic interests closely related to his personality are taken into account can the structure of his conduct of life be understood throughout all social spheres and corresponding conclusions for the future reached.

Although it is impossible to establish a *general* relationship between criminality and patterns of relevance (see Sect. 2.2.3.1 above) - as opposed to the criteria of the cross and the longitudinal section and delinquency - there are certain patterns of relevance which are characteristic of the various forms of development in life and life-styles (see Sect. 2.3.2 below). Therefore, if, in addition, some corresponding patterns of relevance occur in the *individual case* which should be assigned to one of the categories on the basis of the examination of the cross and the longitudinal section, these patterns supplement the criminological picture of the individual offender in the context of his social relationships. (Moreover, the patterns of relevance are of particular importance in connection with considerations concerning differentiated interventions - see Sect. 2.4.2 below.)

Despite its quite considerable *actual* importance for a subject's organization of life, the **value orientation** plays only a minor role within the framework of a diagnostic classification. Some indications can be given as to which value orientation normally goes together with a certain development in life; yet they must be limited to only a few impressions. Consequently, the value orientation - in connection with the patterns of relevance - can help complete the picture obtained in the examination of the cross and the longitudinal section but cannot modify this picture oriented to "hard facts" in any significant way. The value orientation is of special importance mainly for a differentiated therapy or a pedagogic influence on a subject. In some cases, additional psychological tests can be useful (see Sect. 2.4.2 below).

2.3.2 Criminality in the Life of the Offender in the Context of His Social Relationships

The following categories sketch various forms of developments in life where criminality occupies a particular position. These categories are oriented to the position of the offense in the longitudinal section of life - for purely pragmatic reasons; yet they *always take into consideration all three criteria of reference of the Criminological Triad.* Each of these forms has a special nature with respect to the individual criteria of reference and is marked in particular by characteristic forms of all three criteria of reference. These categories are in no way a definitive typology; there are a number of other forms - as it were intermediate ones - beyond the forms described in the following. Moreover, the basic forms presented can also fuse (for example, "criminality in the course of personality maturation" can turn into a "development toward criminality during adulthood" - see also Sect. 2.3.2.3 below) or can occur one after another (a "continuous development toward criminality beginning during early youth" can - e.g., after a stay in prison and a subsequent long-term social rehabilitation - be followed by "criminality despite no other social conspicuousness").

In assigning a subject's development in life to a category, his delinquency is only a point of reference in time. The diagnosis on the basis of the criteria of reference of the Criminological Triad takes place *exclusively* on the basis of the findings of the analysis of *social behavior.* Consequently, the fact of recidivist delinquency alone is no sufficient indication of a more or less continuous development toward criminality or a temporary "criminal period" during a phase in life; no more does the circumstance of an isolated (first) offense alone exclude the possibility of an already present or expected continuous development toward criminality (and further offenses) - and the assignment to this category. General social behavior alone is decisive for the assessment and the diagnostic classification.

This is not contradicted by the fact that the *criminological analysis* of the last offense and previous delinquency (see Sect. 2.2.1.2 above) is useful to supplement this diagnostic classification and offers useful indications for the assessment of an offender in the context of his social relationships. This holds in particular for the *kind of delinquency,* though not in the sense of a precise qualification according to criminal law. Thus, in the following, certain offenses and forms of committing offenses can be described which occur more frequently if a corresponding life pattern and development in life occur. Nevertheless, this does not decisively influence or even determine the various forms of courses. In a continuous development toward criminality, for example, property and fraudulent offenses occur most frequently (see Sect. 2.3.2.1 below), but this does not exclude other kinds of offenses.

The various pictures of criminorelevant developments in life and life-style are a differentiated **measure for the diagnostic classification** of the behavior and the development in life **of the subject to be assessed.** The **procedure** of starting with *the position of the offense in the longitudinal section of life* has proved successful in practice: The individual behavior profile of the subject to be assessed is related to the specific forms of the longitudinal section of the respective type of course. In this way it is possible to obtain a rough classification. In particular, the categories which are clearly out of the question can be excluded. If, for example, there are obvious tendencies toward the O-ideal-typical pole in an individual profile of behavior, criminality as a sudden event and criminality despite no other social conspicuousness can be excluded. Then it must be *weighed* to what extent the *individual profile of a subject's behavior,* the O- or G-criteria determined in the analysis of his cross section of life, and his *patterns of relevance* and *value orientation* correspond to the *characteristic forms of the categories which have not yet been excluded.* Often, an individual subject cannot simply be assigned to one category, particularly since a classification should never be "forced." In such cases, the *tendencies* toward one or the other category should be discussed.

However, the diagnosis is not limited to this rough classification. It also considers the points where a subject *deviates* from the specific forms and the characteristic aspects of the corresponding category as well as the points which occur in a *particularly pronounced way.* These "special aspects" (see Sect. 2.3.3 below) of a specific case are the foundation of the *individual prognosis.*

Exceptionally, a case does not "come out" at all, not even in such a way that it lies between two categories, and remains *entirely open* with respect to a differential diagnosis. If this occurs, it must be examined whether the offender exhibits mental abnormality and whether a psychiatric expert must be called in.

The *diagnosis* on the basis of the criteria of reference of the Criminological Triad leads to the following **result:** As a rule, it is possible to assign a subject to one of the categories below; this classification weighs the special nature of the individual case and is yet more or less unambiguous (if necessary, the points of view in an individual case differing from the characteristic forms must be indicated). If a classification is impossible, it must be considered why the subject cannot be assigned to one of the categories in the context of his longitudinal and his cross section of life, patterns of relevance and value orientation, and to which categories he comes closest.

2.3.2.1 The Continuous Development Toward Criminality Beginning During Early Youth

The continuous development toward criminality beginning during early youth - as an ideal type - is characterized by O-ideal-typical behavior which is as early and as marked as possible throughout *all* social spheres in the **longitudinal section.** Decisive for this development is the complementary development in the *spheres of performance and leisure,* which ultimately leads to an almost total collapse of the structuring of all social spheres (see Part III, Sect. 4.4.2).

In the **cross section,** during the period preceding the last offense, there is usually a *criminovalent constellation* where all four criteria are very marked - often for quite some time before the offense was committed. Additionally, there is a varying number of further O-criteria.

The development in the longitudinal section and the criminovalent constellation in the cross section are mainly decisive in assessing a continuous development toward criminality. Yet there are also several **patterns of relevance** which are characteristic of this development and occur as a rule: Of great importance for these subjects are "freedom" (from any ties), diversity, unrest, and adventure; the atmosphere of "shady" pubs and bars and particularly the "milieu" of large cities and its members attract the subject; the immediate satisfaction of momentary desires and spontaneous needs dominates clearly. These aspects reflect an "unchecked living in the immediate present" which repeatedly leads these persons to commit offenses.

In contrast, it is often impossible to find **values** which the subject orients himself to. Frequently, there is no orientation at all. There are at least no socially sound values which the subject considers binding and which structure his life.

Although the criteria decisive for a continuous development toward criminality are therefore criteria of general social behavior, this does not mean that *earlier offenses* - and related punishments - are of no importance for the assessment of the individual case. On the contrary, they can help complete the picture. It is certainly possible to determine a continuous development toward criminality on the basis of social behavior even when there has been no delinquency yet, i.e., when the assessment relates to a *first* offense. However, there is usually conspicuousness in the form of "offenses" long before the first offense which is punished according to criminal law, often during childhood, i.e., at a time when, by nature, not all behavior patterns which indicate a continuous development toward criminality are fully present. Consistently, these "offenses" continue during youth in the form of punishable acts. In the course of time, a certain routine and increasing persistency can frequently be determined in the sphere of delinquency which are practically analogous to the subject's increasing social conspicuousness (see Sect. 2.2.1.2 above). The extensive social conspicuousness throughout all social spheres mostly corresponds to a relatively widespread criminality including many kinds of offenses. Often, the actual situations in life out of which offenses are committed show an "unchecked living in the immediate present" which can be found in the subject's entire life pattern. They show the subject's attempt to satisfy spontaneous wishes and needs arising from the moment without his considering negative consequences, possibly precisely by committing offenses.

Similar to earlier offenses, *earlier sanctions* can also help complete the examination of social behavior, though not in the sense that sanctions play an important role in a continuous development toward criminality. In contrast, imprisonment, whether in the form of a prison sentence (for juveniles) or committal to a reform school, usually does not occur until *after* a marked continuous development toward criminality and after repeated offenses and punishments.

The **further course** of such a continuous development toward criminality is generally *unfavorable*. The longer such a development has persisted and the further back the criminovalent constellation can be traced in time, the less favorable is the *prognosis*.

Particularly because the offenses are closely intertwined with the subject's orientation in life and do not occur more or less "at random" but are logically consistent with his life-style, a fundamental change of life-style is necessary to prevent further offenses. As the subject's life-style largely corresponds to his intentions, he is rarely truly willing to change.

Yet a continuous development toward criminality in this marked form rarely lasts an entire lifetime. It is not yet possible to make any valid statement on the *end of a "criminal career."* It can often be observed, however, that such a career tends to end during a subject's thirties or forties. This can be indicated by an increasing duration of intervals during which a subject does not commit any offenses (and is therefore not punished). However, what is ultimately decisive in this respect must remain open for the time being.

2.3.2.2 *The Development Toward Criminality Beginning During Adolescence or the Early Years of Adulthood*

The subjects with a development toward criminality beginning during adolescence or the early years of adulthood do not become conspicuous in the **longitudinal section** in the sense of O-ideal-typical behavior until their late teens or twenties (see Part II, Sect. 4.4.3). Although their conspicuousness occurs mainly in the *spheres of leisure and contacts* first, it rapidly spreads to the *sphere of leisure* and quickly leads to a complete neglect of corresponding requirements. In this development, as in a continuous development toward criminality beginning during early youth, there is an almost total collapse of the structuring of all social spheres immediately before the offense.

Consequently, in the **cross section** of the period before the offense, the differences between the early and the late development toward criminality have largely disappeared. There is the same inner logical consistency in the development, which mainly comes to a drastic head through the comprehensive neglect of the sphere of performance. Thus, in the end, there is a marked *criminovalent constellation* as well as a series of other O-criteria.

At the same time, it is possible to observe a change in the **patterns of relevance,** which is relatively easy to delimit, at least with respect to the way they are expressed: At juvenile age, the patterns of relevance - possibly under the influence of external factors of order - are often first concentrated on an adequately structured and productive leisure organization suited to the age of the subject, on strong ties to friends or on training and work. In the course of time, the subject's interests lead in another direction; his leisure behavior in particular changes entirely in orientation. Finally, there is a fundamental change of the subject's entire life pattern. At the end of this development, his dominating patterns of relevance are similar to those in the continuous development toward criminality beginning during early youth.

It is difficult to determine a similar change in the **value orientation:** During the (early) youth of the subject, i.e., when he is usually still socially inconspicuous, it is difficult to establish a marked value orientation with any certainty - which is not unusual at this age. Later on, there are no socially sound values (any longer), and there is often a total lack of any orientation in this context as well (see Sect. 2.3.2.1 above).

For this position of the offense as well, the *sphere of delinquency* exhibits parallels to the subject's general social behavior: There are usually no "offenses" worth mentioning during childhood and no developments comparable to those in a continuous development toward criminality in the sphere of delinquency (such as seizing good opportunities in the immediate social environment). In this context, offenses are usually more serious from the (late) beginning and are planned more carefully and committed more purposefully than those in a continuous development toward criminality. Besides the situations in life described above (Sect. 2.3.2.1), unrealistic aspirations in life frequently play a considerable role for the commission of offenses.

Thus, at the end of such a late but rapid development toward criminality beginning during adolescence or the early years of adulthood, there are no differences between this development and the continuous development toward criminality beginning during early youth. The **further course** is similar to that of the continuous development toward criminality beginning during early youth, and the *prognosis* is *unfavorable.*

2.3.2.3 Criminality in the Course of Personality Maturation

In criminality in the course of personality maturation, there are only certain *temporary* kinds of conspicuousness in the **longitudinal section,** which can be relatively easily delimited as "development specific".

Moreover, the corresponding conspicuousness does not concern all social spheres, but only *some* of them: It occurs mainly in the *sphere of leisure* and is to a large degree *limited* to this sphere. *Requirements in the sphere of performance are mainly still met,* or there have only been irregularities at the most for a short time during the period in which the offense was committed. There is no conspicuousness in the sphere of abode, and strong contacts and ties with the family are kept up to a certain extent. Despite a corresponding leisure organization and partially considerable conspicuousness in this social sphere - often together with a group of friends who are similarly conspicuous - the subject rarely turns to the criminality-prone "milieu." Nonetheless, in connection with corresponding contacts and alcohol or drug consumption in particular, the subject's specific leisure behavior leads to the situations out of which offenses are committed.

Thus, there is no criminovalent constellation in the **cross section** but no criminoresistant one either. Insofar as any *O-criteria* occur, they appear as a product of this phase of maturation and development and usually occur for a short time only. Frequently, there are more or less pronounced G-criteria during the period preceding the offense.

During this *phase of partial social conspicuousness,* therefore, the subject's life pattern is contradictory and disharmonious from a criminological point of view. This can be expressed to a certain extent by a discrepancy and possibly even contrary orientation in the **patterns of relevance** on the one hand and the **value orientation** on the other. However, it is difficult to recognize the patterns of relevance at all for a subject with such a development. At this age, temporary preferences and intentions which come more from outside, e.g., from certain contact persons and the subject's general company, can become dominant for a certain time; they can even appear "artificial." Often, the orientation of leisure toward a certain group of acquaintances becomes so relevant that the patterns of relevance which used to be important are (temporarily) supplanted. In contrast, the value orientation - which is often still largely unconsolidated and also open to influences from outside, according to the age of the subject - often tends more toward an inconspicuous social life even during the period of increased social conspicuousness.

The commission of *offenses* is also frequently closely connected with the subject's group of acquaintances and their organization of leisure: Offenses are often committed jointly without any detailed planning and purposefulness. Individually, however, the subjects would probably never have committed the offenses. The subjects' delinquency can include serious offenses or whole series of offenses, which occur only under the influence of the group or certain members of the group. Insofar as a subject commits an offense alone, he simply seizes good opportunities (e.g., for an offense against property). Occasionally, the loot is not even used but hoarded somewhere for no apparent purpose or thrown away carelessly. The offenses can also express a certain pleasure in disturbing, annoying, or sometimes destroying; equally, unchecked affects and aimless aggression tendencies, e.g., anger and annoyance because of an argument, can lead to an offense, e.g., damage to property or bodily injury.

In view of the characteristic forms of social behavior and delinquency, puberty is basically the period during which offenses are committed "in the course of personality maturation." As a rule, it can be assumed that the phase of puberty is completed toward the end of one's teens. Yet, on occasion, a development can occur at the beginning or in the middle of one's twenties which is comparable to criminality in the course of personality maturation and appears as a *variant shifted in time*. Apart from age, there are no differences between the original and the variant. After a period of partial social conspicuousness, particularly in the sphere of leisure, during which delinquency occurs, the subject returns to his earlier socially inconspicuous life pattern.

The **further course** of criminality in the course of personality maturation is *generally favorable*. The shock of having committed an offense, the impression made by sanctions and other effects of offenses, the consolidation of the subject's system of values, or the completion of the biological phase of maturation lead the subject to deal with his conspicuousness and offenses. Consequently, the conspicuousness and offenses disappear completely (and often all of a sudden). The following social (re)integration of the subject picks up the thread of his earlier inconspicuous life pattern - occasionally with changes corresponding to the phase of life he has reached.

Yet, in criminality in the course of personality maturation, the subject's *further development can also be unfavorable*. Whether development is unfavorable depends decisively on how one manages to see the subject through the phase of maturation, which obviously involves an acute danger of criminality. It is usually not advisable to attempt this by imposing a prison sentence (for juveniles). Particularly for subjects who have never become conspicuous before this phase of maturation, tendencies toward socially conspicuous behavior are often reinforced by a stay in prison and by the influence of fellow prisoners (who are often older). Furthermore, there is the danger of the subject establishing corresponding contacts (and exchanging addresses) in prison. Consequently, when the subject has problems after being released from prison, he visits these "buddies" (or they him) and then runs into difficulties again. In this respect as well, the subjects differ from subjects of their age with a continuous development toward criminality, who usually live in an entirely different social environment.

Occasionally, the social conspicuousness and criminality which initially appears as a criminality in the course of personality maturation turns into a development toward criminality. Such a **further development toward criminality** is usually announced by the onset of serious conspicuousness in the sphere of performance. Instead of the initially minor neglect of this sphere, which the subject was aware of, which he felt embarrassed about, and which was a burden to him, the subject becomes increasingly indifferent to the requirements of normal working life. Gradually, there is a considerable neglect of the sphere of performance, which leads to the subject losing his job and to a total disorder in the course of his days. At this point at the latest, there is a marked *criminovalent constellation*. Although such a development does not always take place dramatically, but frequently rather slowly, it can usually be recognized easily with some experience. Consequently, in some cases, it is possible to stop the development by intervening resolutely.

2.3.2.4 Criminality Despite No Other Social Conspicuousness

In criminality despite no other social conspicuousness, there is *none of the considerable conspicuousness* in the **longitudinal section** which is characteristic of the developments presented above and which points to criminality or causes it to be expected in the future.

In the **cross section,** there is no criminovalent constellation. At best, there is one or the other *O-criterion*. Frequently, however, there are several *G-criteria* or even a *criminoresistant constellation*. Therefore, these aspects of the Criminological Triad are not very informative.

Yet the offense, as opposed to the offense in "criminality as a sudden event" (see Sect. 2.3.2.5 below), is not an entirely extraordinary event in the continuity of life of the offender. The (occasional) moving in a certain borderland of criminality in part of his life, particularly in connection with his work, belongs to the normal conduct of life of the offender. This indicates that there are certain **patterns of relevance** relating, for instance, to economic success, a high standard of living, or one's own business (or its continued existence), etc., as well as a one-sided orientation to entirely predominant **values** which distinguish the offender from nonoffenders: For example, there can be unscrupulous striving for power and profit, excessive careerism, or heedless selfishness - which is often only related to the corresponding partial sphere - connected with a lack of binding, socially sound measures of values, e.g., correct business dealings with third persons, honesty in contacts with business partners and colleagues, etc. The decisive characteristic, therefore, is that certain *values* which are also valid in the general population *are emphasized in a one-sided way and pursued unrestrictedly* without being controlled by other values. In order to realize these values and patterns of relevance, which dominate everything else (in connection with the corresponding personality traits - concerning "unscrupulous personalities", see GÖPPINGER 1980, p. 209ff.), the possibility of violating a law even seriously is accepted. Even if the advantages expected to be gained by committing the offenses are not planned in all detail, they are usually directly intended. To this extent, the *offense* is connected with the subject's way of life in an "instrumentally rational" way.

Characteristically, the subjects attempt to make more of opportunities than they can if they act honestly. This includes certain irregularities in connection with occupation, e.g., billing too many hours of work, billing old exchanged parts as new ones, or even risky business ventures, which can lead into the field of white-collar crime.

The ubiquitous petty offenses (e.g., shop-lifting, evasion of entrance fees, avoiding payment on public transportation) or (minor) customs and tax offenses are also frequently committed out of a life pattern containing no social conspicuousness in the sense of the criteria elaborated here. Such offenses often go together with a value attitude which considers the violation of law a "peccadillo" and "plays down" the damage and thus the degree of injustice of the offense by pointing out the wealth or anonymity of the victim (department stores, government).

Finally, this category also includes the offenders who occasionally commit only bodily injury (with intent). As a rule, they exhibit no conspicuousness in the spheres of performance, leisure or contacts. In the situations leading to violent arguments, they occasionally demonstrate behavior which suggests the frequently rather direct way persons going through puberty solve conflicts. Thus, these offenders differ from the above offenders in their patterns of relevance and their value orientation.

As a whole, therefore, this category includes a broad spectrum of offenses ranging from petty offenses, profit offenses, white-collar crime, offenses against the environment up to corruption in public life on the one hand and certain cases of bodily injury on the other.

After committing the offense, the offender generally remains socially inconspicuous in the **further course** of his life. However, a prolonged stay in prison can destroy his social integration and thrust him into a marginal social position.

The question of *further offenses* must be separated from further *social* inconspicuousness for this category in particular. As the offenses are usually committed out of a one-sided orientation to individual values and patterns of relevance, the *prognosis* is not uniform and depends on the individual case and the kind of offense: For some offenders, the fact that the offense has been discovered, the imposition of a sanction, or other social effects (e.g., the damage to the subject's reputation among acquaintances, business partners, or colleagues) can prevent further offenses. Other offenders - entirely unimpressed by the above - continue moving in the borderland of criminality, either because they (and their environment) still regard certain offenses as "peccadillos" or because they are not willing to give up or push back the one-sided values and patterns of relevance which led to the offense.

2.3.2.5 Criminality as a Sudden Event

In criminality as a sudden event as an (ideal-typical) extreme case, it can be assumed that there are no indications or tendencies in a subject's social development and conduct of life in the **longitudinal section** which can be related to criminality. Thus, generally, the subject is to a large degree socially inconspicuous or completely *socially integrated.* This does not mean that there was no conspicuousness at all in the past; however, it cannot be related directly to the current offense (for details, see Part III, Sect. 4.4.4).

The "break" which the offense constitutes in the life of the offender becomes apparent in particular in the **cross section:** It is marked by G-criteria, and there can even be a criminoresistant constellation.

The subject's **patterns of relevance** and his **value orientation** also show him to be a socially integrated person for whom the (serious) violation of a law is basically not to be expected.

The **further development** and *prognosis* are normally favorable: The offense or its consequences constitute a break in the continuity of the offender's social life; apart from the one-time (possibly serious) offense, the offender with criminality as a sudden event is and remains socially inconspicuous. The legal punishment of the offense or other consequences and effects of the commission of the offense, however, can tear the offender out of his social integration. But even after long-term sentences in prison, such offenders largely remain resistant to "negative" influences and also differ from the majority of prisoners in their behavior in prison. Similarly, after being released from prison, they cope with the difficulties and problems of social reintegration and find their way back.

2.3.3 "Special Aspects" in the Life of the Offender, Particularly in View of Prognosis and Interventions

The first part of the criminological diagnosis, the assessment on the basis of the criteria of reference of the Criminological Triad, is supplemented by considerations concerning those aspects in an offender's life which characterize him in a particular way in the context of his social relationships and, in part, point to his criminologically relevant "weak" and "strong points." In the individual case, these "*special aspects*" differentiate or modify within narrow limits the prognosis given by the classification on the basis of the criteria of reference of the Criminological Triad (see Sect. 2.4.1 below). Above all, however, they provide indications for promising interventions and treatment (see Sect. 2.4.2 below).

The points of view covered by the "special aspects" have already crystallized in the criminological analysis or assessment on the basis of the criteria of reference of the Criminological Triad. Yet not all particularities which are of considerable importance in the everyday life of an offender have necessarily entered this comparison, in some cases because they were of no importance for the classification according to the criteria of reference of the Criminological Triad. Therefore, it is necessary to review the life of the offender from a criminological perspective and to extract the points which characterize him and his behavior in everyday life in particular (with some experience, these points can often be recognized in the course of the investigations). In the same way, it must be examined whether it is possible to extract certain (possibly recurring) situations and phases - in the sense of special social conspicuousness and criminality or special social adaptation, or in the sense of conflict situations (and coping with these situations) or situations where decisive "switches" were shifted.

These "special aspects" differ from subject to subject precisely because they are related to individual behavior. Consequently, they cannot be concretized in detail with respect to their content (for examples, see Case A., Appendix, Sect. 4.2). Only some indications are provided to show which points of view come into consideration.

In the following, the "special aspects" are divided into "internal" and "external" aspects. "Internal" aspects are the points which relate more to the offender, "external" aspects the points which relate more to his social environment. In no way does this mean that these aspects are to be regarded as causes, particularly since, in this respect, it is impossible to distinguish between "cause" and "effect." Important is the purely pragmatic consideration *whether the interventions should affect* the subject or his environment or both.

The **"internal aspects"** become apparent, for example, in *recurring behavior patterns and reactions* which have been determined in the longitudinal section, in the *criteria* which have become apparent in the cross section analysis, in the special weight of one or the other *pattern of relevance,* and in the effects of the *value orientation* and the *attitudes* which become apparent in the value orientation, but also in the subject's *overall orientation in life.*

Examples are a paradoxical expectation of adaptation, a low tolerance for stress and a lack of endurance, which have repeatedly led to conflicts at work; an inadequately high level of aspirations, which is closely related to the commission of offenses against property; a demand to be free from any ties, which characterizes the subject's behavior in all social spheres; a one-sided emphasis on certain values, which sooner or later, leads to offenses; a short perspective in time, "living in the immediate present," being suggestible and easy to tempt, etc. - or the fact that the values determined are basically oriented toward a socially inconspicuous life, that there is a marked willingness to bear responsibility, a long-term differentiated plan for life with definite aims, etc.

The life of the offender and his behavior can (also) be marked by certain "**external aspects**," such as the *nature of his environment* (e.g., his attachment to the "asocial" "milieu" from childhood to the present - or the "integration" in a socially integrated family which the subject finds support in), *certain contacts* (e.g., a peer group of particular importance for the subject recently), or a *certain person of reference* (e.g., a person of authority whom the subject obeys and to whom he submits himself), as well as considerable debts to be paid, a handicap due to a physical impairment, or the necessity to support siblings under age or parents in need of care, etc.

Important in the "special aspects" is, on the one hand, to what extent these points of the past and present *can also take effect in the future*. On the other hand, it must be examined whether, and if so, to what extent and with which measures, these aspects can usually be *changed:* Considering the "internal aspects," to which degree must certain behavior patterns, reactions, attitudes, etc., which have been decisive in a criminological respect and thus mainly for social conspicuousness (and subsequently criminality), be reckoned with in the future? Similarly, for the "external aspects," it must be considered to what extent the offender is still exposed to situations, which, for example, triggered or reinforced certain reactions leading to criminality, and whether or to what degree these aspects can be changed.

It is no less important to examine which of the "internal" and "external aspects" have had a particularly stabilizing effect and to what extent they can be reckoned with in the future - with the consequence that precisely these aspects must be used in a purposive "therapeutic" respect (in the widest sense). Basically, it can be assumed that the "external aspects" are not as persistent as the "internal" ones, which are usually closely related to the personality of the offender (for details, see Sect. 2.4.2 below).

Additionally, it is useful to consider what was of *no importance* in the life of a subject or in his orientation in life, in order to obtain a differentiated overall criminological picture of the offender with regard to prognosis and interventions. This covers, on the one hand, points which are normally the foundation of an inconspicuous, integrated social life in the community (e.g., regular, continued work, a somewhat structured course of a day), but which do not agree with the interests and intentions of the subject or which he has neglected and "bypassed" more or less consciously. On the other hand, points of view may *not* have been *relevant* to him which, for example, characterize a life with particularly marked social conspicuousness (for instance the conspicuousness typical of a continuous development toward criminality). Important indications of what has been **"non-relevant"** - in the form of a "counterexamination" - are the O- and G-criteria of the cross section analysis which obviously do *not* occur for the subject concerned.

The **result** of the examination of the "special aspects" of an individual case consists of a series of aspects which show specific "weak" and "strong points" of the offender. These are of some importance for prognosis and of considerable importance for possible interventions and therapeutic efforts.

2.3.4 The Offender in the Context of His Social Relationships During Imprisonment

The criminological diagnosis presented up to this point normally relates to the time a subject committed his last offense (see Sect. 2.2 above). If the subject was imprisoned in the meantime, however, this may have been years ago. Therefore, for an *up-to-date* assessment of the offender in the context of his social relationships, it may be necessary to take into account his further development during imprisonment as well. It must be examined whether there have been any *fundamental changes* - under consideration of the particularities of imprisonment - in the subject's behavior structure and his orientation in life during imprisonment. It is of particular importance to observe the further development of the criminologically relevant "weak" and "strong points" which characterized the subject's earlier life in freedom (see Sect. 2.3.3 above).

Such changes take time - in imprisonment as in freedom. It is usually impossible to speak of fundamental changes during imprisonment unless a change in behavior has lasted for several years. Therefore, a separate examination of the offender in the context of his social relationships during imprisonment is necessary, in particular for prisoners who have spent several years in prison; these offenders - because of the normal processes of maturation or aging, possibly also because of certain changes in personality - are most likely to demonstrate corresponding changes in their behavior and their orientation in life which can be of importance in their everyday life after being released. In contrast, such changes are unlikely during short-term imprisonment, lasting only a few months, for example.

The points of view in the *assessment* of behavior during imprisonment are similar (in a formal respect) to those in the analysis of behavior in freedom - adapted to the special situation of imprisonment. For example, the *analysis* of behavior during imprisonment *in the longitudinal section* cannot simply be related directly to the contrasting presentation of the O- and the G-ideal-typical behavior in freedom (see Part III, Sect. 2.2); yet it provides important *indications* for estimating behavior during imprisonment and for recognizing changes in one of the directions - against the background of the subject's behavior in freedom.

Despite differing *external* conditions at work, *behavior at work* and *attitude toward work* show as broad a spectrum during imprisonment as that in freedom: At one end, there are the prisoners who "shirk" work by staying away from work on the pretext of being ill and by continuously applying for transfers, who generally seize any opportunity to stay away from work, and who usually perform poorly at work. At the other end, there are the prisoners who work intensively, meet requirements, or are even interested in their work, as monotonous as it appears to them in the beginning.

The special nature of imprisonment precludes pronounced O-specific leisure behavior. Nevertheless, the differences in *leisure behavior* during imprisonment are quite impressive: Some prisoners simply kill time, while others try to use their time in a meaningful and productive way by setting themselves certain tasks within the framework of the possibilities available. Yet, in assessing leisure behavior during imprisonment, one ought not to be tempted to conclude that a subject has fundamentally changed his orientation because he demonstrates - a frequently only superficial - commitment (which is entirely irrelevant for life in freedom). This apparent commitment and interest are frequently due only to the fact that such leisure activities are immediately available in the institution. Often, the subject's participation in structured or productive activities which impose certain demands on him also depend on the extent to which other less demanding, more distracting leisure activities are available.

Although the *sphere of contacts* is also marked by the special situation of imprisonment in many respects, there are parallels with behavior in freedom. Contacts in the institution, i.e., those with fellow prisoners and with the staff of the institution, as well as those with the outside world, offer a broad spectrum: They can be purely utilitarian ones, for example, or strong ones, which can be of considerable importance for a socially inconspicuous and noncriminal life after being released.

Finally, the way the subject *prepares for his release* and what *plans he makes for the future* are also particularly revealing. Some prisoners prepare themselves in a useful way: They try to find a stable job and an ordered place to live, establish strong ties to other persons, etc. Others do not prepare for their release in any specific way. These subjects usually want to "recuperate" from being imprisoned and enjoy unrestrainedly their freedom among their old "buddies" and women in the familiar "milieu."

It is usually relatively easy to recognize the *tendencies* of a subject toward one or the other direction during imprisonment by analyzing his further behavior in the various social spheres differentiatedly. At the same time, insights are obtained regarding the extent to which the behavior of the subject during imprisonment and his earlier behavior and way of life in freedom square, and what has changed. Apart from this analysis, it is also useful to examine the earlier **internal (and external) aspects:** Individual attitudes and tendencies previously reflected in certain O- or G-criteria can also be expressed during imprisonment in modified form. A comparison of the **patterns of relevance** and the **value orientation** before and during imprisonment can also help to complete the overall picture of the offender in the context of his social relationships during imprisonment. Yet, particularly in this respect, the limitations posed by imprisonment leave the subject only a relatively small scope to develop freely.

The **result** of the analysis of behavior during imprisonment is usually an assessment of whether there have been considerable changes in an offender's orientation in life *as compared with his earlier behavior in freedom,* of which problematic points have subsided and which have not, and of which new problems have developed - under consideration of the modifications that are due to the situation of imprisonment. For a *final assessment,* however, the subject's *previous extramural behavior* must be *emphasized.*

If, on the basis of any changes, *conclusions* are to be reached with regard to later behavior in freedom, it is advisable to refer back to *earlier terms of imprisonment* (in particular when the conclusions are particularly "positive"). Often enough, it appears that a subject demonstrated "positive" changes similar to those during his current imprisonment and that these changes had practically no effects in view of social (and criminal) inconspicuousness after he was released. In such cases, the current changes should be viewed somewhat skeptically: Often, the prisoners who have been imprisoned frequently or for a long period adapt particularly well to the situation of imprisonment and are able to behave correspondingly inconspicuously or in accordance with house rules without changing their later behavior in freedom. They also know which explanations go over well with experts or judges. These are frequently also the offenders who have no resistance at all to *any* influences and who let themselves be "tempted" by other people and situations, in as well as out of prison.

2.4 Conclusions

2.4.1 Prognosis

The criminological diagnosis of the offender in the context of his social relationships lays the foundation for *prognostic conclusions,* into which all criminologically relevant particularities and nuances of the individual case enter. This diagnosis offers the possibility of making a prognosis tailored to the individual offender and thus of creating the basis for corresponding legal decisions. In contrast to these categorical decisions, however, the criminological prognosis is only a probability statement; there is no absolute certainty in forecasting future behavior or developments.

For the prognosis, one first assesses criminologically the offender in the context of his social relationships as he currently is. Then one considers what his further development may be like from a criminological perspective, or how he may behave in the future with respect to recidivism. The *individual prognostic statement* is the result of three steps - which must be kept apart mentally - but which *overlap in fact:*

First step: Starting point is the "general" prognosis, i.e., the prognosis which is "typical" for the category to which the subject was assigned.

Second step: The deviations of the specific behavior of the subject from the characteristic forms of the corresponding category lead to the "individual basic prognosis."

Third step: The probable effects of (future) measures and other reactions lead to the "treatment" or "intervention prognosis."

Assigning a subject to one of the categories of the position of the offense in the longitudinal section of life on the basis of the Criminological Triad - **as the first step** - implies a **"general prognosis."** This is a consequence of the development expected in the individual category (for details see Sect. 2.3.2 above).

For example, if a 24-year-old subject demonstrates a continuous development toward criminality and a criminovalent constellation which has been present for some time, as well as patterns of relevance and a value orientation matching his life pattern, the result of assigning the subject's specific development to the category "continuous development toward criminality beginning during early youth" is a "general prognosis," which in this case is always unfavorable (see Sect. 2.3.2.1 above).

In the **second step,** which includes the examination of the particularities of the individual case, a differentiation is made which leads either to the "general prognosis" being confirmed - the usual case - or to its being modified within certain limits. The major indications for the **"individual basic prognosis"** are mainly the deviations of the individual case from the characteristic forms of the category the subject was assigned to and the "special aspects"; they contain the criminologically relevant "weak" and "strong points" of the offender and also point to the special external circumstances which are of importance in the prognosis for this specific offender (see Sect. 2.3.3 above and Case A., Appendix, Sect. 5)

As a rule, however, it is *practically impossible* for a "general prognosis," particularly an unfavorable one, to be *decisively changed* on the basis of certain deviations from the corresponding category or individual "internal" or "external aspects." The changes can concern only nuances, which, however, must be given special attention, particularly as regards specific interventions (see Sect. 2.4.2 below).

This second step, i.e., the consideration of the particularities of the individual case within the framework of the individual basic prognosis, is of *fundamental importance* whenever the "general prognosis" remains unclear because it is impossible to assign a subject to a certain category with some certainty. In these cases especially, the "internal" and "external aspects" can provide important indications of criminologically relevant relationships between general social behavior, certain attitudes, values, etc. and the offense, and thus allow individual conclusions for the prognosis.

Thus, a diagnosis on the basis of the Criminological Triad can remain open as to whether a subject exhibits criminality in the course of personality maturation (shifted in time) or - in view of considerable conspicuousness in the sphere of performance - a beginning development toward criminality. If so, the deviations of the individual case from the two categories and the "special aspects" usually enable one to make a differentiated prognosis, which - also without unambiguously assigning the case to one of the two categories - shows the essential points where interventions are necessary and possible (see Sect. 2.4.2 below).

The second step is of similar importance when the diagnosis indicates *criminality despite no other social conspicuousness.* This category allows for *no* clear "general prognosis" (see Sect. 2.3.2.4 above). Particularly in this context, the weighting of the "special aspects" in view of the commission of the earlier offenses usually allows individual prognostic conclusions.

Finally, besides the consideration of the particularities of the individual case, the importance of the individual basic prognosis also lies in statements on the *kind of offenses to be expected* for the individual.

For each prognosis, future developments and changes must also be taken into account in the diagnosis; in principle, a (criminological) prognosis can never simply be unchanging and static. Particularly in *legal practice,* therefore, the *effects* which the authorities' reaction or the measures taken within the framework of this reaction can have must be incorporated into the diagnosis in the **third step.** These have an influence on the prognosis and can even modify it. Such a *change of the prognosis by specific interventions* is exactly the aim of certain measures and forms of punishment. Therefore, a "recidivism prognosis" cannot be made without regard for a "treatment prognosis" or an **"intervention prognosis."** Thus, for example, it is possible to reduce the danger of recidivism decisively and improve the prognosis correspondingly by issuing an appropriate order in connection with probation or parole. The aim of the criminological assessment is precisely to contribute to the task of finding the reaction in the framework of the legal possibilities which is most likely to reduce the risk of recidivism (see Sect. 2.4 below and Case A., Appendix, Sect. 5).

Such specific effects must be distinguished strictly from the more or less unintended, incidental effects which the police interrogation, trial, or conviction, etc. may have. Even if no formal punishment or measures are imposed, a subject and his behavior can be affected, particularly where a subject who has never been in court before is concerned. Besides, the commission of an offense can affect him in other ways, for example through the reactions of his social environment.

2.4.2 Interventions (and Treatment)

The criminological diagnosis allows more than a mere prognosis. It also offers *specific indications for - specifically criminologically indicated - interventions.*

On the basis of the criminological diagnosis, **social workers,** for example in their work with juveniles, in the probation service, as juvenile court assistants, or within the framework of their activities in prisons, are able to recognize the criminologically relevant "weak points" of an offender and can try to influence them specifically. Moreover, such considerations are also important in **legal practice,** for example when a judge has to decide whether an intervention of some kind is necessary or useful to achieve a preventive effect.

Insofar as interventions are necessary and useful, one must basically attempt to **overcome or steer in a socially sound direction the behavior patterns and the underlying patterns of relevance and attitudes which tended to be conducive to criminality.** As the criminological diagnosis shows not only an offender's difficulties and problems, but also his "strong" points, it is frequently possible to tackle his criminologically relevant "weak" ones by supporting his behavior patterns which tend more toward social inconspicuousness.

The starting point for any kind of intervention is the current life pattern of the subject as shown by the criminological examination. Important indications are provided in particular by the "special aspects": They show which recurring behavior patterns must be given special attention and which situations which were still open to various developments or which difficulties led the subject to swerve from the social order and thus, ultimately, to commit an offense ("internal aspects" -

see Sect. 2.3.3 above). At the same time, they also point to possible influences on the subject from outside ("external aspects" - see Sect. 2.3.3 above).

Some "external" and - to a lesser degree - "internal aspects" can be countered to a certain extent, possibly even changed. Others must, at least in the short run, be accepted as unchanging. For example, the criminological effects of a pattern of relevance which only reflects certain interests can be influenced by shifting these interests to another area (see Sect. 2.2.3.1 above). Equally, certain behavior patterns can be modified: Budgeting, for example, can be practiced; a paradoxical expectation of adaptation can be tackled inside certain limits; a neglect of the sphere of performance by unexcused absences, nonemployment, etc. can be influenced by corresponding efforts. "Internal aspects," in contrast, which express basic determining intentions, are practically impossible to change fundamentally with the limited means available, for example, in probation service or traditional imprisonment. Characteristics such as restlessness and a permanent need for activity, the need to play a central role and to have a "reputation," etc. can be guided into a socially sound direction, for example by the subject taking up an occupational activity which matches these characteristics. Yet a fundamental change is only rarely possible with the limited means of legal practice in the widest sense: This is also true for certain values and attitudes (e.g., the scrupulousness with which a subject pursues individual aims without any consideration for others).

There are similar differences for the "external aspects." On the one hand, a subject's environment with its particularities and rules must be accepted as given: For example, as difficult as it can be for a subject to adapt and to cope with difficult situations, one must start from the fact that any kind of job basically requires a certain degree of adaptation and the ability to cope with difficulties with superiors and fellow employees. Consequently, one has to start with the subject and practice the necessary abilities for these external circumstances. On the other hand, it can be useful, for example, to take a juvenile out of the strained, no longer sound situation in his family of orientation and thus to change his environment.

Of great importance for such interventions are the "strong points" of the subject, which must be used skillfully. For example, for a juvenile subject who remained socially inconspicuous as long as he found support and guidance in the authority of a certain person of reference, it can be useful to find a corresponding environment and person of reference again.

Basically, in the consideration of future interventions, one should always check the subject's past to see whether there were *essential changes* in *one* social sphere (both in the direction of social conspicuousness and marked social adaptation) at some time and then to examine what changed in the *remaining* social spheres (at the same time or immediately before) and whether this may be related to the changes determined first. It is frequently possible to find parallels with other changes during an entire phase of life and thus valuable indications for future interventions.

There is a *broad spectrum of sanctions and differentiated reactions* for such specific interventions in **legal practice.** However, for many reasons, one does not always take full advantage of these possibilities. Particularly important are *mea-*

sures which relate to life in freedom. From a criminological perspective, interventions relating to extramural behavior seem most useful and should therefore be emphasized: The subject must first and foremost prove himself in everyday life in freedom. This does not mean that imprisonment cannot be used for interventions in the sense of *training* or even be the occasion for a *therapy* (see below). For example, social training during imprisonment occasionally allows the taking of first steps toward changes in freedom. A *treatment* in the strict sense is out of the question for the majority of subjects, because of the limited possibilities of treatment in imprisonment.

From a criminological perspective, general *corrective measures for juvenile delinquents,* as well as the various ambulant measures among the manifold *possibilities of sentencing and punishment* according to (juvenile) criminal law, provide a large scope for useful interventions. On probation or parole, the threat of a prison sentence being executed puts a certain pressure on the subject to follow the order. (Another, altogether different problem is the lack of time in practice to devote oneself to the subject and to supervise him appropriately. This particular problem could be solved to a certain degree by using the available capacity more economically by concentrating on the subjects for whom it appears especially useful from a criminological perspective.)

The judge's selection of such measures, and their most effective application through individual instructions and aids, naturally depends on the special nature of the individual case, which becomes apparent in the criminological diagnosis. Nonetheless, it is possible - starting from the various positions of the offense or delinquency in the life of an offender (see Sect. 2.3.2 above) - to provide rough *indications.*

In practice, one will initially concentrate on offenders who commit **offenses in the course of personality maturation.** Here, in particular, a differentiated diagnosis can show which subjects do not require any intervention and for which subjects an intervention is decisive for whether their delinquency will remain temporary or whether it will continue (see Sect. 2.3.2.3 above). Correspondingly, one will attempt to guide the subject through the phase which obviously poses a greater danger of criminality by individual supportive measures. In particular, one must avoid a neglect of the sphere of performance; any existing tendencies toward and beginnings of O-ideal-typical behavior must be tackled. Further efforts must be concentrated on providing for a certain structure in leisure or maintaining any existing structure and, if necessary, breaking off any contacts with persons who harbor a danger of criminality, in particular "milieu" contacts.

In such developments, *ambulant measures* which do not go together with a prolonged imprisonment and do not tear the subject out of his social integration are particularly appropriate. Moreover, the execution of a prison sentence (for juveniles) is not advisable, because the subject runs the risk of developing closer contacts with persons from the "milieu," who could have a correspondingly negative effect on him.

Also at the **beginning of a continuous development toward criminality beginning during early youth** (see Sect. 2.3.2.1 above) and - possibly - at the **beginning of a**

development toward criminality beginning during adolescence or the early years of adulthood (see Sect. 2.3.2.2 above), it is possible to exert a certain influence on the expected further course, particularly when a subject still demonstrates a somewhat structured course of a day. For these subjects, it is important to keep an eye on practically all social spheres, though the intervention will generally have to concentrate on creating a firm order in the spheres of performance and abode. Ambulant interventions are often sufficient, providing their fulfillment can be adequately monitored. A more comprehensive intervention can also be indicated in the form of a stay in a reform school, committal to a foster family, or - in exceptional cases - a prison sentence (for juveniles), especially when adequate supervision by the family of orientation or another person cannot be guaranteed (thus, when there are unfavorable "external aspects" in this respect which cannot be changed in any other way).

A further emphasis for such interventions lies with the subjects who have showed prolonged marked tendencies toward O-ideal-typical behavior in connection with repeated offenses and stays in prison and could thus put an end to their "criminal careers." Here, a differentiated criminological analysis can provide indications, possibly of minor changes during the recent past, which should be encouraged if the subject shows clearly by his own efforts that he wishes to change his life-style.

Yet one must be aware that it is practically impossible to put a final end to a prolonged criminal career *at once*. Even for a subject who makes a serious effort to lead a socially inconspicuous life there is no guarantee of success. Usually, he commits a - usually relatively minor - offense after an unusually long period without offenses - as compared with his previous situation. If the court considers this recidivism aggravating and imposes a prison sentence without probation, the subject's previous efforts usually collapse entirely and he is certain to continue his criminal career. In contrast, examples from our own experience have shown that the subjects managed not to commit any more offenses under the influence of the probation officer despite the new offense - providing it was punished with a prison sentence suspended on probation - and to gain a foothold in occupational life with a good social integration.

In contrast to the aforementioned groups, the starting points for promising interventions for subjects whose delinquency must be considered **criminality despite no other social conspicuousness** (see Sect. 2.3.2.4 above) do not lie in their general social behavior, which is mainly inconspicuous, but in certain patterns of relevance, in their value orientation or "internal" and "external aspects." The social disapproval expressed in punishment as such or the illustration of the social and legal risks of the punishment of their incorrect behavior can suffice to cause corresponding changes. This is not so for the small group of offenders who commit exclusively bodily injury: Here, behavior modification is generally indicated and certainly promising.

Subjects who demonstrate **criminality as a sudden event** (see Sect. 2.3.2.5 above) are socially integrated; any intervention aimed at their social behavior is superfluous. Here, it can even be necessary to prevent social disintegration which can occur through the consequences of the offense or the legal sanctions.

Interventions aimed at the life-style of an offender, insofar as they are possible within the framework of probation service, supervision of conduct, or traditional methods of imprisonment, however, can be successful only if the patterns of relevance and the value orientation of the individual subjects favor a socially inconspicuous life or are at least not opposed to such a life. These interventions are usually of *no assistance* in connection with recidivist offenders who demonstrate a **prolonged (continuous) development toward criminality** and have been imprisoned *repeatedly and for many years* without showing any indications of changing their life-style. Here, the possibilities of intervention end for those without psychological or psychiatric training.

A criminological examination and a differentiated criminological diagnosis are also absolutely necessary for psychologists or persons with corresponding basic psychological training *to conduct correctly a therapy* aimed at *changing* a subject *fundamentally*. Any treatment which goes beyond mere behavior modification is arduous, because the subjects frequently lack the immediate pressure of suffering, which is essential for any therapy. The socially conspicuous life-style and corresponding patterns of relevance are not a burden to the subject but usually correspond to his intentions. At the most, the subject feels his occasional imprisonment to be an adversity. However, he seldom relates imprisonment to his life pattern. Changes in the subject's way of living and a new outlook on life usually mean great sacrifices and privations and are therefore not at all desired.

A therapy for offenders who have been socially conspicuous for a prolonged period can therefore be successful at best with respect to long-term possibilities of intervention. For this purpose, the entire repertoire of *treatment and therapy in psychology* must be utilized. It is always *necessary* to make a *criminological diagnosis as well* to show systematically the specific criminological points of view and problematic areas in an individual case.

That therapeutic efforts have had limited success with offenders to date is not least due to the fact that, to treat recidivist offenders, therapists have used methods which were developed in psychology or psychotherapy with persons who were *not* (recidivist) offenders and which therefore largely disregard specifically criminological problematic areas and aspects. Thus, elaborating specific useful methods of intervention and treatment and delimiting them - under consideration of the knowledge of Applied Criminology - is a new field of activity of great practical importance. This refers mainly to the sciences related to criminology, especially psychology.

3 General Explanations on the Presentation of a Criminological Assessment

In everyday legal practice, the investigations and the assessment are usually *not* recorded differentiatedly. However, recording the investigations and the assessment remains necessary until sound experience in using the instruments of Applied Criminology has been acquired. Moreover, in practice, the investigations or the criminological assessment are recorded in writing whenever, as is common, the findings are passed on to others.

In a written procedure, especially in the preparation of a **criminological expertise,** the following *pattern of investigation and assessment* (see below) has proved successful. It takes into account the fact that the individual social spheres of the subject are first examined separately in the criminological analysis.

To facilitate orientation, it is advisable to have a short, possibly tabular *survey of personal record* of about one page precede the written assessment.

In the presentation of the *investigations,* the entire information from all sources is summarized and handled under the title "*Information from the Records and Direct Investigations*" (see Case A., Appendix, Sect. 2). In principle, all information and facts which are of importance for a criminological assessment are taken into consideration. On the basis of this information, it must be possible for anyone who is familiar with the criteria of analysis and diagnosis to obtain a picture of the subject and thus to duplicate the assessment of the expertise. It is considerably easier to make an assessment when the relevant facts and other information of the corresponding sphere are assigned when recording the investigations. As certain facts can be relevant in more than one sphere, a certain amount of repetition is inevitable. However, this can usually be circumvented by using cross-references.

Written recording of the investigations according to systematic points of view of order also serves as a means of *self-supervision,* in particular if a subject shows an eventful life history. Furthermore, a written record - even if it comprises only a short sketch or key words - offers some protection against neglecting an important point or even an entire social sphere in the exploration.

The entire account of the investigations should always be a purely descriptive "statement of facts" *without* any value judgment and *without* any interpretation. It would be a fundamental error to incorporate any (premature) opinion or any other kind of comment which should be expressed in the analysis and diagnosis alone (see also Sects. 2.1 and 2.1.1 above).

The presentation of the *criminological analysis and diagnosis* is oriented to the actual procedure as described above (see Sects. 2.2 and 2.3 above). The *conclusions* in view of prognosis and intervention follow from the criminological diagnosis, in particular from the presentation of the "special aspects," which again lead to answers to the questions to be covered in the expertise.

In the criminological assessment of persons who have been *imprisoned* for a long period at the time of the assessment (i.e., as a rule for several years), it is advisable to *divide* the criminological diagnosis into two parts (see below): First -

as in the usual procedure - a diagnostic assessment of the (previous) behavior of the subject *in freedom up to the last offense* or up to imprisonment is made on the basis of the criteria of reference of the criminological triad. Subsequently, the offender's behavior *during imprisonment* in the various social spheres is analyzed and *compared* with or contrasted to his behavior *in freedom*. Previous and current patterns of relevance and value orientation are also compared. On the basis of this contrasting examination, the *current "special aspects"* in the life of the offender can be estimated.

Survey

The assessment of the offender in the context of his social relationships according to the comparative analysis of individual cases based on ideal types

	See (Part, Sect.)
I Survey of Personal Record	
II Information from the Records and Direct Investigations	IV, 2.1
1 General Social Behavior	
1.1 Childhood and Child Rearing (Family of Orientation)	
1.2 The Sphere of Abode	
1.3 The Sphere of Performance	
1.4 The Sphere of Leisure	
1.5 The Sphere of Contacts	
1.6 The Family of Procreation	
1.7 Alcohol and Drug Consumption	
2 The Sphere of Delinquency	
2.1 Previous Offenses, Convictions, and Sentences Served	
2.2 Last Offense(s)	
2.2.1 The Period Immediately Preceding the Offense	
2.2.2 The Event of the Offense	
2.2.3 The Period Following the Offense	
3 Behavior in the Penal Institution[1]	
4 Orientation in Life (Perspective in Time and Value Orientation)	
III Data Analysis	IV, 2.2
1 The Analysis of the Longitudinal Section of Life	IV, 2.2.1.1
1.1 Behavior in the Various Social Spheres	
1.1.1 Child Rearing[2]	III, 2.2.1
1.1.2 The Sphere of Abode and Living	III, 2.2.2
1.1.3 The Sphere of Performance	III, 2.2.3
1.1.4 The Sphere of Leisure	III, 2.2.4

[1] Behavior in the penal institution should be considered only if the *term of imprisonment* was a prolonged one (see Sect. 2.3.4 above).

[2] The short term "child rearing" was chosen for practical reasons. The correct term in full is: the subject's behavior in connection with parental child rearing during childhood and youth.

1.1.5 The Sphere of Contacts	III, 2.2.5
1.1.6 The Family of Procreation	III, 2.2.5.4
1.2 The Sphere of Delinquency	IV, 2.2.1.2
2 The Analysis of the Cross Section of Life	IV, 2.2.2
2.1 The O-Criteria[3]	III, 3.3.3.1 and 3.3.3.3
2.2 The G-criteria[4]	III, 3.3.3.2 and 3.3.3.3
3 Patterns of Relevance and Value Orientation	IV, 2.2.3
3.1 Patterns of Relevance	III, 5
3.2 Value Orientation	III, 5
IV The Criminological Diagnosis	IV, 2.3
1 Assessment on the Basis of the Criteria of Reference of the Criminological Triad	IV, 2.3.1 and 2.3.2
- The Position of the Offense in the Longitudinal Section of Life	
- The Criminorelevant Constellations	
- Patterns of Relevance and Value Orientation	
2 "Special Aspects" in the Life of the Offender, Particularly in View of Prognosis and Interventions	IV, 2.3.3
V Conclusions in View of Prognosis and Interventions	IV, 2.4

Only for prisoners who have been interned for several years:

(I to III, see above)

IV The Criminological Diagnosis

1 Assessment on the Basis of the Criteria of Reference of the Criminological Triad
- The Position of the Offense in the Longitudinal Section of Life
- The Criminorelevant Constellations
- Patterns of Relevance and Value Orientation

2 The Offender in the Context of His Social Relationships During Imprisonment in Comparison with His Previous Behavior — IV; 2.3.4

3 "Special Aspects" in the Life of the Offender, Particularly in View of Prognosis and Interventions

V Conclusions in View of Prognosis and Interventions

[3] "O" stands for offender

[4] "G" stands for general

Appendix – The Criminological Assessment of a Case

Preliminary Remarks

The attempt to illustrate how to proceed in the assessment of an individual case entails certain difficulties. For *didactic reasons,* it is unavoidable to present the assessment, i. e., the analysis of the investigations and the criminological diagnosis, as differentiatedly as possible and to show the individual considerations which are essential in estimating and evaluating a certain behavior. However, this may lead to considerable *misunderstandings* concerning the **amount of time required** to conduct a criminological assessment in practice. Therefore, a comment in advance in this respect.

In the **beginning,** when assessing a subject on the basis of the method described here, one should examine the case *not only in one's mind* as systematically as it is done in the case presented here, but also *in writing,* even and in particular if one has *many years of experience* (and corresponding - subjective - points of view for the assessment). In this way alone can one guarantee the self-control necessary for a systematic assessment and acquire the necessary security to apply the instruments in practice.

Finally, when one has *mastered* the method and disposes of wide experience in handling the instrument, one can simply go through the various stages of the analysis up to the diagnosis in one's mind and put into writing - besides the result, i. e., the diagnostic assignment and the "special aspects" - only certain particularly important or unclear points. As a rule, one usually does not need more than one hour to assess a subject, particularly since one can refer to information which is available anyhow (i. e., information in records) from one's own investigations.

In the following, a relatively simple case from the broad spectrum of possibilities of practical application and appearances of developments in life and delinquency is presented and assessed: For *didactic reasons,* the case is one which does not simply "come out," in particular to show that a classification on the basis of the criteria of reference of the Criminological Triad cannot be "forced" and is not even necessary to gain knowledge which can be used in practice. On the basis of a case like the following one, the considerations which are absolutely necessary to make a differentiated assessment can be demonstrated especially clearly.

In contrast, the assessment of developments in life where the characteristic forms of the various courses occur almost in full, i. e., in a marked continuous development toward criminality beginning during early youth or in criminality with no other social conspicuousness, usually pose no difficulties and do not need to be presented separately (for examples, see Part III, Sects. 4.4.2, 4.4.3, 4.4.4, 4.4.5, and 4.4.6).

1 Survey of Personal Record

July 1960	A. was born. He grew up in his socially inconspicuous parents' home.
1966-1975	A. went to the *Grundschule* and *Hauptschule* and had a long-standing friendship with a schoolmate.
September 1975-January 1979	A. completed his apprenticeship as a precision mechanic; he regularly worked out at a body-building club during leisure time; he had various girlfriends and became engaged.
January 1979-March 1980	A. was employed as a milling worker and set-up man; he pursued hobbies and spent time with his fiancee during his leisure.
From February 1980 on	A.'s stepfather stayed in a hospital and sanatorium for a prolonged period; he died in May 1980.
Since February 1980	A. spent an increasing amount of his leisure time in pubs, discotheques, and bars in the "milieu" of the large city.
April - early May 1980	A. no longer worked after giving notice.
May/June 1980	A. was employed as a mechanic; he repeatedly stayed away from work unexcused, performed poorly at work, and lost his job.
Summer 1980	A. stole money from the family and stole rides; his fiancee broke their engagement.
July/August 1980	A. went on a "tour" to Frankfurt, Hannover, and Hamburg with a "buddy" to "see something of the world"; he possessed arms illegally.
September 1980	A. returned home.
From October 1980 on	A. was regularly employed; he initially still spent his leisure time mainly in pubs, bars, and discotheques.
November/December 1980	A. committed four burglaries to finance his visits to bars.
Since November 1980	A. spent most of his leisure time together with his girlfriend.
January 1981	Time of assessment.

2 Information from the Records and Direct Investigations[1]

2.1 General Social Behavior

2.1.1 Childhood and Child Rearing (Family of Orientation)[2]

A. was born as an illegitimate child in R-city on July 27, 1960. His father was a locksmith, his mother initially worked as a saleswoman. After A.'s birth, his mother took care of him and ran the household. His parents married in 1963. His sister, 4 years younger, also came from this marriage. His parents were divorced in 1969 at the request of his mother because of the persistent extramarital relations of his father. In July 1970, A.'s mother married Z., a butcher who was 20 years older. A. had a brother, 10 years younger, by this marriage. The economic circumstances of the family were always ordered; the family had a good reputation.

A. grew up with his parents. Child rearing was mainly the task of his mother. According to his mother, A. had posed no difficulties as a child and had always been quite well behaved. His stepfather had a good relationship not only with his own son but also with A. and his sister. The children were everything for him; he took very good care of them. The children also liked him, though he was strict and emphasized orderliness. There were no difficulties worth mentioning at home during A.'s apprenticeship either.

In early February 1980, A.'s stepfather had a heart attack. Subsequently, he spent 6 weeks in a hospital and a prolonged period in a sanatorium. According to A.'s mother, A. changed entirely during this time. He no longer listened to her and became fresh and rebellious. He was almost never at home in the evening and roamed about. There was really no way she could influence him anymore though she tried again and again.

A.'s stepfather died on May 18, 1980, after a second heart attack. After his death, the family did not receive any pension for a long time, and their savings were almost used up. In spite of this, A. did not support his mother and even caused additional debts by buying an expensive leather jacket on his mother's account. Perforce, she paid the bill (see also Sect. 2.2.1 below).

Since he came back home in September 1980 (see Sect. 2.1.2 below), he has paid for his room and board regularly and has also paid more attention to his mother, brother, and sister.

---

[1] The information collected in the direct investigations is based on the indications of the subject and his mother. On the problem of the correctness of such information, see Part IV, Sect. 2.1, and in particular Sect. 2.1.2.

[2] Although the subject's behavior is central to the criminological analysis, it is usually useful to provide a short overview of the family background of the subject.

2.1.2 The Sphere of Abode

A. first lived with his parents in R-city. In 1968, when his father changed jobs, the family moved to S-city. From October 1970 on, i.e., after his mother remarried, the family lived in a well-furnished, well-cared-for five-room-apartment in T-city. A., like his brother and sister, had a room of his own, which he was largely free to arrange.

After he had difficulties at home and at work during the spring and summer of 1980, A. decided to "see something of the world" in mid-July 1980 when a "buddy" he had recently gotten to know suggested leaving. (Answer to the question: What kind of buddy was that?) "He was a real super guy! He just came and asked, you want to come, and I went along. I had enough of everything anyway and wanted to go away." First, they hitchhiked to Frankfurt and stayed there for about 2 weeks, sleeping outside in sleeping bags. In early August 1980, they went to Hamburg to sign onto a ship. But this was not as easy as they had imagined. Finally, they hitchhiked to Hannover. In Hannover, they also slept outside at first, then in the apartment of some "buddies" they had gotten to know. Finally, they spent a few days with two girls they had picked up in a discotheque. According to A., the whole affair had become boring after a short time. His "buddy" had still wanted to see some "action" and suggested going to Berlin. But he had no longer been "keen on traveling all over the place" and had hitchhiked home, while his "buddy" had gone on to Berlin. In early September 1980, he turned up at his mother's place and has been living at home again since.

2.1.3 The Sphere of Performance

A. performed well in the *Grundschule* and *Hauptschule* in spite of changing schools frequently. He never had to repeat a year and only played truant once or twice. After completing the *Hauptschule* in September 1975, he started an apprenticeship as a precision mechanic on his own initiative on the advice of an acquaintance. He liked both his apprenticeship and vocational school. His performance was slightly above average up to the second year of his apprenticeship; he even received a prize for his work records, a subject he liked especially well. His behavior toward his superiors and fellow employees was impeccable. He handed in his entire apprentice's payment at home, keeping only some pocket money. Toward the end of his apprenticeship, however, he found it more and more difficult to complete his occupational training as he no longer liked it in the company. Exactly why this had been so, he couldn't say. He had simply been "fed up" with everything. Nonetheless, he took the final apprenticeship examination on January 12, 1979, and passed with barely average results.

He went to the employment office to find a new job even before the examination. On January 21, 1979, he started as a milling worker for a company which manufactured cameras and optical equipment in T-city. Later on, he worked there as a set-up man. There were no difficulties at first, though A. was sometimes tardy. According to his mother, who knew him, the master craftsman had the impression that the job overtaxed A. somewhat, which made him lose interest in his work. By mid-February 1980, A. gave notice as of March 31, 1980. According to A., he didn't like it anymore. Afterward, he did not work for about one month. At first, he did not look for a new job at all. But since his mother, his fiancee (see Sect. 2.1.5 below), and his stepfather (during sporadic visits at the clinic) urged him to look for a new job, he did so. To his own surprise, he found a job as a mechanic in a machine factory in T-city by the beginning of May 1980. He did not make a very positive impression during the first few weeks. He repeatedly stayed away from work unexcused or came to work much too late and without having slept enough after making a night of it (in the old town of the nearest large city). Correspondingly, he produced "scrap metal" and was advised to give notice at the end of the month.

He had been definitely "through" with it then, especially since he had trouble at home and with his fiancee again. In mid-July 1980, he went on a "tour" and "stayed above water" in Frankfurt by doing temporary work at the central market. When he did not succeed in signing onto a ship in Hamburg and his money ran out, he and his "buddy" took their belongings to a pawnshop; among them was a valuable watch he had inherited from his stepfather. In Hannover, they "sponged on" their acquaintances and the two girls.

When he came back home, he was able to start working as a mechanic in a company in T-city on October 1, 1980, where he is still working. By doing overtime, he makes about DM 1300 net a month. He hands in DM 500 a month at home and has used part of his first wages to pay the obligations and the fine the court imposed on him (see Sect. 2.2.1 below). Moreover, he has bought a second-hand car in the meantime, for which he still has to pay eight installments of DM 400 each.

2.1.4 The Sphere of Leisure

At school age, he did "the usual" during his leisure time: He played with friends from school and from the neighborhood, spent time with his parents or brother and sister, or often did handicrafts with his stepfather.

From the beginning of his apprenticeship on, he went to a body-building club regularly twice a week and occasionally went to have a beer together with some friends afterward. Body-building was very important for him then; he practiced no other sports. In the evenings, he either watched television at home or went to a discotheque or to the movies. He was always back home by 11 p.m. at the latest. He also listened to pop music for hours in his room.

When he worked for the camera producer, he started filming (cinefilm). Cutting the films and making soundtracks took up a large amount of his leisure time. At that time, he also often spent the evenings or the weekends with his fiancee.

In February 1980, he went to the old town of S-city with a fellow employee. According to A., the "milieu" of taverns, discotheques, and bars had been "really super." During the following weeks, he spent practically every evening there until midnight ("until the last streetcar"). In the beginning, he went together with his fellow employee, later on, alone. In the meantime, he had gotten to know some "buddies." He always met one or the other of them by chance somewhere in the old town and went to bars and discotheques with them. During the time he was unemployed (April/May 1980), he usually slept until noon, went to the "Espresso", a disreputable bar near the train station of T-city, in the afternoon and on to S-city in the evening, where he roamed about the old town with some "buddies," often until early in the morning. During this period, he often took a taxi home, and his previous wages, unemployment benefits and even his savings rapidly went "down the drain." He cut out his body-building entirely and had almost no time for his fiancee.

When he was on his "tour" in the summer of 1980, he was usually in the center of a large town together with his "buddy," "hung around" amusement arcades, and spent the day any which way; he had always met someone, and it had always been eventful.

After returning to T-city in September 1980, he frequently spent the evenings in the pubs and bars of the old town of S-city again but was regularly back home by midnight. In late November 1980, he got to know his current girlfriend F. In the period that followed he spent almost every evening and particularly the weekends with F. They went to discotheques, to the movies, or did something else. But he still met his "buddies" from the old town and even sees them occasionally at present, though much less frequently than a few months ago. He spends most of his time with his girlfriend. They are on the road with his car a lot, simply "driving around."

2.1.5 The Sphere of Contacts

A. had a good relationship with his stepfather, whose death affected A. deeply. His relationship with his mother was a little more reserved, particularly after his stepfather's death. Yet he called home repeatedly during the time he was on his "tour." Somehow, his conscience had bothered him when he had thought of his mother.

Besides the children he knew from school or from the neighborhood, A. had a close friend for many years while he went to school. Shortly after he left school, the friendship broke up. (Answer to a question:) "There was no special reason; we just didn't get along anymore." During his apprenticeship, he had a close friend in the body-building club for a short time. This friend already had "quite a record" and was committed to a home again after several offenses. During the past few years, he had had no particular close friend, only contacts with one or the other fellow employee after working hours. For the rest, he had found a large number of "buddies" recently in the old town of S-city.

He had first close contacts with a girl of his age at the age of 14. This friendship lasted only a few months. At the age of 15, he had his first intimate experiences with an 18-year-old girl. In the following period, he had a number of short-term acquaintances, including sexual contacts. In the spring of 1979, he became engaged to V., who, according to his mother, was a "decent girl from a respectable family." V. broke the engagement during the summer of 1980 since A. was leading a disorderly life. "That hit me hard somehow, but then it was all the same." Since November 1980, he has had a close relationship with F., with whom - according to A. - he gets along very well. "It's a real super relationship, it really gets under my skin."

2.1.6 Alcohol and Drug Consumption

According to A., he was not "into" drugs. Yet he could hold quite a lot of alcohol and had been rather "tight" several times. (Answer to a question:) during the spring and summer of 1980, more than once a week, recently not as frequently; he mainly drank beer and whiskey. He had started smoking at the age of 16 and smoked about two packs of cigarettes a day.

2.2 The Sphere of Delinquency

2.2.1 Previous Offenses, Convictions, and Sentences Served

As a child, he had surely been up to some pranks, but he could not remember any details. There had not been anything "serious."

According to his mother, he had secretly stolen household money more than once, and the small savings of his brother and sister as well as the money his mother kept for emergencies, about DM 100, had not been safe from him either. A. confirmed this.

To date, he has appeared in court three times: The first time was at the age of 16. It happened together with his friend from the body-building club. They had gone to a pub for a quick beer after a workout, and his friend had suggested "organizing" some cigarettes on the way home. They had smashed a cigarette machine with a cramp iron they had found at a construction site nearby and had stolen 10 packs of cigarettes. He was sentenced to work for the Red Cross eight times on Saturdays. (According to the extract from the juvenile record, a warning and a juvenile court order to work.)

The two other cases occurred during the summer of 1980: In July 1980, he had been caught on a streetcar using the monthly card of his fiancee V. He had made the first name on the card partly illegible with a razor blade. He was punished with a fine of DM 1200 in November 1980. (According to the case record, he was sentenced to a fine of 30 daily rates of DM 40 each for forgery of documents and continued fraud.)

In August 1980, he was arrested together with some "buddies" in a summerhouse near Hannover. They had wanted to stay the night there but had "banged away" with a revolver he had "organized" at the train station in Frankfurt and had foolishly drawn attention to themselves. He had to pay DM 800. (According to the case record, paying DM 800 to a charitable institution because of illegal possession of arms.)

2.2.2 Last Offenses[3]

According to the investigation records, A. spent three Saturday evenings in various taverns in T-city together with the two co-accused X. and Y. (November 15 and 22, and December 6, 1980). Toward midnight, they decided to go to the "Lido" or the "Maxim", both disreputable nightclubs. As they were "hard up," they had to get money.

At the suggestion of A., they went to the machine factory where A. had worked for a short time in May/June 1980 twice and to the company where he had completed his apprenticeship once. They entered the office and canteen buildings through a window, searched the buildings and stole DM 800, DM 500, and DM 150 from strongboxes, as well as 200 packs of cigarette and eight bottles of schnapps. They divided the loot fairly; the money was usually used up during the same night in bars and discotheques.

On a Saturday (November 29, 1980), A. went out with his girlfriend. After he brought her home, he suddenly had the idea of getting some money. He broke into the company where he had completed his apprenticeship and tried to break open the safe in the pay office with a drill he had fetched from the workshop. As this had made a considerable amount of noise, he gave up.

A. was found out after the police caught the co-accused X. and Y. in the very act of burglarizing.

2.3 Orientation in Life

Depending on how things went, he would stay at his current job. Furthermore, he had to reckon with a draft order in the spring of 1981. He spent almost all his leisure time with his girlfriend at present and wanted to continue doing so. However, he was not yet thinking of getting married; he had to lay a solid foundation first and "be something." The relationship with F. was so good that he had no doubts she would stand by him even if he had to go to prison. For the future, he saw a certain obligation in caring for his mother and his brother and sister, who didn't have anyone to look after them since his stepfather had died.

[3] See Part IV, Sects. 2.2.1.2 and 3. In simple cases, it can be useful to do without a distinction between the "period immediately preceding the offense," the "event of the offense," and the "period following the offense" in favor of a comprehensive presentation; nonetheless, the various periods should still be taken into consideration.

3 Data Analysis[4]

3.1 The Analysis of the Longitudinal Section of Life[5]

3.1.1 Behavior in the Various Social Spheres

3.1.1.1 Child Rearing[6]

A.'s behavior tended rather clearly toward the G-ideal-typical pole during childhood and youth: A. obviously adjusted himself to his (ordered) family of orientation and also accepted a certain supervision. Not until adolescence and after the hospitalization and death of his stepfather were there unambiguous tendencies toward the O-ideal-typical pole insofar as A. avoided any influence of and supervision by his mother. Even since A.'s return home, no influence of his mother worth mentioning can be determined.

3.1.1.2 The Sphere of Abode and Living[7]

Up to the age of 20, A.'s sphere of abode and living was marked by the socially inconspicuous, ordered home of his parents. From the spring of 1980 on, there were increasing tendencies toward O-ideal-typical behavior: A. used the sphere of living of his parents only as a place to sleep, and this sphere receded entirely into the background temporarily during the summer of 1980. A.'s breaking away from home in search of adventure led from an immediate social environment to the large city - for A. an anonymous environment. There was a (merely short) period of roaming about more or less without a fixed abode connected with houselessness and entirely interchangeable temporary places to sleep with any kind of acquaintances. Yet A. kept up some contact with his family (telephone calls). Thus, there was no final separation from home despite the very strong O-ideal-typical tendencies. A.'s return home obviously tends in the G-ideal-typical direction since he clearly came home on his own initiative. Even if the sphere of living of the parents' home no longer played an essential role, e.g., as a place of leisure, there have been relatively obvious tendencies toward the G-ideal-typical pole since September 1980.

3.1.1.3 The Sphere of Performance[8]

A.'s behavior in the sphere of performance also clearly tended toward the G-ideal-typical pole at school age and the age of occupational training. Although A. saw his

[4] On the procedure of analysis, see Part IV, Sect. 2.2.
[5] On the procedure of analysis of the longitudinal section of life, see Part IV, Sect. 2.2.1.
[6] For the criteria of assessment, see Part III, Sect. 2.2.1.
[7] For the criteria of assessment, see Part III, Sect. 2.2.2.
[8] For the criteria of assessment, see Part III, Sect. 2.2.3.

difficulties through at work toward the end of his apprenticeship (i. e., his behavior belonged more to the G-ideal-typical pole), these difficulties can also be regarded as first, though not yet pronounced signs of tendencies toward the O-ideal-typical pole coinciding with A.'s further behavior in the sphere of performance.[9]

From the spring of 1980 on, A.'s behavior in the sphere of performance tended more and more toward O-ideal-typical forms: A. terminated his employment contract seemingly spontaneously and planlessly out of a general listlessness, his next job did not follow the old one immediately, his attitude at work was marked by disinterest; and, finally, he no longer worked regularly for several weeks. Yet he still earned part of his living at temporary jobs during this phase of entirely irregular working behavior.

Since the fall of 1980, there has been an opposite tendency pointing in the direction of G-ideal-typical behavior: A. has been working regularly again.

3.1.1.4 The Sphere of Leisure[10]

A.'s leisure behavior showed a similar development: During childhood and youth, A.'s behavior pointed more or less clearly to the G-ideal-typical side with respect to availability, structure and course and place of leisure.

A fundamental change in the direction of O-ideal-typical behavior started in early February 1980: A. first extended his leisure time at the expense of the period of rest and sleep, and, after a short time, also at the expense of the sphere of performance. Even at the job starting in May 1980, A. repeatedly extended his leisure time at the expense of the sphere of performance. Finally, by the summer of 1980, leisure totally dominated the entire course of a day during the period of A.'s almost complete nonemployment. At that time, A. favored unstructured leisure activities which took place away from home, had unpredictable courses, and were obviously "milieu"-oriented.

This kind of leisure organization was also of central importance in the fall of 1980, when A. was working regularly again, though the course of his leisure activities was no longer entirely unpredictable, particularly with respect to time. A. extended his leisure time at the most at the expense of the period of rest and sleep and no longer at the expense of the sphere of performance. As A. worked overtime, there was even a certain limitation of leisure time.

Not until the end of November 1980 does there seem to be a partially structured organization of leisure oriented toward spending time with a definite person: his acquaintance with F. This leisure organization inside certain limits in view of time, space, and persons seems to have become more important; thus, A.'s sphere of leisure has shown certain G-ideal-typical forms again.

---

[9] Because of a lack of information, this could not be determined clearly. However, it is not of decisive importance for the present assessment.

[10] For the criteria of assessment, see Part III, Sect. 2.2.4.

3.1.1.5 The Sphere of Contacts[11]

With respect to given contacts, A.'s behavior during childhood and youth belonged to the G-ideal-typical pole. This tendency became particularly obvious in the relationship between A. and his stepfather, while the relationship between A. and his mother receded into the background in comparison. A.'s relationship with his family of orientation became obviously utilitarian during the spring and summer of 1980, i.e., after the absence and death of his stepfather (A. even stole from his family repeatedly) and thus tended toward the O-ideal-typical pole. Yet A. never severed all contacts with his family, not even in July and August 1980. To what extent ties with his mother, brother, and sister played a certain role in A.'s coming back home in September 1980 remains unclear. Yet A.'s return home does not seem to have occurred chiefly for material reasons. This became apparent in A.'s other behavior (e.g., his paying for room and board at home). Recently, therefore, there have been certain tendencies toward G-ideal-typical forms in A.'s given contacts.

A.'s self-chosen contacts with friends and acquaintances also pointed in the G-ideal-typical direction during childhood and youth. However, a first prolonged contact with an apparently somewhat conspicuous person of A.'s age from the body-building club occurred at the beginning of his apprenticeship. This contact led to A.'s first offense. A marked change in the direction of the O-ideal-typical pole, however, did not occur until the beginning of 1980: "Milieu"-oriented and entirely interchangeable contacts with "buddies" gained more and more importance. In this context, it became apparent that A. is to a certain extent suggestible. These contacts correspondingly affected the remaining social spheres and increasingly determined A.'s entire life pattern, leading him to commit offenses. As these contacts played a considerable role for A. until quite recently, it cannot yet be estimated to what extent A.'s new relationship with F. can bring about a change (particularly since A. committed his last offense immediately after spending an evening together with F.).

A.'s sexual contacts cannot be classified unequivocally: On the one hand, there were A.'s relatively early first sexual intercourse and frequent, possibly very frequent changes of sexual partners, which pointed in the direction of O-ideal-typical behavior. On the other hand, the more stable, long-term relationships with V. and F. obviously tend toward the G-ideal-typical pole.

3.1.2 The Sphere of Delinquency[12]

While "offenses" during childhood can be disregarded, a comparison of A.'s earlier offenses and the pending offenses (fall 1980) shows that the way A. committed his offenses became considerably more purposeful: A.'s first offense (stealing cigarettes at the age of16) may well be characterized by the joint commission of the

---

[11] For the criteria of assessment, see Part III, Sect. 2.2.5.

[12] For the criteria of assessment, see Part IV, Sect. 2.2.1.2.

offense, and A. may have even been only a hanger-on.[13] A.'s stealing from his family during the summer of 1980 was not very purposeful: Apparently, he simply seized good opportunities in the immediate social environment.[14] The - apparently recurring - stealing of rides and manipulations to this end (forgery of documents), in contrast, exhibit a methodical, considered procedure. A.'s last offenses, obtaining money in a methodical, well-considered way to finance an expensive leisure organization, were even more purposefully committed. It is particularly worth noting that A.'s last offenses took place at a time when he was working regularly and earned relatively good wages. The offense against the Weapons Act *(Waffengesetz)* cannot be qualified in any detail.[15]

3.2 The Analysis of the Cross Section of Life[16]

In the following, the interval for the cross section is the period from A.'s return home in September 1980 to his last offenses in early December 1980.[17]

3.2.1 O-Criteria[18]

A *neglect of the sphere of work and performance as well as of family and other social obligations* cannot be determined for the interval of the cross section: A. obviously worked regularly and did not neglect his obligations toward his family of orientation in any serious way. For example, he regularly paid for his room and board at home. In contrast, there are numerous indications of this criterion from February to August 1980 (frequent job changes and nonemployment, not supporting or helping his mother, sister, or brother, stealing from the family, inconsiderateness toward his fiancee, etc.)

There was also no unequivocal *deficient relationship to money and property* during the interval of the cross section. This criterion, however, did occur during the spring and summer of 1980 (Indications of this are A.'s expensive visits to pubs and bars or buying an expensive leather jacket without being willing to guarantee a regular income; pawning the last possessions of the family, particularly the heirloom of his stepfather, etc.).

---

[13] It is assumed that A. committed the offenses he is accused of the way they are described in the investigation records.

[14] Only the criminological perspective is concerned here; the moral reprehensibleness of stealing the money A.'s mother had saved for emergencies is of no importance in *this* connection. However, in view of A.'s value orientation at that time, this theft provides some insights (see Sect. 3.3.2 below).

[15] Not all offenses can be assessed reliably from a criminological perspective with the criteria elaborated and presented up to this point. This is particularly true for any kind of offense pertaining to law on supplementary penalties, not to the heart of general criminal law (see also Part IV, Sect. 1.3).

[16] On the procedure, see Part IV, Sect. 2.2.2.

[17] The starting point for the analysis of the cross section are all four pending offenses, the period between the first and the last offense being considered in the analysis of the cross section as well.

[18] On the criteria to be examined and related explanations, see Part III, Sect. 3.3.3.

Unstructured leisure behavior cannot be unequivocally assumed despite A.'s still frequent visits to the old town of S-city during the interval of the cross section: These visits to the "milieu," as opposed to earlier visits, apparently remain inside certain time limits, and leisure time is partially limited by overtime work. The criterion applies without reservations during the spring and summer of 1980.

During the interval of the cross section, there are some indications of a certain planning in life for the first time in a long while. This is also due to A.'s coming back home and taking up a regular job. Yet - under consideration of A.'s age - a wellconsidered and sound planning in life may still be absent. The criterion *absence of planning in life* applies without reservations during the spring and summer of 1980 (as opposed to previous years).

During the spring and summer of 1980, there are also indications of a *low tolerance for stress* (repeatedly giving up regular work); during the interval of the cross section, however, there are no longer such indications.

At least since the spring of 1980, there is a more or less pronounced *demand to be free from any ties.* However, this is expressed in A.'s leisure behavior only during the interval of the cross section, as opposed to the earlier period.

Despite A.'s frequent visits to pubs and bars, there are insufficient indications of *uncontrolled, excessive alcohol consumption.*

3.2.2 G-Criteria[19]

Neither during the interval of the cross section nor during the period reaching back to the spring of 1980 are any of the G-criteria unequivocally apparent. Although there are recent indications of a *fulfillment of social obligations* and *strong ties,* e.g., with his girlfriend and his mother, these tendencies do *not* yet suffice to assume either one of these criteria.

In earlier years, in contrast, there are rather clear indications of several G-criteria, such as *fulfillment of social obligations,* an *adequate relationship to money and property, attachment to a well-ordered home (and family life), dedication to and satisfaction from work, commitment to the affairs of persons and institutions,* and *strong ties.*

3.3 Patterns of Relevance and Value Orientation

3.3.1 Patterns of Relevance[20]

Since the spring of 1980, A. has exhibited a considerable striving for "freedom" (from any ties), which is entirely opposed to the earlier integration in his parents' home. In this context, his visits to the *"milieu" of bars, discotheques, and nightclubs (of large cities)* and *spending time with "buddies"* started to play a dominating role and almost became A.'s entire purpose in life for a certain time.

---

[19] On the criteria to be examined and related explanations, see Part III, Sect. 3.3.3.

[20] On the assessment of the patterns of relevance, see Part IV, Sect. 2.2.3.1.

Although A. pushed his parents' home into the background during the spring and summer of 1980, the actual importance of his *parents' home* becomes apparent in his coming back to his ordered home after a short time of going out "into the wide world." Generally, it seems that certain *ties* with a definite person (formerly stepfather and V., now F. and probably also his mother) are of some importance, despite the aforementioned pattern of relevance.

3.3.2 Value Orientation[21]

A.'s value orientation seems to be as conflicting as his patterns of relevance. There are practically no indications of any somewhat stable system of values, particularly since A. has shown tendencies toward both sides in his behavior, at least recently:[22] On the one hand, he practically abandoned himself to an "unchecked living in the immediate present" and had no scruples about stealing the money his mother had put aside for emergencies or the money his sister and brother had saved, for example. On the other hand, he showed obvious indications of a basically ordered life in the past (e.g., completing an apprenticeship, a basic willingness to work, the relationship with his fiancee). Yet his returning home and starting to work again during the fall of 1980, which was his own decision, do permit concluding that the values relevant to him during childhood and youth are still - or again - of some importance. Thus, at present, he still seems to have a certain notion of responsibility, e.g., toward his mother; his remark that he had to be something and had to lay a solid foundation before he could marry also point in this direction.

[21] On the assessment of the value orientation, see Part IV, Sect. 2.2.3.2.

[22] In no way are the values and value orientation expressed by a subject in the exploration, for example, solely decisive for the assessment of the value orientation; the value orientation can also be expressed in the actual behavior of a subject. Furthermore, in the analysis of the value orientation, the actual behavior of a subject should always be compared with the values and value orientation he expresses.

4 The Criminological Diagnosis[23]

4.1 Assessment on the Basis of the Criteria of Reference of the Criminological Triad[24]

A.'s *longitudinal profile* shows pronounced tendencies toward the G-ideal-typical pole in all social spheres during childhood and youth. From the spring of 1980 on, i.e., when A. was 19, there were obvious tendencies toward O-ideal-typical behavior in the spheres of leisure and contacts. These tendencies rapidly characterized the sphere of performance as well and, during the summer of 1980, temporarily even the sphere of abode. During this phase of pronounced O-behavior, A. stole from the family, committed fraud in connection with forgery of documents, and committed the offense against the Weapons Act.

From September 1980 on, however, there were increasing changes in the spheres of abode and performance in the direction of G-ideal-typical behavior and first indications of similar changes in the spheres of leisure and contacts. Nevertheless, the pending offenses took place precisely during the period when A.'s general social behavior went partially in the direction of the G-ideal-typical pole. This longitudinal profile cannot be easily assigned to any one position of the offense in the longitudinal section of life: The pronounced tendencies toward O-ideal-typical behavior in all social spheres during the summer of 1980 point to a development toward criminality beginning during adolescence or the early years of adulthood. Yet, despite the last offenses, there are tendencies toward the O-ideal-typical pole only in the spheres of leisure and contacts during the fall of 1980. Since these tendencies are obviously becoming less strong, this points more to criminality in the course of personality maturation.

The impression which arises on the basis of the longitudinal profile is supported by the *examination of the cross section:* While there was no criminovalent constellation during the fall of 1980, the period of the pending offenses, this was not so during the summer of 1980. During this period, there was a neglect of the sphere of work and performance as well as of family and other social obligations, a deficient relationship to money and property, unstructured leisure behavior, and an absence of planning in life. Consequently, A. stole from his family and committed the forgery in connection with fraud. In September 1980, A. avoided the almost compelling need to commit further property or fraudulent offenses to keep up a corresponding life-style by returning home and starting to work again. Thus, A.'s parents' home ultimately had the function of a safety net, which possibly prevented him from lapsing further into criminality (against property).

---

[23] On the procedure of criminological diagnosis, see Part IV, Sect. 2.3.

[24] On the criteria of reference, see Part IV, Sect. 2.3.1.

This - changing - life pattern corresponds to A.'s *patterns of relevance:* A.'s striving for "freedom" (from any ties) and his orientation toward "milieu" contacts determined his life-style at that time and were also particularly conducive to the commission of offenses later on. On the other hand, during the fall of 1980, i.e., when A. committed the pending offenses, other patterns of relevance more favorable to a socially inconspicuous life were already gaining importance without having yet replaced the earlier patterns of relevance, particularly the "milieu" contacts. A.'s *value orientation* appears as unconsolidated and changing as his patterns of relevance, though they may well tend in a socially sound direction.

In conclusion, it can be said that, despite the pronounced tendencies toward the O-ideal-typical pole throughout all social spheres during the summer of 1980 and the criminovalent constellation present at that time, A. exhibits *criminality in the course of personality maturation*[25] shifted in time. On the one hand, the tendencies toward O-ideal-typical behavior were mainly limited to the spheres of leisure and contacts in November and December 1980, and, recently, there has no longer been a criminovalent constellation. On the other hand, A.'s return to an ordered social life and his more and more obvious tendencies toward G-ideal-typical behavior, especially in the sphere of performance - as compared with the summer of 1980 - are of essential importance. On the whole, a considerable number of indications show that the phase of A.'s comprehensive orientation toward O-ideal-typical behavior during the summer of 1980 was an episode, and not the beginning of a development toward criminality.

4.2 "Special Aspects" in the Life of the Offender, Particularly in View of Prognosis and Interventions[26]

A.'s suggestibility, which has recently been shown more than once in connection with his contacts with "buddies" and the "milieu," the absence of sound planning in life corresponding to his age, and the lack of a clear value orientation are the "*internal aspects*" which must be taken into consideration. A.'s return home in September 1980, when he withdrew from the influence of his "buddy," and his most recent behavior are indications that values which can be regarded as requirements of an ordered social life are certainly not unfamiliar to him. Furthermore, in view of possible interventions, there are A.'s basic willingness to work and his ability and willingness to establish strong ties with another person.

"*External aspects*" are, on the one hand, A.'s parents' home, his relationship with his mother and, more recently, that with his girlfriend. On the other hand, there is the attraction of the criminality-prone "milieu" and corresponding contacts - though it seems to be declining at present.

---

[25] This position of the offense in the life of an offender is in no way limited to the period of puberty; it can also occur in later years, when it can be a variant, considerably shifted in time - see Part III, Sect. 4.4.5.

[26] On the assessment of the "special aspects," see Part IV, Sect. 2.3.3.

Against the background of the "internal aspects," which are still open both to a socially sound and to a criminality-prone life, both "external aspects" were brought to bear in a pronounced way during the past year in particular: After the illness and death of A.'s stepfather, who apparently provided clear guidelines for A.'s life ("strict and emphasized orderliness"), A.'s demand for "freedom" (from any ties) and his demand for "unchecked living in the immediate present", together with his orientation toward the criminality-prone "milieu" manifested themselves fully. Recently, in contrast, former relationships have been more important again, i.e., A.'s parents' home, his ties with a definite person (mother, girlfriend) and regular work, i.e., an on the whole socially sound life.

5 Conclusions in View of Prognosis and Interventions[27]

The position of delinquency in A.'s life can be considered criminality in the course of personality maturation (shifted in time) although, no more than a few months ago, there were obvious indications of a development toward criminality in A.'s general social behavior. Thus, the *general prognosis* is rather favorable. However, this estimation depends, even more than in the cases of criminality in the course of personality maturation which occur generally, on specific interventions considering the still existing signs of a danger of criminality, particularly A.'s being influenced by his "buddies" and the "milieu" *(individual basic prognosis).* It is of decisive importance to sever any remaining ties with the "milieu" on the one hand, and to encourage A.'s basic willingness to work, which has become apparent during the past few months, and strengthen his ties with his parents' home and his girlfriend (or another confidential person) on the other hand. This could contribute to a certain planning in life in the long run and influence his general orientation in life. As has become apparent, A. can be induced to lead a socially sound life by relatively strict guidance (formerly that of his stepfather). Yet his striving to be free from any ties and his still unconsolidated value orientation are jeopardizing elements, particularly if he turns back to the "milieu" and corresponding contacts. But A.'s behavior during the past months has shown that he himself tends to more inconspicuous contacts and that his value orientation corresponds more to socially accepted values. On the whole, therefore, it should be possible to guide A. back to a socially sound life. A certain integration, for example the relationship with F., may well be of great importance *(intervention prognosis).*[28]

---

[27] On the fundamental principle, see Part III, Sect. 2.4.

[28] Here, the criminological assessment in the strict sense ends. Which measures should be taken according to (juvenile) criminal law must be decided by the competent institution, see also Part IV, Sect. 2.4.2.

References

Baker D, Telfer MA, Richardson CE, Clark GR (1970) Chromosome errors in men with antisocial behavior. Comparison of selected men with Klinefelter's syndrome and XYY chromosome pattern. JAMA 214: 869-878

Bock M (1983) Kriminologie als Wirklichkeitswissenschaft. Duncker and Humblot, Berlin

Bohm E (1967) Psychodiagnostisches Vademecum, 2nd edn. Huber, Bern

Bresser PH (1965) Grundlagen und Grenzen der Begutachtung jugendlicher Rechtsbrecher. de Gruyter, Berlin

Buikhuisen W (1979) Kriminologie in biosociaal perspektief. Kluwer, Deventer

Centro Nazionale di Prevenzione e Difesa Sociale (1969) Recidivismo e giovani adulti. Rome

Conger JJ, Miller WC (1966) Personality, social class and delinquency. Wiley, New York

Dolde G (1978) Sozialisation und kriminelle Karriere. Eine empirische Analyse der sozio-ökonomischen und familialen Sozialisationsbedingungen männlicher Strafgefangener im Vergleich zur Normal-Bevölkerung. Minerva, München

Exner F (1939) Kriminalbiologie in ihren Grundzügen. Hanseatische Verlagsanstalt, Hamburg

Ferguson T (1952) The young delinquent in his social setting. Oxford University Press, London

Ferracuti F, Dinitz S, Acosta de Brenes E (1975) Delinquents and nondelinquents in the Puerto Rico slum culture. Ohio State University Press, Columbus

Gibbons DC (1977) Society, crime and criminal careers. An introduction to criminology, 3rd edn. Prentice Hall, Englewood Cliffs

Glueck S, Glueck E (1957) Unraveling juvenile delinquency, 3rd edn. Harvard University Press, Cambridge

Glueck S, Glueck E (1974) Of delinquency and crime. A panorama of years of search and research. Thomas, Springfield

Göppinger H (1960) Der Verkehrssünder als krimineller Typus. In: Mezger E, Würtenberger T (eds) Kriminalbiologische Gegenwartsfragen 4. Enke, Stuttgart, pp 76-85

Göppinger H (1970) Neuere Ergebnisse der kriminologischen Forschung in Tübingen. In: Göppinger H, Witter H (eds) Kriminologische Gegenwartsfragen 9. Enke, Stuttgart, pp 70-91

Göppinger H (1971 a) Interdisciplinary criminological research in Tübingen. Methodological problems and experience. (Japanese, with a short introduction translated by K Miyazawa). Hogaku-Kankyu (Journal of Law, Politics and Sociology of the Law Faculty of the Keio University in Tokyo), Tokyo

Göppinger H (1971 b) Problems of interdisciplinary research in criminology. Law and State 3: 22-44

Göppinger H (1974) Practically oriented research about the offender and his spheres. Indian J Criminol 2 (1): 11-21

Göppinger H (1975) Criminologia. (Spanish translation of the 2nd edn. of Kriminologie). Reus, Madrid

Göppinger H (1978) Specific criminological methods for the diagnostic recording of the offender in his social interdependencies and for prognostic statements on his social dangerousness. Human Aggression and Dangerousness. Overview of Ongoing Research in the Basic Sciences in Connection with the Treatment and Rehabilitation of Delinquents. Fifth international seminar in comparative clinical criminology, June 13-15, 1977, Montreal

Göppinger H (1980) Kriminologie, 4 th edn. Beck, München

Göppinger H (1983) Angewandte Kriminologie und ihre Bedeutung für die forensische Psychiatrie. In: Gross G, Schüttler R (eds) Empirische Forschung in der Psychiatrie. Schattauer, Stuttgart

Göppinger H (1985) Angewandte Kriminologie. Springer, Berlin Heidelberg New York Tokyo

Haberlandt WF (1970) Cytogenetische Untersuchung einer auslesefreien Population von Kriminellen und einer vergleichbaren Kontrollserie. In: Göppinger H, Witter H (eds) Kriminologische Gegenwartsfragen 9. Enke, Stuttgart, pp 142-154

Healy W, Bronner AF (1926) Delinquents and criminals. Their making and unmaking. Judge Baker Foundation Publication 3, New York
Healy W, Bronner AF (1936) New light on delinquency and its treatment. Yale University Press, Westport, Conn
Hindelang MJ, Hirschi T, Weis JG (1981) Measuring delinquency, vol 123. Sage Publications, Beverly Hills
Jaspers K (1963) General Psychopathology (Translated by J Hoenig and MW Hamilton), 7th edn. University of Chicago Press, Chicago
Johanson E (1981) Recidivistic criminals and their families: morbidity, morality and abuse of alcohol. A longitudinal study of earlier youth prison inmates and of a control group and their families in three generations. Scand J Med 27. Almqvist & Wiksell, Stockholm
Jörgensen G (1969) Verbrechen als Schicksal. Zur Problematik der XYY-"Super"-Männer. Dtsch Ärzteblatt 66: 483-484
Kaiser G (1967) Probleme interdisziplinärer empirischer Forschung in der Kriminologie. Monatsschr Kriminol Strafrechtsreform 50: 352-366
Kerner HJ (1972) Alkoholgenuß und Rauschmittelgebrauch bei Kriminellen. Vergleich mit sozial nicht auffälligen Personen. In: Turčin R et al (eds) Psihopatske Ličnosti, Izdanje Psihijatrijske Bolnice Vrapče, Svezak V, Zagreb
Keske M (1979) Der Anteil der Bestraften in der Bevölkerung. Ein Überblick über nationale und internationale Prävalenzraten. Monatsschr Kriminol Strafrechtsreform 62: 257-272
Keske M (1983) Die Kriminalität der "Kriminellen". Eine empirische Untersuchung von Struktur und Verlauf der Kriminalität bei Strafgefangenen sowie ihrer Sanktionierung. Minerva, München
Klein-Vogler U, Haberlandt W (1974) Kriminalität und chromosomale Konstitution. Ergebnisse einer genetischen Untersuchung von drei Populationen Krimineller und einer Vergleichsserie aus der Durchschnittsbevölkerung. Monatsschr Kriminol Strafrechtsreform 57: 329-337
Kleining G, Moore H (1968) Soziale Selbsteinstufung (SSE). Ein Instrument zur Messung sozialer Schichten. Kölner Z Soziol und Sozialpsychol 20: 502-552
Kofler R (1980) Beruf und Kriminalität. Eine empirische Untersuchung der Zusammenhänge zwischen Beruf und Straffälligkeit bei den Probanden der Tübinger Jungtäter-Vergleichsuntersuchung. Minerva, München
Lempp R (1978) Frühkindliche Hirnschäden. Die Bedeutung eines frühkindlichen exogenen Psychosyndroms für die Entstehung kindlicher Neurosen und milieureaktiver Verhaltensstörungen, 3rd edn. Huber, Bern
Lewis DO, Shanok SS (1977) Medical histories of delinquent and nondelinquent children. An epidemiological study. Am J Psychiatry 134: 1020-1025
Lienert GA (1967) Testaufbau und Testanalyse, 2nd edn. Beltz, Weinheim
Lin ST (1972) Diebstahlsdelikte von Jungtätern. Diss Tübingen
Loomis SD (1967) EEG abnormalities as a correlate of behavior in adolescent male delinquents. Am J Psychiatry 121: 1003-1006
Maschke W (1986) Das Umfeld der Straftat. Ein erfahrungswissenschaftlicher Beitrag zum kriminologischen Tatbild. Beiträge zur empirischen Kriminologie. Göppinger H (ed). Minerva, München
McCord W, McCord J (1959) Origins of crime. A new evaluation of the Cambridge-Somerville youth study. Columbia University Press, New York
McCord W, McCord J (1960) Origins of alcoholism. Stanford University Press, Stanford
Otterström E (1946) Delinquency and children from bad homes. A study of their prognosis from a social point of view. Diss Stockholm
Petrilowitsch N (1966) Abnorme Persönlichkeiten, 3rd edn. Karger, Basel
Pongratz L, Hübner HO (1959) Lebensbewährung nach öffentlicher Erziehung. Luchterhand, Berlin
Powers E, Witmer H (1951) The Cambridge-Somerville youth study. An experiment in the prevention of delinquency. Columbia University Press, New York
Robins LN (1966) Deviant children grow up. A sociological and psychiatric study of sociopathic personality. Williams and Wilkins, Baltimore
Rosenquist CM, Megargee EJ (1969) Delinquency in three cultures. University of Texas Press, Austin
Rusell DH, Bender FH (1970) Legal implications of the XYY syndrome. Semin Psychiatry 2. Grune & Stratton, New York, pp 40-52

Sack F (1969) Probleme der Kriminalsoziologie. In: König R (ed) Handbuch der empirischen Sozialforschung, vol 2. Enke, Stuttgart, pp 961-1049
Schindhelm M (1972) Der Sellin-Wolfgang-Index - ein ergänzendes Maß der Strafrechtspflegestatistik. Enke, Stuttgart
Schmehl, H-H (1980) Jugendliche und heranwachsende Straftäter während ihrer Ausbildung. Eine Untersuchung über die Bedeutung schulischer und beruflicher Ausbildung für die Legalbewährung. Beschreibung einer Gruppe von Straffälligen und einer Vergleichsgruppe. Minerva, München
Schmidt G, Sigusch V (1971) Arbeiter-Sexualität. Eine empirische Untersuchung an jungen Industriearbeitern. Luchterhand, Neuwied
Schneider K (1980) Klinische Psychopathologie, 12th edn. Thieme, Stuttgart
Schöch H (1976) Ist Kriminalität normal? Probleme und Ergebnisse der Dunkelfeldforschung. In: Göppinger H, Kaiser G (eds) Kriminologie und Strafverfahren. Kriminologische Gegenwartsfragen 12. Enke, Stuttgart, pp 211-228
Schulz H, Mainusch G (1969) Beitrag der klinischen Elektroencephalographie zur forensischen Begutachtung. Psych Neurol med Psychol 21: 266-275
Sellin T, Wolfgang ME (1964) The measurement of delinquency. Wiley, New York
Statens offentliga utredningar (1971) Unga lagöverträdare I. Undersökningsmetodik Brottsdebut och återfall. Stockholm
Statens offentliga utredningar (1972) Unga lagöverträdare II. Familj, skola och samhälle i belysning av officiella data. Stockholm
Statens offentliga utredningar (1973a) Olofsson B (ed) Unga lagöverträdare III. Hem, uppfostran, skola och kamratmiljö i belysning av intervju-och uppföljningsdata. Stockholm
Statens offentliga utredningar (1973b) Ahnsjö S (ed) Unga lagöverträdare IV. Kroppslig - psykisk utveckling och status i belysning av föräldra-intervju och uppföljningsdata. Stockholm
Statens offentliga utredningar (1974) Humble K, Settergren-Carlson G (eds) Unga lagöverträdare V. Personlighet och relationer i belysning av projektiva metoder. Stockholm
Stutte H (1974) Neurotische Dissozialität auf dem Boden eines Thersites-Komplexes. Prax Kinderpsychol Kinderpsychiatr 23: 161-166
Szewczyk H (1974) Untersuchungen zur kriminellen Entwicklung Jugendlicher. Szewczyk H (ed) Kriminalität und Persönlichkeit. Psychiatrisch-psychologische und strafrechtliche Aspekte, 2nd edn. Fischer, Jena, pp 15-34
Traulsen M (1976) Delinquente Kinder und ihre Legalbewährung. Eine empirische Untersuchung über Kinderdelinquenz, spätere Straffälligkeit, Herkunft, Verhalten und Erziehungsmaßnahmen. Lang, Frankfurt
Vetter K (1972) Elektroencephalographische Untersuchungen und ihre Bedeutung in foro. Göppinger H, Witter H (eds) Handbuch der forensischen Psychiatrie, vol 2. Springer, Berlin Heidelberg New York, 1511-1519
Weber M (1968) Economy and society. An outline of interpretive sociology, vol 2 Roth G, Wittich C (eds) (translated by E Fischoff et al). Bedminster Press, New York
Weber M (1973) Gesammelte Aufsätze zur Wissenschaftslehre, 4th edn. Mohr, Tübingen
Wechsler D (1964) Die Messung der Intelligenz Erwachsener, 3rd edn. Huber, Bern
West DJ (1969) Present conduct and future delinquency. First report of the Cambridge study in delinquent development. Heinemann, London
West DJ (1982) Delinquency. Its roots, careers and prospects. Heinemann, London
West DJ, Farrington DP (1973) Who becomes delinquent? Second report of the Cambridge study in delinquent development. Heinemann, London
West DJ, Farrington DP (1977) The delinquent way of life. Third report of the Cambridge study in delinquent development. Heinemann, London
Wiener JM, Delano JG, Klass DW (1966) An EEG study of delinquent and nondelinquent adolescents. Arch Gen Psychiatry 15: 144-176
Wittmann H-J (1980) Zur Bedeutung der Ehe für die Bewährung von Straffälligen. Z Strafvollzug Straffälligenhilfe 29: 204-208
Wolfgang ME, Figlio RM, Sellin T (1972) Delinquency in a birth cohort. The University Press, Chicago
Wulf BR (1979) Kriminelle Karrieren von "Lebenslänglichen". Eine empirische Analyse ihrer Verlaufsformen und Strukturen anhand von 141 Straf- und Vollzugsakten. Minerva, München

Subject Index

(Note: the page numbers in italic give the location, where the subject is discussed in most detail)

MIX
Papier aus verantwortungsvollen Quellen
Paper from responsible sources
FSC® C105338

If you have any concerns about our products,
you can contact us on
ProductSafety@springernature.com

In case Publisher is established outside the EU,
the EU authorized representative is:
Springer Nature Customer Service Center GmbH
Europaplatz 3, 69115 Heidelberg, Germany

Printed by Libri Plureos GmbH
in Hamburg, Germany